THE PLASMA PROTEINS:
Structure, Function, and Genetic Control
Second Edition
Volume 2

When the first edition of THE PLASMA PRO-TEINS was published some fifteen years ago, *Nature* hailed it as "a major contribution to the literature on proteins," and the *Quarterly Review of Biology* commented, "This treatise . . . is likely to stand for a good many years to come as the most authoritative survey of the whole field of plasma proteins . . . it is indispensable for workers in this field."

The long-awaited second edition of THE PLASMA PROTEINS has now been completely rewritten by an international group of eminent contributors under the editorship of Frank W. Putnam. Incorporating all the major developments that have occurred within the last fifteen years, THE PLASMA PROTEINS (Second Edition) is the only comprehensive, integrated, up-to-date treatise on blood plasma proteins. It fully covers the structure, function, and genetic control of blood proteins, with special emphasis on their clinical relevance.

This new edition of THE PLASMA PROTEINS will be of great value to biochemists, immunologists, clinical chemists, hematologists, geneticists, biologists, and medical researchers.

MA PROTEINS:
unction, and
trol
ion

NK W. PUTNAM
BN: 0-12-568401-0

The
Plasma Proteins

Structure, Function,
and Genetic Control

Second Edition / Volume II

Contributors

George J. Doellgast

Russell F. Doolittle

John R. Clamp

William H. Fishman

David Gitlin

Jonathan D. Gitlin

M. D. Poulik

Frank W. Putnam

Robert F. Ritchie

M. L. Weiss

The Plasma Proteins

STRUCTURE, FUNCTION,
AND GENETIC CONTROL

Second Edition / Volume II

Edited by

FRANK W. PUTNAM

Distinguished Professor of Molecular Biology and Zoology
Professor of Biochemistry (Medical Sciences)
Indiana University, Bloomington, Indiana

Academic Press
NEW YORK SAN FRANCISCO LONDON 1975
A Subsidiary of Harcourt Brace Jovanovich, Publishers

ACADEMIC PRESS, INC.
111 Fifth Avenue, New York, New York 10003

United Kingdom Edition published by
ACADEMIC PRESS, INC. (LONDON) LTD.
24/28 Oval Road, London NW1

Library of Congress Cataloging in Publication Data

Putnam, Frank W   ed.
        The plasma proteins : structure, function, and
genetic control.

        Includes bibliographies and index.
        1.   Plasma proteins.   I.   Title.   [DNLM: 1.   Blood
proteins.   QY455 P715]
[QP99.3.P7P87 1975]   612'.11   75-3970
ISBN 0−12−568402−9 (v. 2)

To Dorothy

Contents

4 Structure and Function of Glycoproteins

John R. Clamp

5 Tissue-Derived Plasma Enzymes

William H. Fishman and George J. Doellgast

6 Fetal and Neonatal Development of Human Plasma Proteins

David Gitlin and Jonathan D. Gitlin

7 Genetic Alterations in the Plasma Proteins of Man

David Gitlin and Jonathan D. Gitlin

8 Automated Immunoprecipitation Analysis of Serum Proteins

Robert F. Ritchie

List of Contributors

Numbers in parentheses indicate the pages on which the authors' contributions begin.

George J. Doellgast (213), Cancer Research Center, Tufts University School of Medicine, Boston, Massachusetts

Russell F. Doolittle (109), Department of Chemistry, University of California, San Diego, La Jolla, California

John R. Clamp (163), Department of Medicine, University of Bristol School of Medicine, Bristol, England

William H. Fishman (213), Cancer Research Center, Tufts University School of Medicine, Boston, Massachusetts

David Gitlin (263, 321), Department of Pediatrics, University of Pittsburgh School of Medicine, Pittsburgh, Pennsylvania

Jonathan D. Gitlin (263, 321), Department of Pediatrics, University of Pittsburgh School of Medicine, Pittsburgh, Pennsylvania

M. D. Poulik (51), Department of Immunochemistry, William Beaumont Hospital, Royal Oak, Michigan, and Department of Pediatrics, Wayne State University, School of Medicine, Detroit, Michigan

Frank W. Putnam (1), Department of Zoology, Indiana University, Bloomington, Indiana

Robert F. Ritchie (375), Rheumatic Disease Laboratory, Maine Medical Center, Portland, Maine

M. L. Weiss (51), Department of Immunochemistry, William Beaumont Hospital, Royal Oak, Michigan, and Department of Anthropology, Wayne State University, Detroit, Michigan

Preface

In the fifteen years that have elapsed since the first edition of this treatise was published the alphabet of the plasma proteins has expanded from α-, β-, and γ-globulins to an evergrowing list limited only by the sensitivity of methods of detection and the zeal of the investigator. Excluding hormones, tissue-derived enzymes, and erythrocyte components, plasma contains more than 100 proteins, many of which do not as yet have recognized functions. Some of the interacting components are multienzyme systems such as the complement pathway, blood coagulation, and the fibrinolytic and kininogen systems. Other plasma protein systems of great physiological and medical importance include the immunoglobulins, lipoproteins, transport proteins, and proteinase inhibitors. In addition, there are innumerable α- and β-glycoproteins of unknown function and hundreds of trace and ultratrace components. Many of the latter are transient indicators of disease, tissue damage, and cellular changes. More than 100 genetic variants of human plasma proteins are known and also many examples of hereditary deficiency diseases. The range of normal concentration of individual plasma proteins spans six logs from albumin to IgE.

How to cover the explosive development in knowledge of plasma proteins in a comprehensive integrated way without being encyclopedic was a continuous challenge to me over the past decade. For some years I felt the best way to attain integration was to completely rewrite the second edition myself. I undertook to do so, and this explains why, in somewhat unusual fashion, about one-third of the chapters are authored by the editor. However, the rate of progress in plasma proteins outstripped my pen. As each chapter was completed, its predecessors had to be rewritten. Inexorably, I was driven to call on friends throughout the world to bring their expertise quickly to my rescue. They responded nobly, and met short deadlines at sacrifice of other commitments. In less than a year from the target date for receipt of manuscripts, Volumes I and II were in proof and Volume III well advanced. This cooperation assures balance, simultaneity, continuity, and a degree of up-to-dateness that could not be achieved by any single author. At the same time integration was achieved by exchange of outlines and manuscripts among the contributors.

The purpose of this treatise is to describe the plasma proteins in a systematic integrated fashion. The intention is to present first the perspectives and a global look at plasma proteins, then a series of chapters on the well-characterized major proteins, followed by comprehensive chapters on integrated systems of plasma proteins. The emphasis is on structure, function, and genetic control rather than on metabolism and biosynthesis. Clinical relevance is introduced in terms of principles rather than detail. Where the information is known, emphasis is on human proteins, for the same principles apply throughout the animal kingdom. However, where more is known about animal proteins, as in some phases of blood coagulation, these are used as examples.

Unlike the first edition, which came at a time when plasma proteins were the focus of development of new techniques, the second edition does not emphasize methodology. However, one comprehensive new approach is introduced in the chapter on automated immunoprecipitation, and Volume III will have a chapter on plasma protein fractionation by the foremost exponents in the field. It is hoped that "The Plasma Proteins" will be an open-ended treatise, and that future volumes will include a number of short contributions on specialized topics that are incompletely developed in Volumes I to III. The future volumes will also focus more on the clinical significance of human plasma proteins, on methods of measurement and evaluation, and on the comparative biochemistry and evolutionary development of plasma proteins.

The first phase of my writing was done at Cambridge University with the aid of a Guggenheim Fellowship, followed by a second period at Cambridge as an Overseas Fellow of Churchill College, under the sponsorship of the Winston Churchill Foundation. Thanks are due these foundations, and also to Churchill College and the Laboratory of Molecular Biology which provided support, facilities, and amenities.

As editor, I owe thanks to many for advice, encouragement, and help: first, to the many new contributors to the second edition and to the four from the first edition who are again represented; to the late Kurt Jacoby and to the staff of Academic Press for early encouragement and enduring patience; to my secretarial staff, Liz Frederick, Judy Johnson, and Cathy Rogers, who accepted responsibilities and showed interest beyond their duties; and most of all to my wife, Dorothy, for years of encouragement, gentle persistence, and much personal sacrifice during a period of illness, fortunately overcome as this volume was about to be published.

Frank W. Putnam

Contents of Other Volumes

1 / Haptoglobin

Frank W. Putnam

I. Introduction

The haptoglobins (Hp) are a family of glycoproteins found in the α_2-globulin fraction of many mammalian species and were so named by their discoverers Polonovski and Jayle (1938, 1940) because of the ability of haptoglobin to form specific stable complexes with hemoglobin (haptein = to bind). An earlier name is seromucoid $\alpha 2$. In plasma the hemoglobin is derived from erythrocyte breakdown. Although a number of proteins bind hemoglobin, haptoglobins do so far more strongly than any other plasma protein. Owing to its common molecular variations in man as a protein with similar function and structure the name haptoglobin may be used both in the singular and in the plural.

The biological function of haptoglobin is to bind hemoglobin in a one-to-one ratio yielding a relatively high molecular weight complex. This prevents undue loss of iron through urinary excretion, for haptoglobin is the major factor regulating the renal threshold for hemoglobin. This also protects the kidney from damage by hemoglobin. The oxygenated but not the reduced form of hemoglobin is bound. Under certain conditions the haptoglobin–hemoglobin complex (Hp-Hb) exhibits peroxidase activity; this property provides one method for the quantitative estimation of haptoglobin. However, the peroxidase activity may not be an essential attribute of haptoglobin but rather a function of the hemoglobin and the ionic environment of the Hp-Hb complex. The Hp-Hb complex is taken up by the reticuloendothelial system. Haptoglobin, however, is not a true transport protein because it does not return to the circulation since the entire Hp-Hb complex is metabolized. Thus, haptoglobin is one of the triumvirate of plasma proteins involved in the conservation and transport of hemoglobin and its metabolites, the others being transferrin for transport of iron, and hemopexin for heme.

In 1955 Smithies demonstrated by starch gel electrophoresis that there are three major haptoglobin types (or groups); these are now designated Hp 1-1, Hp 2-1, and Hp 2-2. The three types, which are differentiated by their complex electrophoretic patterns, were at first thought to represent phenotypic expression of only two autosomal genes (Smithies and Walker, 1956). However, the multiple bands obtained for the phenotype Hp 2-1 did not agree with the pattern expected for a heterozygote of the Hp^2 and the Hp^1 genes. Dissociation of haptoglobin into its constituent polypeptide chains by reduction and alkylation in 6 M urea showed that there were two kinds of chains, α and β, and that variations in the structure of the α chain were the cause of the differences in electrophoretic patterns of the intact molecules. Two subtypes of the hpα^1 chain were identified, hpα^{1F} and hpα^{1S}; each contains 84 amino acid residues, but they differ by a single amino acid substitution, lysine in hpα^{1F} for glutamic acid in hpα^{1S} at position 54. The hpα^2 chain has 143 amino acids and has an internal duplication in sequence of a large segment of the hpα^1 chain. Progress has been made in sequence analysis of the hpβ chain; 171 of the 300-odd residues have been reported by Kurosky *et al.* (1974, 1975).

Great interest was aroused in the genetics of human haptoglobin when it was shown that the α chain had two alternative forms, one of which represented a partial internal gene duplication of the other. A large number of variant haptoglobin phenotypes have been described in man. Some involve quantitative variations in the expression of $Hp\alpha$ genes; other represent changes in the structural genes. The structural basis of most of these genetic variants has yet to be elucidated; however, numerous studies of the population genetics and geographic distribution of polymorphic haptoglobins have been reported. Haptoglobin typing has also proved useful in forensic medicine.

Although there is a wide range in normal haptoglobin concentration (40–180 mg/100 ml), haptoglobin levels are fairly constant in healthy individuals. However, because there is a marked decrease in inflammation, liver damage, hemolytic episodes, and other diseases, there is much clinical interest in the measurement of haptoglobin. Hereditary deficiencies in haptoglobin synthesis (hypohaptoglobinemia) are common in the Black race. A variety of methods for the measurement of haptoglobin have been reported, and an automated procedure is now commercially available. More widespread application of quantitative haptoglobin determinations may be expected in the future. See Ritchie, Chapter 8.

Because of great interest in the physiological role, clinical significance, structural variation, and population genetics of haptoglobin, many papers and quite a few reviews have been written on one or more of these subjects. Among the earlier reviews are those of Smithies (1959a, 1964), Nyman (1959a), Harris *et al.* (1959), Barnicot (1961), Galatius-Jensen (1960, 1962), Jayle (1962), Jayle and Moretti (1962), Laurell (1960), Laurell and Grönvall (1962), Prokop and Bundschuh (1963), and Parker and Bearn (1963). More recent reviews include a comprehensive coverage of the physical, chemical, and physiological properties of haptoglobin in the monograph by Schultze and Heremans (1966), a brief review by Javid (1967), a monograph by Kirk (1968), Sutton (1970), and several reviews by Giblett (1968, 1975). The monograph by Pintera (1971) has almost 700 references and gives a complete review of the literature to 1971. Excellent chapters on the formal genetics of the human haptoglobin system are to be found in the monographs by Giblett (1969) and Kirk (1968), both of whom give a tabular summary of the geographic distribution of haptoglobin genes, as well as an extensive bibliography. Hence, this subject will only be summarized briefly in this chapter.

II. Purification and Properties

A. Qualitative Detection and Identification of Common Phenotypes

The distinguishing characteristic of haptoglobin is its ability to form a specific stable complex with hemoglobin, and as a result haptoglobin is usually detected as the Hb-Hp complex. Haptoglobin was discovered by Polonovski and Jayle (1939) owing to the peroxidase activity of this complex, and this property provides an indirect but accurate method of estimating serum haptoglobin level. However, haptoglobin is now most commonly detected by methods of electrophoresis which combine a molecular sieving effect and thus permit identification of haptoglobin types. In 1955 by use of starch gel electrophoresis Smithies discovered the three major haptoglobin types or groups now designated Hp 1-1, Hp 2-1, and Hp 2-2. In the starch gel medium the haptoglobin types are separated on the basis of their molecular size as well as by their charge differences. The original horizontal procedure has been modified by many authors with the aim of increasing the resolution and of adaptation to the routine comparative analysis of many sera. Poulik (1957) added the principle of electrophoresis in a discontinuous buffer system which promotes finer resolution of many serum proteins including the separation of free hemoglobin from the Hp-Hb complex. Smithies (1959b) introduced vertical starch gel electrophoresis to enhance resolution of many serum protein components including haptoglobins. Polyacrylamide gel is often employed in place of starch gel because of better reproducibility of the gel and the wider range of sieving effect. Because of interest in the physiological role, clinical significance, and genetic polymorphism of the haptoglobins many modifications of the electrophoretic methods have been developed, including use of a variety of discontinuous buffer systems.

These have been summarized and compared critically in the monograph by Pintera (1971); directions for the most common procedures are also given by Giblett (1969). The resolution of the principal haptoglobin types in the presence of other serum components is illustrated in Fig. 4 of Chapter 1, Volume I. Schematic diagrams of the starch gel electrophoretic patterns of haptoglobin phenotypes and subtypes are given later.

The more common haptoglobin types can also be differentiated by immunoelectrophoresis in agar gel by the method introduced by Hirschfeld (1959, 1960) which gives a simultaneous resolution of the Gc system. Medicolegal techniques for the identification of blood include enhancing the specificity of the peroxidase test for blood by the addition of haptoglobin; for Hp typing of old dry blood samples the immunoelectrophoretic method is preferred.

The hereditary haptoglobin types are ascertained by starch gel or polyacrylamide gel electrophoresis of whole serum in discontinuous buffers of alkaline pH (ca. pH 8.6) and are visualized with staining by appropriate procedures. In contrast, the haptoglobin subtypes described later are determined by gel electrophoresis of the purified haptoglobins in acidic buffers (pH 4.9) containing 8 M urea after reduction and alkylation to separate the α and β polypeptide chains. Thus separate procedures are required to determine Hp types and subtypes.

A schematic diagram of the common Hp types is given in Fig. 1 taken from Giblett (1969). Type 1-1 migrates as a single band in starch or polyacrylamide gel electrophoresis, but type 2-2 migrates as a series of up to 12 bands, the concentration of which is related to the rate of migration. The heterozygous type, Hp 2-1, resembles 2-2 in having a

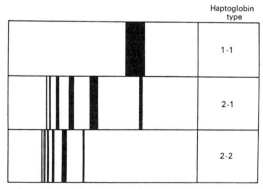

Fig. 1. Diagram of starch gel electrophoretic patterns of the three common human haptoglobin types. The origin is on the left, and migration is from the left toward the anode on the right (from Giblett, 1969).

series of bands but with different migration rates, although the fastest band is like that of 1-1. Type 2-1 (modified), later illustrated, shows the same general pattern as the usual 2-1 type, but the concentrations of the components differ, i.e., the two fastest moving bands are increased, and the others are decreased. When complexed with hemoglobin, the individual haptoglobin components migrate more slowly, but the general appearance of the patterns is unchanged. This indicates that the heterogeneous patterns are a function of the haptoglobin structure rather than a result of complex formation. Polyacrylamide gel gives patterns similar to those of starch gel with many bands likewise appearing in the Hp 2-1 and Hp 2-2 phenotypes (Pastewka *et al.,* 1973).

Heterogeneity of haptoglobin 1-1 has been demonstrated by electrophoresis of serum in starch gels at pH 4.9 in a discontinuous buffer containing borate but no urea (Fagerhol and Jacobsen, 1969). Eight protein zones are obtained, but the zones disappear if boric acid is replaced by other acids in the buffer. Hence the zones represent borate complexes that probably involve the carbohydrate groups. In contrast, the heterogeneous types 2-1 and 2-2 seen in alkaline gels are not artifacts but represent a series of polymers (see below).

B. Quantitative Determination of Haptoglobin

Whereas qualitative detection of haptoglobin types is of interest chiefly for studies of population genetics, the quantitative estimation of total serum haptoglobin is significant because of the physiological role of haptoglobin and its changing level in various diseases. The values are usually expressed as the hemoglobin-binding capacity per 100 ml which is abbreviated HbBC. Almost all of the analytical methods for measurement of haptoglobin concentration depend on the change in properties of the two components of the Hb-Hp complex, and most of the methods utilize hemoglobinometry of some kind. In a detailed discussion of various analytical techniques Pintera (1971) lists six properties employed for the estimation of haptoglobin; of these, the first two are the most frequently used:

(1) The ability to enhance the peroxidatic activity of hemoglobin
(2) Changes in electrophoretic ability
(3) The changed precipitation by Rivanol
(4) The increase of molecular weight displayed in gel filtration
(5) The protection of spectral properties against denaturation
(6) Immunochemical properties—the only way of specifically distinguishing unbound haptoglobin

Jayle's original peroxidase method (1951) has been widely applied and remains a standard procedure, but it has been modified by use of a variety of electron donors (Nyman, 1959a; Connell and Smithies, 1959) and an automated method for patient screening (Burrows and Hosten, 1966). The method depends on the enhancement of the peroxidase activity of hemoglobin when it is complexed with haptoglobin. The affinity of Hp for Hb is so high that there is no free Hb until all the Hp is saturated. An excess of hemoglobin is added to the serum to be analyzed, and the Hp-Hb content is measured from the peroxidase activity.

Results similar to the peroxidase method are given by procedures using electrophoresis to separate the Hp-Hb complex from free hemoglobin (Laurell and Nyman, 1957). Acrylamide gel, starch gel, paper, cellulose acetate, etc., may be used as carriers. The hemoglobin present in the complex and in the free form is measured in various ways such as by staining followed by photoelectric scanning (Hommes, 1959; Javid and Horowitz, 1960; Rowe, 1961; Smith and Owen, 1961; Ferris *et al.*, 1966; Tarukoski, 1966) or from its radioactivity when using hemoglobin labeled with radioactive iron-59 (Sass and Spear, 1962). Bernier (1967) has described a very rapid method for determination of serum haptoglobin levels based on high voltage electrophoresis in agar gel and benzidine staining. The electrophoretic determination of Hp as the hemoglobin complex is described by Malin *et al.* (1972). Gel filtration on Sephadex G-100 has been used as an alternative procedure to separate the Hp-Hb complex and free Hb with measurement of the hemoglobin by the usual procedures (Ratcliff and Hardwicke, 1964; Killander, 1964; Hodgson and Sewell, 1965). Roy *et al.* (1969) have described a simple method for the quantitative determination of haptoglobin based on the fact that haptoglobin protects hemoglobin from acid denaturation.

Quantitative immunochemical methods can also be applied for the direct determination of haptoglobin (Kluthe *et al.*, 1965). The antisera may be polyvalent and react with all types of haptoglobin or monovalent and react with individual types. The availability of commercial polyvalent sera specific for human haptoglobin has prompted the exploration of radial immunodiffusion methods applicable to routine assay. Though these methods are promising, some problems have been experienced because of the slower diffusion of the Hp 2-1 and Hp 2-2 polymers and also because of differences in antigenic determinants of the various Hp types (Pintera, 1971). Automated immunoprecipitation is likely to be the method of choice for the future (see Chapter 8 by Ritchie).

C. Purification of Haptoglobin

Haptoglobin is prepared from pooled human plasma (Laurell, 1959) or from haptoglobin-containing fractions obtained by the Cohn ethanol fractionation scheme (Pavliček and Kalous, 1964). Since haptoglobin represents less than 2% of the total plasma proteins, other body fluids that are rich in haptoglobin may sometimes be used, such as ascitic fluid or the urine of patients suffering from lipoid nephrosis who may excrete large amounts of haptoglobin if it is the monomeric type Hp 1-1. In animals the amount of haptoglobin in plasma may be increased by injections that precipitate an acute phase reaction. Several methods of purifying haptoglobin have been described since the original procedure of Jayle and Boussier (1954); these are based on selective adsorption by an anion-exchange resin (Connell and Smithies, 1959) or chromatography on DEAE-cellulose (Laurell, 1959; Connell and Shaw, 1961), or a combination of ammonium sulfate and Rivanol precipitation with zone electrophoresis (Schultze *et al.*, 1963). In pooled plasma the various types of haptoglobin may be separated by fractional precipitation with ammonium sulfate (1.9–2.2 M) followed by preparative zone electrophoresis (Herman-Boussier *et al.*, 1960a) or by chromatography on DEAE-cellulose (Steinbuch and Quentin, 1961; Smith *et al.*, 1962) or DEAE-Sephadex (Hamaguchi, 1969). Pintera (1971) gives a table modified from Cloarec and Moretti (1965) that summarizes the procedures used by various workers. For detailed procedures for the isolation of human haptoglobin and for its location in various plasma fractionation schemes see Pintera (1971) and Chapter 8, Volume III.

The isolation of pure haptoglobin types requires a combination of procedures; gel filtration on Sephadex G-200 facilitates the separation of the monomer Hp 1-1 from the Hp 2-1 and 2-2 polymers (Gordon *et al.*, 1969). Crystallization of human Hp 1-1 has been accomplished after a purification scheme involving precipitation first with Rivanol and then with ammonium sulfate followed by preparative zone electrophoresis and gel filtration (Haupt and Heide, 1970).

The purification of animal haptoglobins may require different procedures for each species; as an example see the method for the isolation of canine haptoglobin described by Dobryszycka *et al.* (1969). Haptoglobin as usually purified is free of hemoglobin; the Hp-Hb complex may also be prepared but since the complex is difficult to dissociate, the procedure is not used for the isolation of haptoglobin.

The monomeric unit of human haptoglobin is composed of four polypeptide chains: two α chains and two β chains which are joined by disulfide bonds (Shim and Bearn, 1964; Malchy and Dixon, 1973a,b; Malchy *et al.*, 1973). The α and β chains are dissociated by reduction with mercaptoethanol in the presence of 8 *M* urea followed by alkylation with iodoacetamide or similar alkylating agents with separation by starch gel electrophoresis (Smithies *et al.*, 1966; Connell *et al.*, 1966). For preparative purposes the haptoglobin is reduced in the presence of 5 *M* guanidine and the chains are separated by gel filtration on Sephadex G-200 in the presence of guanidine to minimize aggregation (Gordon *et al.*, 1968; Barnett *et al.*, 1972). The separation of the chains is illustrated schematically in a later section.

D. Physicochemical Properties

Haptoglobin is an α_2-globulin with an electrophoretic mobility of 4.5 Tiselius units at pH 8.6 in 0.1 ionic strength buffer and an isolectric point of pH 4.1. It has the expected solubility being precipitated at about 2 *M* ammonium sulfate, and as a glycoprotein it is soluble in the perchloric acid fraction (0.6 *M*). Actually, the monomeric Hp 1-1 is somewhat more soluble than the polymeric Hp 2-2, for the latter is precipitated at 1.8–2.2 *M* ammonium sulfate and the former at 2.0–2.4 *M*. This illustrates the frequent qualification that must be made about the molecular kinetic properties of this heterogeneous protein because of the existence of allotypes with numerous polymeric forms.

From the physicochemical point of view only Hp 1-1 appears to be a homogeneous protein. It migrates as a single band in starch gel electrophoresis, and, whether complexed with hemoglobin or not, it sediments as a single symmetrical peak in the analytical ultracentrifuge. In contrast, haptoglobin type 2-2 sediments as an asymmetrical peak, and type 2-1 gives evidence of at least three ultracentrifugal components (Bearn and Franklin, 1958, 1959). The heterogeneous types are stable polymers and are not artifacts, but 2-1 cannot be produced simply by mixing 1-1 and 2-2 (Connell and Smithies, 1959).

Although it was well established that Hp 2-2 consists of a series of polymers, the exact nature of the individual components was unknown until Fuller *et al.* (1973) unravelled the complex subunit composition of the polymers. Because of the characteristic spacing of the multiple bands in starch or acrylamide gel electrophoresis, it was assumed they represented a polymeric series. However, several investigators held different views regarding the number of α and β polypeptide chains in the polymers, e.g., whether each successively larger polymer was due to addition of one β chain (Sutton, 1970), a half-molecule (Marnay, 1961), or one monomeric molecule (Shim and Bearn, 1964). Until the advent of detergent gel electrophoresis, it was not possible to calculate the molecular weights accurately from the distance moved since differences in charge would also affect the mobility. Many attempts to determine molecular weight differences by analytical ultracentrifugation also failed because of inability to separate the polymers. The solution to this problem was achieved by Fuller *et al.* (1973) who isolated six discrete Hp 2-2 polymers from a series of 12 to 14 by polyacrylamide gel electrophoresis. Quantitative amino terminal analysis and amino acid analysis showed that each polymer consisted of α^2 and β polypeptide chains in a 1:1 ratio. Molecular weight determination by SDS acrylamide gel electrophoresis and by ultracentrifugal analysis showed that each polymer differs from the next member in the series by an average increment of 54,500. This is the approximate size of a subunit consisting of an α^2 chain (17,300) and a β chain (40,000). Differential reduction with mercaptoethanol proved that the α^2/β subunits are joined together through disulfide bonds to form the polymers. The six polymers isolated conformed to the series $\alpha_3\beta_3$, $\alpha_4\beta_4$, . . ., $\alpha_8\beta_8$ and ranged in theoretical molecular weights from 171,000 to 456,000. Hence, it is clear that the physical constants of Hp 2-2 represent average values; this explains some of the large discrepancies in molecular parameters reported for Hp 2-2.

The differences in the patterns of Hp 2-1 and 2-2 have been elucidated by Javid (1964) who confirmed the hypothesis of Allison (1959) and Parker and Bearn (1963) that the $Hp^{\alpha 1}$ gene product (the α^1 chain of lower molecular weight) is incorporated into the polymers formed by the $Hp^{\alpha 2}$ gene product (the α^2 chain of higher molecular weight which is responsible for the polymerization phenomenon). Thus, the molecular chain formula for Hp 1-1 is $(\alpha^1\beta)_2$, that of Hp 2-2 is $(\alpha^2\beta)_n$ where n is a series. The hypothetical formula of Hp 2-1 would include hybrid polymers of these two such as $(\alpha^1\beta)_m \cdot (\alpha^2\beta)_n$. The polymer model for Hp 2-1 is thus similar to the polymer model for Hp 2-2 (Barnett *et al.,* 1975).

A round number of 100,000 is generally cited for the molecular weight of the homozygote haptoglobin 1-1 (Pintera, 1971; Schultze and Heremans, 1966). This is based on sedimentation-diffusion data and on the hemoglobin-combining capacity (Herman-Boussier, 1960). A value of $98,770 \pm 2270$ is given for Hp 1-1 by Cheftal and Moretti (1966) and Moretti *et al.* (1966). A figure close to 100,000 is also in accord with sequence data and with molecular weight determinations on the individual chains. The molecular weight of the α^{1S} chain calculated from sequence data is 9304, and the molecular weight of the β chain determined from ultracentrifugation is 42,582 (Black *et al.,* 1970), which gives a sum of 103,772 for the four-chain monomer. Since one molecule of Hp 1-1 binds one molecule (or two half molecules) of hemoglobin (Laurell, 1960), the complex has a molecular weight of about 165,000. The average molecular weight of the hemoglobin-free polymers is about 400,000 for Hp 2-2 and 220,000 for Hp 2-1 (Herman-Boussier *et al.,* 1960a,b; Smithies, 1959a). These data, though approximate are in accord with the heterogeneous starch gel patterns observed for types 2-1 and 2-2 that indicate that these haptoglobins form stable polymers. The lower molecular weight of Hp 1-1 explains its excretion in amounts up to several grams a day in nephrotic urine (Guinand *et al.,* 1956; Marnay, 1961) and its readier excretion in normal urine compared to types 2-1 and 2-2 (Berggård and Bearn, 1962).

Although there is good agreement in the molecular weight calculated from the physical constants of haptoglobin type Hp 1-1 ($D_{20} = 4.7$ Fick units and $s_{20,\,w} = 4.45$ S) and the molecular weight calculated from structural data, there is a serious discrepancy in the partial specific volume for which various authors give a range of from 0.660 (Waks and Alfsen, 1968) to 0.770 (Cheftel *et al.,* 1960). The latter value is much too high for a glycoprotein and the former is unusually low. Since the calculation of molecular weight from the sedimentation and diffusion constants is strongly dependent on the partial specific volume, a serious error may occur if the value used is off in even the second decimal place. This indicates that a careful redetermination of the partial specific volume and other physical constants ought to be done in order to calculate the molecular weight of Hp 1-1 more precisely.

Although the various types of haptoglobin differ in migration rate in starch gel or acrylamide gel electrophoresis because of the retardation of polymeric forms, Hp 1-1 moves only slightly faster than Hp 2-2 at pH 8.6 in free boundary electrophoresis where molecular weight has no effect. The isoelectric points of the several types are likewise similar, being pH 4.2–4.25 for Hp 1-1 and pH 4.1–4.2 for Hp 2-2 (Herman-Boussier *et al.,* 1960b).

E. Molecular Conformation

Very little is known about the molecular conformation of the monomeric form of haptoglobin (i.e., Hp 1-1) or about the variety of polymeric forms of Hp 2-1 and Hp 2-2. Although Hp 1-1 has been crystallized (Haupt and Heide, 1970), detailed X-ray diffraction studies have not yet been reported. However, small angle scattering measurements of Hp 1-1 indicate a volume of $165,000 \pm 20,000$ Å with an equivalent ellipsoid of rotation with half axes $a = 14$ Å and $b = 56$ Å (Waks *et al.,* 1969). The results of optical rotatory dispersion studies of Hp 1-1 and Hp 2-2 at pH 5.5 suggest that neither type is in the α-helix or random coil configuration and that some other kind of structure may be present

(Waks and Alfsen, 1966). From the circular dichroism spectra in the 200–240 nm region Hamaguchi (1969) has concluded that the helical content is negligible in all three types of haptoglobin but the β structure is present. The circular dichroism spectra indicate that Hp 1-1 and Hp 2-2 differ significantly in conformation and that Hp 2-1 more closely resembles 2-2.

The rather anomalous titration behavior of haptoglobins between pH 3 and pH 9 (Waks and Alfsen, 1966) is followed by an apparent reversible dissociation into identical subunits from pH 9.0 to 11.5 (Waks *et al.*, 1967). Although ultracentrifugal analysis indicates that alkali alone induces dissociation into identical subunits of molecular weight of 40,000 (Waks and Alfsen, 1968), this does not accord with the observation of other workers that reducing agents such as mercaptoethanol are required to achieve dissociation by disruption of interchain disulfide bonds (Connell *et al.*, 1962; Shim and Bearn, 1964; Barnett *et al.*, 1972). Furthermore, Malchy *et al.* (1973) have shown that the half-haptoglobin molecule is obtained by selective cleavage of a $21\alpha–21\alpha$ disulfide bond. Undoubtedly this question will be cleared up by the sequence analysis now underway by Barnett *et al.* (1972) and Kurosky *et al.* (1974). Haptoglobin is easily denatured especially at acidic pH. Acidification of whole serum only to pH 4.2 is said to denature 80% of the haptoglobin in 30 min (Connell and Shaw, 1961).

The spontaneous refolding of human haptoglobins after extensive reduction and dissociation has been reported by Bernini and Borri-Voltattorni (1970). They reduced Hp 1-1 and 2-2 with mercaptoethanol in 8 M urea or 6 M guanidine leading to the liberation of 18 and 24 SH groups/mole of protein, respectively. Removal of denaturing agents and reoxidation in the presence of O_2 and a catalytic amount of thiol was followed by restoration of the chemical and immunological properties of the native protein with a yield of 60 to 90% under the most favorable conditions. The ease of reassembly of this multichain molecule is surprising and suggests the importance of chain pairing in the folding of the protein during biosynthesis.

F. The Haptoglobin–Hemoglobin Complex

Since complex formation with hemoglobin is the characteristic physicochemical and physiological property of haptoglobin, the nature of the interaction has been widely studied. Although the mechanism of the interaction of human haptoglobin and hemoglobin A has partially been elucidated, the nature of the binding sites on haptoglobin and of the bond or bonds linking Hp and Hb is still unknown.

Haptoglobin combines stoichiometrically with Hb A to form a stable undissociated complex of one mole of Hp and one mole of Hb. Hp binds so tightly to Hb that the reaction is considered to be essentially irreversible. That the heme part is unimportant in the linkage is shown by the fact that haptoglobin combines with globin but does not combine with either heme or myoglobin (Javid *et al.*, 1959; Nyman, 1959b; Wheby *et al.*, 1960) or with deoxyhemoglobin (Giblett, 1969). The haptoglobin complex formed with oxyhemoglobin is essentially irreversible (Nagel and Gibson, 1971); however, the oxygen equilibrium of the combined Hb is greatly altered (Nagel *et al.*, 1965). The combination is not species-specific, for human haptoglobin can combine with various animal hemoglobins (Makinen *et al.*, 1972; Cohen-Dix *et al.*, 1973) as avidly as with human fetal hemoglobin or with certain abnormal hemoglobins (Nagel and Ranney, 1964). Indeed, rat hemoglobin forms microcrystals with human Hp 1-1 and 2-2 (Waks *et al.*, 1968). Although the reaction of human haptoglobin with hemoglobin has a very broad species specificity, very distantly related hemoglobins, such as those of the frog or carp, do exhibit weaker binding than mammalian hemoglobins, which appear indistinguishable from human Hb in this interaction (Cohen-Dix *et al.*, 1973).

The α chain of hemoglobin is essential for normal binding to haptoglobin as shown by the fact that Hb Barts (a β chain tetramer) and isolated Hb β chains that have been reacted with mercuribenzoate have only a very low affinity for haptoglobin. Yet, when α chains reacted with mercuribenzoate are added to the mixture in sufficient amounts to fill half the sites, the binding of both the α and β chains of Hb proceeds normally to full saturation of the haptoglobin (Nagel and Gibson, 1967; Chiancone *et al.*, 1966; Alfsen *et al.*, 1970).

Laurell (1960) and Laurell and Grönvall (1962) were the first to suggest that the binding of Hb to Hp occurs through the α,β dimer of hemoglobin. Their experimental data indicated that the interaction between Hp and half-Hb molecules at neutral reaction is stronger than the interaction between the two halves constituting the whole hemoglobin molecule and thus that the fully saturated simplest haptoglobin (1-1) binds two halves of a hemoglobin molecule instead of one unsplit Hb molecule (Laurell, 1960). A number of other authors have described an Hp $\cdot \frac{1}{2}$Hb intermediate complex (Hamaguchi and Sasazuki, 1967; Ogawa *et al.*, 1968; Peacock *et al.*, 1970). Studies cited above on the interaction of isolated Hb chains with Hp have confirmed this viewpoint. Waks *et al.* (1969) have described two complexes of Hp 1-1 and Hb having a 1:1 stoichiometry designated Cx and Cd for which they propose different conformations. Kawamura *et al.* (1972a,b) have also made kinetic studies of the intermediate and saturated forms of human Hp-Hb complexes.

A detailed kinetic analysis of the reaction between deoxyhemoglobin, which does not bind to haptoglobin, and a haptoglobin solution saturated with carbon monoxide indicated that the hemoglobin tetramer is incapable of binding haptoglobin and its dissociation to dimers is a prerequisite for the reaction (Nagel and Gibson, 1971). Study of the reaction of isolated α- and β- hemoglobin chains toward haptoglobin half-saturated by α chains or Hb A led to the conclusion that haptoglobin probably contains four binding sites, two for each hemoglobin α,β dimer. The two pair of sites appeared to be independent but within each pair a strong interaction exists between the α-specific site and the allosterically induced β site. Nagel and Gibson (1971) write the reaction as

$$\tfrac{1}{2}Hp + \alpha\beta \rightarrow \tfrac{1}{2}Hp\alpha\beta$$

and give a rate constant of about 5.5×10^5 M^{-1} sec^{-1}. In this proposed mechanism the haptoglobin molecule binds an α,β dimer at its α-specific site thereby inducing an allosteric change in the haptoglobin molecule, a process which creates a β-binding site probably in close proximity to the α-binding site.

The formal relationship of the binding of two half-molecules of Hb by Hp to the binding of two antigenic determinants by a bivalent antibody has been noted by a number of authors (Malchy and Dixon, 1970; Nagel and Gibson, 1971). Black and Dixon (1968) earlier pointed out that immunoglobulins and haptoglobins have a similar subunit structure, each being composed of two pair of polypeptide chains linked together through disulfide bonds; they further suggested that the smaller chains of the two kinds of molecules (the light chains of the immunoglobulins and the Hp α chains) are structurally homologous. However, as seen later, the Hp β chains and the immunoglobulin heavy chains do not exhibit sequence homology. Furthermore, haptoglobin has only a single specificity and is composed of only a few polymorphic forms, whereas highly specific antibody molecules may be induced by immunization with an enormous variety of antigens. The structural diversity of immunoglobulins and the division of their polypeptide chains into variable and constant regions also distinguishes them from the haptoglobins. Another difference is that the association constant of the haptoglobin–hemoglobin complex is several orders of magnitude greater than that of the antibody–antigen complex with the result that the Hb-Hp complex is essentially irreversible whereas the latter complex dissolves in antigen excess.

The nature of the forces involved in formation of the Hp-Hb complex has not been established. The unusual stability of the bond is puzzling. Electrostatic and hydrophobic bonds apparently stabilize the interaction, but sulfhydryl groups and disulfide bonds are not involved. The complementary nature of the interaction of two molecules, each consisting of two pairs of polypeptide chains, may be a significant factor. Calorimetric studies indicate that enthalpy rather than entropy is the driving force of the interaction (Adams and Weiss, 1969). Blocking of the amino groups of haptoglobin by trinitrophenylation reduces the hemoglobin-binding capacity suggesting that the amino groups may be involved (Shinoda, 1965). Canine haptoglobin in which all the accessible tyrosine or tryptophan groups have been blocked by acetylation retains the capacity to react with hemoglobin, but the complex formed between hemoglobin and the modified Hp lacks peroxidase activity (Dobryszycka *et al.*, 1969). However, nitration of the tyrosyl groups of human haptoglobin abolishes both its ability to combine with hemoglobin and to enhance the peroxidase activity of hemoglobin. On the basis of this and other methods of chemical modification of human haptoglobin, Chiao and Bezkorovainy (1972) conclude that tyrosyl groups are the only hemoglobin-binding ligands in haptoglobin whose role is reasonably certain.

Just as IgM antibodies tend to have a lower expressed valence per subunit than do IgG antibodies of the same specificity, one might expect the polymeric types of haptoglobin to have a lower Hb-binding capacity per milligram of Hp because of shielding of some binding sites. Although this effect has been reported by Javid (1965), other authors have concluded that an equivalent amount of hemoglobin is bound per subunit to all the common Hp types when they are fully saturated (Hamaguchi, 1969).

Formation of the Hp-Hb complex leads to significant changes in the properties of hemoglobin. Because conformational rearrangements are involved in the reversible oxygenation of hemoglobin (Perutz, 1970), it is not surprising that the oxygen equilibria are affected by the Hp-Hb complex formation which must induce a profound conformational change in the hemoglobin. The Hp-Hb complex has a high affinity for oxygen but lacks a Bohr effect. Nagel *et al.* (1965) suggest that the haptoglobin binding of hemoglobin probably impairs the separation of hemoglobin into pairs of symmetrical subunits. The heme–heme interaction is decreased resulting in a hyperbolic oxygen-dissociation curve. Circular dichroism (Hamaguchi, 1969), fluorescent probe studies (Russo and Chen, 1974), electron spin resonance spectra (Hamaguchi *et al.*, 1971), and electron magnetic resonance measurements (Makinen and Kon, 1971) of the Hp-Hb complex confirm the conformational change in the bound hemoglobin. Giblett (1975) has suggested that an irreversible fixation of the

COOH-terminal histidine of the β chain of hemoglobin (β-146) may occur in the Hp-Hb complex accounting for the greatly reduced Bohr effect. In hemoglobin this histidine is involved in important salt bridges to Asp-94 in the same β chain and Lys-40 on the adjacent α chain (Perutz, 1970). Although deoxyhemoglobin is not bound by haptoglobin, it will form the Hp-Hb complex after removal of this histidine by carboxypeptidase A (Hb DesHis) (Chianconne *et al.*, 1966). Furthermore, Hb Hiroshima (in which β-146 is aspartic acid rather than histidine) binds Hp quite well when in the deoxy form if also stripped of phosphate (Nagel and Gibson, 1972).

Several authors have proposed that the contact region between the two hemoglobin α,β dimers contains the Hp-binding site (Makinen *et al.*, 1972; Nagel and Gibson, 1972; Cohen-Dix *et al.*, 1974). As a result, the hemoglobin–haptoglobin reaction has been used as a probe for hemoglobin conformation. For example, Nagel and Gibson (1972) used the rate of binding of haptoglobin to demonstrate differences in conformation of native Hb A, deoxy A, deoxy A stripped of phosphate, mixed liganded hybrids, and several abnormal hemoglobins. Waks and Beychok (1974) studied the effect of induced conformational states in human apohemoglobin on the binding of Hp 1-1. The isolated heme-free globin chains (α° and β°) do not measurably combine to form apohemoglobin. However, in the presence of haptoglobin, a stable complex is formed comprising one haptoglobin molecule and $2\alpha^\circ$ and $2\beta^\circ$ chains (Hp-$2\alpha^\circ2\beta^\circ$). The interaction of haptoglobin with apohemoglobin "freezes" the conformational state of the globin and prevents the restoration of native structure usually brought about by addition of heme. Complex formation with hemoglobin greatly enhances the peroxidase activity of hemoglobin, which itself is not a true peroxidase. This activity of the Hp-Hb complex is not dependent on the oxidation state of the heme, for the methemoglobin complex is equally active. Nor does it depend on the integrity of the carbohydrate groups on the haptoglobin, for removal of up to 70% of the sialic acid does not impair the peroxidase activity (Rafelson *et al.*, 1961). On the other hand, this enzyme-like function is reduced by blocking the amino groups of haptoglobin (Shinoda, 1965) and is abolished by completely blocking the accessible tyrosyl or tryptophanyl groups of the haptoglobin prior to complex formation (Chiao and Bezkorovainy, 1972). This shows that the integrity of the haptoglobin protein moiety is essential for the enhanced peroxidase activity.

G. *Immunochemical Properties of Hp and the Hp-Hb Complex*

The qualitative demonstration of human haptoglobin phenotypes by immunoelectrophoresis (Hirschfeld, 1959, 1960) and the quantitative determination of serum haptoglobins by an immunological method (Kluthe *et al.,* 1965) depend on the fact that immunization with human haptoglobin elicits strong specific antisera in nonprimates such as rabbits. Korngold (1963) was the first to demonstrate antigenic differences among human haptoglobins. Hp 2-2 and Hp 1-1 give a reaction of partial identity in immunodiffusion against a hyperimmune antiserum to Hp 2-2. Shim and Bearn (1964) showed that the isolated polypeptide chains hpα^1 and hpβ contain both common and specific antigenic determinants. A number of specific determinants in human haptoglobin have been recognized by various workers—eight in Hp 2-1 and seven in Hp 1-1 (Javid and Fuhrman, 1971). Some are present on the hpα chain and others on the hpβ chain, and allotype haptoglobins such as Bellevue and Marburg have somewhat different determinants (Shim *et al.,* 1967; Javid and Yingling, 1968a,b). No differences between the Hp 1-1 phenotypes (1F-1F) and (1S-1S) were found by Shim and Bearn (1964), but these were distinguished immunochemically by Ehnholm (1968) although they differ by only a single amino acid, an interchange of lysine and glutamic acid at position 54α. All nonhuman primate haptoglobins lack a determinant which depends upon the polymeric configuration of haptoglobin. The nonhuman primates, when ordered in their evolutionary proximity to man, show a progressive decrease in the number of determinants they share with man, but determinants located near the Hb binding site are shared by all the species (Javid and Fuhrman, 1971). In the Hp-Hb complex the hemoglobin blocks several antigenic determinants of the native haptoglobin, 1 mole of hemoglobin being necessary to block the maximum number of antigenic determinants of 1 mole of Hp 1-1. Type-specific antisera can still distinguish Hp 1-1 and Hp 2-2 when it is complexed with hemoglobin (Korngold, 1965). The quality of the antigenic determinants of hemoglobin is not modified in the Hb-Hp complex, but the precipitability with antiserum and inducibility of antibody against Hb are quantitatively modified, both being greater (Tsunoo *et al.,* 1974). The sites on hemoglobin where haptoglobin binds and the sites of antibody binding are completely independent (Cohen-Dix *et al.,* 1973). For the immunochemical characterization of haptoglobin see Chung and Shim (1973).

III. Molecular Structure

A. Chemical Composition

The amino acid composition of human haptoglobin has been investigated by a number of workers with results that are in reasonable agreement (Herman-Boussier et al., 1960a,b, 1962; Heimburger et al., 1964). Little difference was found among Hp 1-1, 2-1, and 2-2, the reason, of course, being that all three share the same β chain, which is the major component and also the fact that the α^2 chain is a partial duplication of the α^1 chain.

In Table I the amino acid composition is given in moles per mole for the α and β chains of human Hp 1-1 and for the whole protein. The composition of the α^{1F}, α^{1S}, and α^2 chains is calculated from their amino acid sequence (Black and Dixon, 1968; Malchy and Dixon, 1973a,b), and data for the β chain and for Hp 1-1 are taken from Barnett et al. (1972) and from Heimburger et al. (1964), respectively. The α chains are unusually high in dicarboxylic acids, unusually low in hydroxyamino acids and leucine, and lack methionine and phenylalanine. In contrast, the latter amino acids are present in the β chain which has an abundance of hydroxyamino acids and leucine and a normal content of aspartic and glutamic acids. Thus the two kinds of chains are somewhat complementary in amino acid composition. From Table I it may be noted that the β chain is almost twice as long as the α^2 chain and nearly four times as long as the α^1 chain. Also, the composition of Hp 1-1 minus that of two β chains approximates that of two α^1 chains indicating a concordance of the analyses of three different sets of workers on the isolated chains and the whole protein.

Animal haptoglobins differ significantly from their human counterpart and also from species to species both in their amino acid composition and their carbohydrate content. Lombart et al. (1965) have reported analyses for the rabbit and rat haptoglobins and Dobryszycka et al. (1969) for the dog. The latter authors have tabulated the data for the three animal species in comparison to man. In all four cases aspartic and glutamic acids account for 19 to 20% of the haptoglobin molecule.

Sialic acid, galactose, mannose, hexosamine, and fucose are present in the animal and human haptoglobins; in human haptoglobin the moles per mole of these sugars are given by Heimburger et al. (1964) as: hexose 43, acetylhexosamine, 24, sialic acid, 17, and fucose, 1. Comparable figures for canine haptoglobin are hexose, 28, hexosamine, 27–28, sialic acid, 13, and fucose, 1 (Dobryszycka et al., 1969). In both cases the ratio of galactose to mannose is approximately 2:1.

TABLE I

Amino Acid Composition[a] in Moles per Mole of the α and β Chains of Haptoglobin and of Hp 1-1

	α^{1S}	α^{1F}	α^2	β	Hp 1-1	2β	Hp-2β	$2\alpha^{1S}$	$2\alpha^{1F}$
Lysine	8	9	15	22	64	44	20	16	18
Histidine	2	2	4	10	23	20	3	4	
Arginine	2	2	4	5	14	10	4	4	
Aspartic acid	15	15	23	28	83	56	27	30	
Threonine	3	3	5	19	44	38	6	6	
Serine	2	2	3	15	40	30	10	4	
Glutamic acid	9	8	16	29	75	58	17	18	16
Proline	7	7	11	13	43	26	17	14	
Glycine	7	7	12	20	51	40	11	14	
Alanine	5	5	8	21	50	42	8	10	
Half-cystine	4	4	7	6	20	12	8	8	
Valine	8	8	12	27	63	54	9	16	
Methionine	0	0	0	4	8	8	0	0	
Isoleucine	3	3	5	13	30	26	4	6	
Leucine	3	3	6	23	53	46	7	6	
Tyrosine	5	5	10	12	34	24	10	10	
Phenylalanine	0	0	0	8	16	16	0	0	
Tryptophan	1	1	2	5	14	10	4	2	
Total	84	84	143	280	725	560	165	168	
$2\alpha + 2\beta$					725				
Molecular weight	9300	9300	17,300	42,580	104,000				

[a] Composition of α^{1F}, α^{1S}, and α^2 chains calculated from amino acid sequence of Black and Dixon (1968). Composition of Hp 1-1 taken from Heimburger *et al.* (1964). Note α^{1F} has lysine at position 54 and α^{1S} has glutamic acid at position 54. Composition of β chain from Barnett *et al.* (1972). The half-cystine content of the α chains is corrected according to Malchy and Dixon (1973a,b). More recent structural studies of Kurosky *et al.* (1975) indicate that the β chain consists of some 310 amino acid residues.

B. Subunit and Polypeptide Chain Structure

Haptoglobin resembles the immunoglobins in subunit structure, for both proteins have a tetrachain structure consisting of a pair of identical smaller polypeptide chains disulfide-bonded to a pair of larger chains. In haptoglobin the small chains — sometimes referred to as the light chains — are the α chains, and the large (or heavy) chains are the β chains. However, to avoid confusion it is best to reserve the use of the terms light and heavy chains for the immunoglobulins. Enough confusion has already resulted from the use of the same symbols, α and β, for the two pairs of polypeptide chains present both in haptoglobin and in hemoglobin, its partner in the Hp-Hb complex, for the α and β chains of these two proteins have no structural relationship.

The working model for the subunit structure of haptoglobin presented by Malchy *et al.* (1973) is a modification of the four-chain structure first proposed by Shim and Bearn (1964) (Fig. 2). The pair of α chains having N-terminal valine are shown on the inside of this schematic model and are joined by disulfide bonds to the larger β chains having N-terminal isoleucine that are pictured on the outside of the model. All of the carbohydrate is attached to the β chains. The number and location of the half-cystine residues and of the disulfide bonds in the α chain are known, but the position of the half-cystines in the β chain is unknown; therefore, the disulfide bonds in the β chain are not correctly shown in the model. From Table I it can be seen that there are four half-cystines in the sequence of the α^1 chain and six are reported from amino acid analysis of the β chain. However, from the partial sequence data in the current literature it is unclear whether there are five or six half-cystines in the β chain. Altogether, five half-cystines have been identified in partial sequences of portions of the β chain by various workers. In a numbering system of the β chain based on alignment to the serine proteases, Cys-168 forms an intrachain disulfide linkage with Cys-182, and Cys-122 represents the only disulfide bridge of the β chain to the α chain (Kurosky et al., 1974). One of the important problems in determination of the primary structure of haptoglobins obviously will be the localization of all the interchain and intrachain disulfide bridges.

The three major types of haptoglobins previously illustrated may be divided into a total of six subtypes on the basis of electrophoretic differences of their component polypeptide chains after reductive cleavage

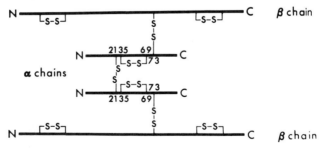

Fig. 2. Working model for the structure of human haptoglobin 1-1 proposed by Malchy *et al.* (1973). The location of the half-cystines and of the disulfide bonds in the α chain is known, but the position of the half-cystines in the β chain is unknown. (Reproduced by permission of the National Research Council of Canada from the *Canadian Journal of Biochemistry* **51**, 265–273, 1973.)

in urea (Connell *et al.,* 1962). The polypeptide chains are joined by disulfide bridges in the native molecule but are dissociated by reduction with mercaptoethanol in 8 M urea and may be separated by electrophoresis in acid-urea starch gel. Despite the multiple bands seen for the subtypes, this method reveals that there are only two kinds of polypeptide chains in haptoglobin, α and β. The haptoglobin subtypes are identified by the pattern of the α polypeptide chain in the urea starch gel. Only the α chain patterns are shown in Fig. 3 because the β chain is identical for all six subtypes. By custom the haptoglobins are designated Hp, the chains hp, and the genes *Hp.* An α chain of a given subtype may be denoted as hp 1α (earlier usage) or hpα^1, and a typical molecular chain formula would be (hp$\alpha^1 \cdot$ hpβ)$_2$ or hp$\alpha^1_2 \cdot$ hpβ_2. The symbol hp indicates the α and β chains are unique to haptoglobin and have no structural relationship to hemoglobin. Other symbols that have been used are α^{1hp} and β^{hp} for the respective chains (Nagel and Gibson, 1971), and chain formulas such as (hp$1\alpha \cdot$ hpβ)$_2$ have been used (Pintera, 1971).

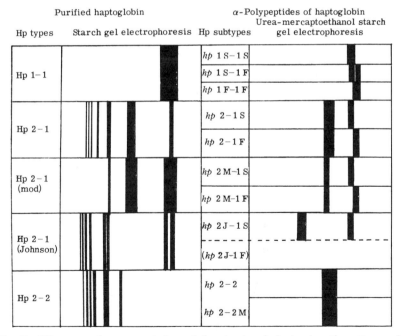

Fig. 3. Diagrammatic representation of the starch gel electrophoretic patterns of the common haptoglobin phenotypes and their respective subtypes. The subtypes of Hp 2-1 (Johnson) have the α chains hp 2J and 1S (from Giblett and Brooks, 1963).

Electrophoresis in acid-urea starch gel demonstrates that there are three common kinds of α chains and that these are responsible for the different starch gel patterns of the three major haptoglobin types. Three allelic genes taken two at a time account for the polymorphism. There are two allelic forms of the hpα^1 chain; the more rapidly migrating is designated hpα^{1F}, and the slower hpα^{1S}. A third form of α chain, hpα^2, is the only α chain present in Hp 2-2, but in Hp 2-1 it is present in combination with either hpα^{1S} or hpα^{1F}. This accords with the hypothesis that the six subtypes of haptoglobin are the phenotypic expression of the combination of three allelic genes Hp^{1F}, Hp^{1S}, and Hp^2. The former are alleles of Hp^2. However, in the absence of reductive cleavage the phenotypes corresponding to the genotypes Hp^{1F}/Hp^{1F}, Hp^{1S}/Hp^{1S}, and Hp^{1S}/Hp^{1F} are indistinguishable since all migrate in alkaline starch gel as the homogeneous band Hp 1-1 (alternative designation = Hp I). Likewise, the phenotypes Hp^2/Hp^{1F} and Hp^2/Hp^{1S} are indistinguishable in the absence of reduction, and they migrate as the multiple bands shown for Hp 2-1.

Haptoglobin is thus polycatenate with one chain (the β chain) common to all forms known except for a few rare genetic variants. Because the β chain does not migrate on starch gel electrophoresis in acid-urea, or migrates very slowly, reductively cleaved haptoglobins yield a pattern characteristic of the α chain. According to the genotype, one, two, or three possible bands may be present. For example, individual donor preparations of Hp 1-1 give either a single fast band (hpα^{1F}) or a single slow band (hpα^{1S}) or both bands in equal amounts. These correspond to the three subtypes Hp 1F-1F, Hp 1S-1S, and Hp 1F-1S, respectively. Hp 2-1 gives hpα^2 and either hpα^{1S} or hpα^{1F}, but not both. Hp 2-2 gives only hpα^2 or a modified form not illustrated in Fig. 3. Family studies (Smithies et al., 1962a,b) indicate that the three subtypes (hp^{1F}, hp^{1S}, and hp^2) are the expression of the three alleles (Hp^{1F}, Hp^{1S}, and Hp^2), each of which gives rise to the corresponding α chain.

Rarer types of haptoglobins may be detected by alkaline starch gel or acrylamide electrophoresis in the same manner as shown in Fig. 3 for the three major types; comparative patterns are illustrated later. Since most of the rarer haptoglobins have not been subjected either to amino acid sequence analysis or fingerprinting, the structural basis of their differences is not known and in some instances the locus of variation has not been assigned to either the α or β chain. An excellent review of the less common haptoglobin types is given by Giblett (1969, 1975) who for convenience divides them into quantitative and qualitative variants. Quantitative variants largely consist of modifications in the Hp 2-1 electrophoretic pattern, and thus affect the α chain. Qualitative variants are very rare, presumably reflect structural changes, and may affect either the α or the β chain (Barnett *et al.*, 1975).

The most common quantitative variants are those designated Hp 2-1(mod). A series of patterns are obtained that differ in the proportion of the slower moving polymeric bands (Fig. 3). Such patterns are found in about 10% of American Blacks and only rarely in persons not of African ancestry (Giblett, 1968). Family studies by Giblett and Steinberg (1960) indicate that an allele Hp^{2M} is responsible for the Hp 2-1(mod) phenotype. The method of subtyping by electrophoresis in an acid-urea starch gel does not distinguish the Hp 2-1(mod) patterns from the Hp 2-1 patterns so no difference in α chains has been identified. The Hp 2-1 (mod) group has been further subdivided by Sutton and Karp (1964) into four subclasses which they consider to be the expression of at least two different alleles that produce different amounts of the $hp\alpha^2$ chain. The cause of this quantitative difference in the $hp\alpha^2$ polymeric bands is unknown. Giblett (1968) suggests that there is some kind of regulation of $hp\alpha^2$ chain biosynthesis, perhaps through a series of Hp structural isoalleles.

Other quantitative variants of Hp 2-1 that have been described include haptoglobin Carlberg (Hp Ca) first reported by Galatius-Jensen (1958b) and later studied by a number of workers, especially Nance and Smithies (1963), and Hp 2-1(Trans) and Hp 2-1(Haw) discovered by Giblett (1964). In the latter cases a cellular mosaicism resulting from double fertilization has been implicated as the probable cause. The mosaicism could lead to the production of Hp 2-1 by one cell population and Hp 2-2 by another, or some transition between the two phenotypes.

Rarer phenotypes, referred to above as qualitative variants, are discussed in a later section, as is the phenomenon of hereditary hypohaptoglobinemia, which affects a surprising proportion of the population in Asiatic and African countries.

C. Primary Structure of Haptoglobin α Chains

The molecular polymorphism of human haptoglobin results usually from genetic alterations in the primary structure of the α chain, the smaller of the two kinds of polypeptide chains in this tetrachain protein. The three common forms of the α chain are closely related in structure; $hp\alpha^{1F}$ and $hp\alpha^{1S}$ contain 84 amino acid residues and have an identical amino acid sequence except that in $hp\alpha^{1S}$ glutamic acid replaces the lysine shown at position 54 in Fig. 4 which gives the amino acid sequence of $hp\alpha^{1F}$. The $hp\alpha^2$ chain is nearly twice as long; it contains 143 residues and consists of portions of the $hp\alpha^{1F}$ and $hp\alpha^{1S}$ chains

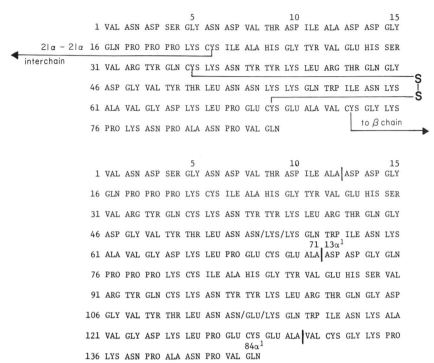

Fig. 4. Amino acid sequence of the α^{1F} chain of human haptoglobin (upper) and of the α^2 chain (lower) based on the sequences of Black and Dixon (1968) as corrected by Malchy and Dixon (1973b). In the slow variant the α^{1S} chain has a substitution of glutamic acid for the lysine in the a^{1F} chain at position 54. The short slant lines at Lys-54 and at Glu-113 in α^2 indicate that lysine is at one of these positions and glutamic acid at the other. The vertical lines in the α^2 chain identify the duplicated segments of the α^1 chain, Asp-13 through Ala-71 and Asp-72 through Ala-130.

joined together. This represents a relatively recent event of nonhomologous unequal crossing-over.

Preliminary studies of the structure of the three frequently occurring α-polypeptide chains of haptoglobin were first reported by Smithies *et al.* (1962b). Peptide maps of the hpα^{1F} and hpα^{1S} chains indicated they differed only by a single peptide spot, designated F and S, respectively. Amino acid analyses suggested the replacement of a single lysine residue in hpα^{1F} by an acidic residue in hpα^{1S}. This was confirmed by partial amino acid sequence analysis by Smithies (1964) and by complete amino acid sequence analysis of the three α chains by Dixon, Black, Wood, Kauffman, Connell, and Smithies. To date, experimental details of the latter work have not been published, but the sequences have been reported in preliminary form by Black and Dixon (1968). The published sequence has been corrected by including a half-cystine at position 73 (Malchy and Dixon, 1973b). The replacement of glutamic acid by lysine accords with the mobility difference of the two α chains in acid-urea starch gels and is consistent with a single nucleotide base change in the codon for glutamic acid, GA_G^A, to that for lysine, AA_G^A. This suggests a relatively recent mutation. Similar exchanges have been reported in the abnormal human hemoglobins.

The haptoglobin α^2 chain yields the same chymotryptic peptides as the α^1 chains, including the F and S peptides, but has one additional peptide known as J peptide, Because the molecular weight of the α^2 chain is almost twice that of the α^1 chain (17,300 vs. 8860 according to molecular weight determinations by the Archibald method), Smithies *et al.* (1962b), suggested that all or part of the amino acid sequence of the α^1 chain occurs twice in the α^2 chain. From partial amino acid sequence data Smithies (1964) proposed that a chromosomal rearrangement of the Hp^{1F} and Hp^{1S} genes had occurred leading to a partial internal duplication yielding the Hp^2 gene. This novel hypothesis was fully substantiated by complete amino acid sequence analysis of the hpα^2 chain. As shown in Fig. 4, the hpα^2 chain consists of the first 71 residues and the last 72 residues of the hpα^1 chain joined together to form a polypeptide of 143 residues. As a result, the sequence from Asp-13 through Ala-71 of hpα^1 and hpα^2 is repeated as Asp-72 through Ala-130 in the hpα^2 chain. Thus, a 59-residue segment is duplicated within the hpα^2 chain. One of the repeated segments is derived from hpα^{1S} and contains glutamic acid as the residue corresponding to position 54 in the hpα^1 chains; the other segment is from hpα^{1S} and contains lysine at the corresponding position. However, for technical reasons, it cannot be decided whether the first part is from hpα^{1S} or from hpα^{1F}.

The hpα^2 chain is the first example of a partial gene duplication that has been fully documented by amino acid sequence analysis. Partial gene duplication has been proposed as an important mechanism for the evolution of proteins (Smithies *et al.,* 1962a; Black and Dixon, 1968). Other examples of internal homology have been described for the hemoglobins, ferredoxins, and the light and heavy chains of immunoglobulins. A more complete discussion of the genetic mechanism of the haptoglobin gene duplication is given in a later section which also reviews the hypothesis of the evolutionary relationship between immunoglobulin light chains and haptoglobin α chains. Other genetic variants of haptoglobin are described in that section also since the structural basis for these variants has not yet been established.

D. Primary Structure of the Haptoglobin β Chain

The hpβ chain is identical in all three common Hp genetic types in its behavior in electrophoresis in acid-urea gels (Smithies *et al.*, 1962b), in antigenic determinants (Shim *et al.*, 1965), and in tryptic peptide maps and amino acid composition (Cleve *et al.*, 1967). The β chain contains about 310 amino acid residues and has all the carbohydrate of the molecule (Cleve *et al.*, 1969, Barnett *et al.*, 1975) and has a molecular weight of about 40,000 (Cheftel and Moretti, 1966).

Altogether about two-thirds of the sequence of the haptoglobin β chain has been reported, but many of the fragments have not yet been placed in order in the sequence. The amino terminal and carboxyl terminal portions of the sequence of the haptoglobin β chain have been published by Barnett *et al.* (1970, 1972). Some peptides containing half-cystine and also a large fragment have been reported by Hew and Dixon (1971), Malchy and Dixon (1973a,b), and Malchy *et al.* (1973). Subsequently Kurosky *et al.* (1974) gave sequence data on some 170 residues including placement of some but not all of the peptides mentioned above. See also Barnett *et al.* (1975) and Kurosky *et al.* (1975).

The preliminary data on the sequence of the hpβ chain suggest a striking homology to the chymotrypsin family of serine proteases rather than to the immunoglobulins as had been expected from the conclusions of Black and Dixon (1968) about the homology of the hpα chain and the light chains of immunoglobulins. The sequence reiteration of residues 2 through 9 at positions 20 through 27 reported previously by Barnett *et al.* (1972) and Kurosky *et al.* (1974) has been corrected by these authors (D. R. Barnett and A. Kurosky, personal communication). The mistaken sequence resulted from a partial cyanogen bromide cleavage at Met-18. The two CNBr fragments co-purified. One fragment started from the N-terminal Ile while the other began at Val-19. The nature of residues 20–27 were such that a low yield of PTH-derivatives was obtained while residues 2–9 were recovered from the contaminating fragment in high yield. The corrected sequence of the hpβ chain is

```
1              5                  10                   15
Ile-Leu-Gly-Gly-His-Leu-Asp-Ala-Lys-Gly-Ser-Phe-Pro-Trp-Gln-
        20            CHO       25                   30
Ala-Lys-Met-Val-Ser-His-His-Asn-Leu-Thr-Thr-Gly-Ala-Thr-Leu
```

Instead of the expected homology in primary structure between the haptoglobin β chain and immunoglobulin heavy chains, unexpected homologies were found between the haptoglobin β chain and corresponding regions of bovine chymotrypsin A (BC-A) and bovine trypsin (BT). These are illustrated below only for the amino terminal octadecapeptides, but a similar degree of homology continues through the first 36 residues of all three chains and through much of the remaining sequence.

```
          1              5                10               15         18
Hp β   Ile-Leu-Gly-Gly-His-Leu-Asp-Ala-Lys-Gly-Ser-Phe-Pro-Trp-Gln-Ala-Lys-Met
BC-A   Ile-Val-Asn-Gly-Glu-Glu-Ala -Val-Pro-Gly-Ser-Trp-Pro-Trp-Gln-Val-Ser -Leu
BT     Ile-Val-Gly-Gly-Tyr-Thr-Cys-Gly-Ala-Asn-Thr-Val-Pro-Tyr-Gln-Val-Ser -Leu
```

A similar homology was apparent on comparison of the C-terminal nonapeptide sequences of the haptoglobin β chain and the same proteolytic enzymes (Barnett *et al.*, 1970, 1972). On the other hand, the sequence shown below does not bear any resemblance to the C-terminal nonapeptide sequences of the μ, γ, or α heavy chains of the immunoglobulins (Putnam, 1972).

```
Hp β   Trp-Val-Glx-Lys-Thr-Ile -Ala-Glu-Asn
BC-A   Trp-Val-Gln-Gln-Thr-Leu-Ala-Ala-Asn
BT     Trp-Ile -Lys-Gln-Thr-Ile -Ala-Ser-Asn
γ      Gln-Lys-Ser -Leu-Ser -Leu-Ser -Pro-Gly
μ      Met-Ser -Asp Thr-Ala -Gly-Thr-Cys-Tyr
α      Met-Ala-Glu-Val -Asp-Gly-Thr-Cys-Tyr
```

Further sequence study of the hpβ chain greatly extended its apparent homology with the chymotrypsin family of serine proteases (Kurosky *et al.*, 1974, 1975). In this study fragments of the hpβ chain totaling some 170 residues were aligned on the basis of residue similarity to the protease chains because the sequence of the hpβ chain was incomplete. In this comparison representing about 60% of the human hpβ chain about 30% of the residues were identical to residues occurring in the sequence of each of the five protease chains, all of which are very homologous to each other (i.e., porcine elastase and bovine chymotrypsin A, chymotrypsin B, trypsin, and the thrombin B chain). In the combined comparison at least one of the proteases had an identical (or chemically similar) residue at two-thirds of the positions compared with the hpβ chain. A pairwise comparison yielding 30% identity in sequence with relatively few gaps inserted to maximize the identity is very impressive indeed. However, the meaning of these apparent homologies will not be clear until the complete sequence is available for the hpβ chain. It should be noted that the sequence similarities occur in the N-terminal regions of the active proteolytic enzymes and not in the N-terminal regions of the corresponding zymogens. Barnett *et al.* (1972) suggest that the similarities in primary structure may indicate that the structural genes for the Hp α and β chains were each derived from ancestral genes common to those for the immunoglobulins and serine proteinases, respectively.

Among the important missing data for the hpβ chain are the location and the kind of disulfide bridges. As was discussed previously, the location and kind of disulfide bridges on the β chain is only partially known. Since only the Hp 2-1 and Hp 2-2 types are polymeric, it may be assumed that one or more of the 3 extra half-cystines in the hpα^2 chain are involved in polymer cross-linking.

E. Glycopeptides and Carbohydrate Prosthetic Groups of the β Chain

All the carbohydrate of human haptoglobin appears to be on the β chain. No qualitative differences with respect to the type of haptoglobin have been found. The carbohydrate content is about 20%, but different values for the distribution of the sugars have been reported by various workers (Heimburger *et al.*, 1964; Cheftel *et al.*, 1960; Gerbeck *et al.*, 1967). Hexose in the form of galactose (5.3%) and mannose (2.5%) is most abundant, and hexosamine and sialic acid are present in nearly equal amounts on a percentage basis—each being about 5.3% (Heimburger *et al.*, 1964). Neuraminidase removes about 70% of the sialic acid both from free haptoglobin and from haptoglobin combined with hemoglobin, but without loss of peroxidase activity. Thus, the susceptible sialic acid residues are not involved in this function (Rafelson *et al.*, 1961). Glycopeptides of two different kinds have been isolated from a pronase digest of human haptoglobin (Cheftel *et al.*, 1965; Gerbeck *et al.*, 1967). As in most pronase glycopeptides, the amino acids are not present in stoichiometric amounts. Aspartic acid is the predominant amino acid in one type of glycopeptide, and the molecular weight calculated on the basis of the aspartic acid content is about 3000 (range of 2750 to 3050). In both types of glycopeptides the carbohydrate content is similar: 5–6 moles of hexose (galactose and mannose), 3–4 moles of *N*-acetylglucosamine, and 0–3 moles of sialic acid. Fucose is present in some glycopeptides but not in others and is present in the whole protein only in small amounts. The glycopeptides appeared to be the same for different haptoglobin genetic types (Gerbeck *et al.*, 1967); similar glycopeptides have been isolated from rabbit haptoglobin (Cheftel *et al.*, 1969). Based on an assumed molecular weight of 100,000, there are 7 oligosaccharide units in human haptoglobin Hp 2-1 and 6 in the rabbit.

The findings cited above raise a number of questions. What is the function of the carbohydrate and what is its role in the heterogeneity of haptoglobin? Since the carbohydrate is supposed to be distributed among the three major haptoglobin types in proportion to their molecular weight (Cheftel *et al.*, 1969), it should not contribute to their heterogeneity. However, incomplete biosynthesis of the oligosaccharides or metabolic degradation through the action of neuraminidase could cause changes in mobility. Further studies on the location of the oligosaccharides on the polypeptide chain would be desirable but will have to await complete sequence determination of the β chain. One carbohydrate has been located at Asn-23 in the N-terminus of the human and dog hpβ chain but is absent in the rat hpβ chain where this residue is glycine (D. R. Barnett and A. Kurosky, personal communication).

IV. Genetics and Population Distribution

A. α Chain Mutations and Gene Duplication

Of the mutations that have produced genetic variation in haptoglobins the most common are those affecting the α chain. The known mutations are of three types: (1) A single-step mutation resulting in the glutamic acid-lysine substitution at position 54 in the α^1 chain that differentiates α^{1S}, which has glutamic acid at this position, and α^{1F}, which has lysine. (2) Chromosomal rearrangement leading to partial gene duplication, which is the logical explanation of the partial duplication of the α^{1F} and α^{1S} sequences in the sequence of the α^2 chain. (3) Alterations in the control of the rate of synthesis of either the α or the β polypeptide chains resulting in reduced haptoglobin synthesis analogous to the hemoglobin thalassemias.

Substitutions involving charged amino acids such as the glutamic acid-lysine interchange should readily be detected through the change in electrophoretic mobility. However, the α^{1F} and α^{1S} phenotypes are detected only after reduction and alkylation of the native haptoglobins followed by gel electrophoresis in media containing urea. This indicates that the change in charge is somehow masked by the interactions with the β polypeptide chain in the native molecule. Other structural variants involving a single amino acid interchange have not been reported for either the α or the β chain.

Haptoglobin is remarkable for being the first example in which a postulated chromosomal rearrangement (Smithies *et al.*, 1962a,b) has been substantiated by amino acid sequence analysis (Black and Dixon, 1968). In the hpα^2 chain the first 71 and the last 72 residues of the hpα^1 chain are joined together to form a single chain of 143 residues (Fig. 4). To explain this Black and Dixon (1968) have proposed a possible mechanism for the nonhomologous synapsis and crossover at the Hp^{1F}/Hp^{1S} locus leading to the juncture at a position corresponding to residues

71–72 in the α^2 chain. Thus, as a result of the asymmetrical alignment at meiosis of an Hp^{1S} and an Hp^{1F} gene followed by an intracistronic cross-over a new gene Hp^{2FS} would arise. Examination of the base sequences corresponding to the amino acid sequences from residues 11–17 and 67–75 shows considerable homology. The failure of normal synapse leading to partial duplication of the α^1 chain should result in the formation of a smaller or "deletion" gene as pictured in Fig. 5. However, just as in the case of Lepore-type hemoglobins where an homologous but unequal crossover is thought to occur, no evidence of the protein product of the deletion gene has been found. Of course, the polypeptide product, if it were formed, would have only 25 residues — the first 12 and the last 13 of the α^1 chain — and because of the presence of only one half-cystine could not form a covalent tetrachain monomer.

Because of the randomness and rarity of genetic events such as the postulated chromosomal breakage and because the α^{2FS} chain appears to be identical in all sera tested, it is assumed that the partial duplication took place but once early in human history in an individual who was heterozygous for hpα^{1S} and hpα^{1F} (Smithies, 1964). Genetic and electrophoretic evidence for the existence of additional alleles of the type Hp^{2SS} and Hp^{2FF} has been adduced by Nance and Smithies (1963), but the gene products have not been examined by amino acid sequence analysis. These new alleles could have originated by unequal crossing-over in Hp^2/Hp^1 heterozygotes, for, as Smithies *et al.* (1962a,b) have pointed out, once the initial partial duplication event occurred, the possibility of

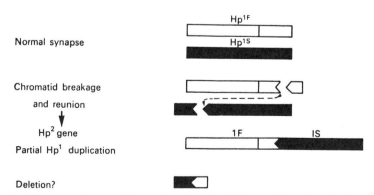

Fig. 5.   Diagram of a possible mechanism for Hp^2 gene formation by breakage of Hp^{1S} and Hp^{1F} at two widely separated regions, followed by reunion. This random event need not depend on homology of the base sequences in the two regions. A second "deletion" gene might also be formed by this mechanism. The vertical line in Hp^{1F} represents the site of base substitution which differentiates it from Hp^{1S}, i.e., the site of the lysine-glutamic acid substitution (from Giblett, 1969).

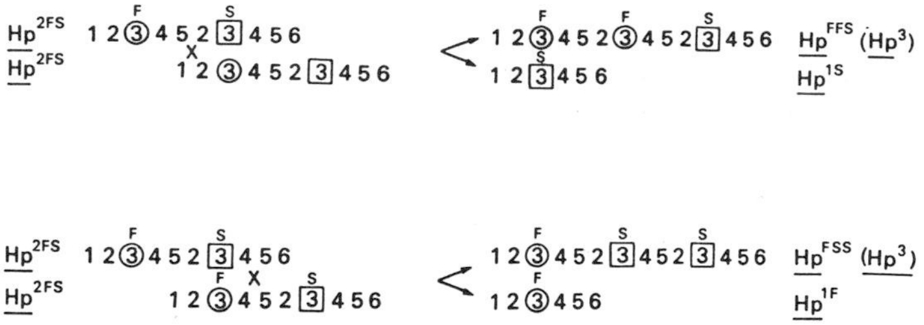

Fig. 6. Diagram of a postulated partial gene triplication, perhaps exemplified by the Hp^J gene, indicated here as Hp^3. Each number represents a segment of DNA in a haptoglobin gene. The single base pair substitution known to exist in Hp^{1F} and Hp^{1S} is shown as being in segment 3 by the circle and the squares, respectively. The two examples of Hp^3 shown vary slightly because of a difference in the site of crossing-over (from Giblett, 1969).

further chromosomal rearrangements was greatly increased. Since the cistron for the hpα^2 chain is nearly twice as long as the cistrons for the hpα^{1S} and hpα^{1F} chains, synapsis of the homologous chromosomes can never be complete in the Hp^2/Hp^1 heterozygote.

Because of the internal homology in the Hp^{2FS} gene, partial triplication can occur in an individual who is homozygous for the Hp^{2FS} gene as is illustrated in Fig. 6 from Giblett (1969). In this case a displaced synapse occurs between two homologous portions of the DNA at different ends of the cistron. As seen earlier in Fig. 3, the rare phenotype Hp Johnson (Hp 2J-1S) on subtyping in alkaline urea gel exhibits an α^{1S} chain and a second chain that moves more slowly than the usual α^2 (Smithies *et al.*, 1962a; Ramot *et al.*, 1962). Several variants of the Johnson type have been reported (Giblett, 1968). The slowly moving hp 2Jα chain is assumed to be of higher molecular weight and thus the possible product of a partial gene triplication. The gene is currently designated Hp^J, but Giblett (1968) points out a better name would be Hp^3 if the triplication hypothesis is borne out by sequence analysis. Of course, by their very nature internal duplications of amino acid sequence are difficult to establish exactly by the customary methods of sequence analysis, e.g., note that the order of the F/S loci is not yet determined in the α^{2FS} chain.

B. Rare Genetic Variants

In addition to the Johnson variant described above, a number of other rare haptoglobin phenotypes have been reported. These are summarized in Table II and some are illustrated in Fig. 7, both of which are taken from Kirk (1968), who gives a detailed description of these unusual phenotypes. In none of these cases has the structural change been deter-

TABLE II

Rare Phenotypes in the Human Haptoglobin System[a]

Abnormal phenotypes observed in starch gel at pH 8.6	Notes	Suggested gene symbol	Genotypic combinations with normal phenotypes	Genotypic combinations with abnormal phenotypes
Hp 2–1 "Carlberg"	Reduced hp 1 synthesis	Hp^{1ca}	Hp^{1ca}/Hp^1	Hp^{1ca}/Hp^{1ca} Hp^{1ca}/Hp^2
Hp 2–1 "Johnson"	a "Triplicated" hp α chain	Hp^J		Hp^1/Hp^J Hp^2/Hp^J Reduced Hp^J/Hp^J synthesis
Hp 1–P Hp 2–P	Observed only on normal gel when complexed with Hb	Hp^P		Hp^P/Hp^P, Hp^P/Hp^{1S} Hp^P/Hp^{1F}, Hp^P/Hp^2
Hp 2–L	Observed only on normal gel when complexed with Hb	Hp^L		Hp^L/Hp^2, Hp^L/Hp^1? Hp^L/Hp^L?
Hp 1–H	Observed on normal gel both complexed and not complexed with Hb	Hp^H		Hp^H/Hp^1, Hp^H/Hp^2 Hp^H/Hp^H?
Hp 2–1(Trans)	Reduced hp 2 synthesis	Hp^{2Tr}	Hp^2/Hp^{2Tr}	Hp^1/Hp^{2Tr} Hp^{2Tr}/Hp^{2Tr} (Hp 0 ?)
Hp 2–1(Haw)	Reduced hp 2 synthesis	Hp^{2Haw}	Hp^2/Hp^{2Haw}	Hp^1/Hp^{2Haw} Hp^{2Haw}/Hp^{2Haw} (Hp 0 ?)
Hp Ab	Reduced hp 2 synthesis	Hp^{Ab}	Hp^2/Hp^{Ab}	Hp^1/Hp^{Ab} Hp^{Ab}/Hp^{Ab} (Hp 0 ?)
Hp 2–1D	Not detectable when complexed with Hb	Hp^{1D}		Hp^{1D}/Hp^{1D}, Hp^{1S}/Hp^{1D} Hp^{1F}/Hp^{1D}, Hp^2/Hp^{1D}
Hp 1–B Hp 2–B	Possibly a 1 α or a 2 α chain mutation	Hp^B		Hp^1/Hp^B, Hp^2/Hp^B Hp^B/Hp^B
Hp 1-"Marburg" Hp 2-"Marburg"	An hp β chain mutation	Hp^{Mb}		Hp^{Mb}/Hp^{Mb}, Hp^1/Hp^{Mb} Hp^2/Hp^{Mb}
Hp 2–1 "Bellevue"	A hp β chain mutation	Hp^{Bell}		Hp^1/Hp^{Bell}, Hp^2/Hp^{Bell} Hp^{Bell}/Hp^{Bell}

[a] Reproduced by permission from Kirk, R. L., "The Haptoglobin Groups in Man. Monographs in Human Genetics," vol. 4 (Karger, Basel, 1968).

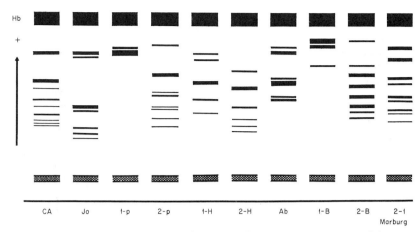

CA   Jo   1-p   2-p   1-H   2-H   Ab   1-B   2-B   2-1
                                                          Marburg

Fig. 7. Diagram of the electrophoretic patterns in starch gel at pH 8.6 of the Hp-Hb complexes from rare phenotypes in the human haptoglobin system. The relative mobility of free Hb is shown at the top. The mobility of Hp 2-1 Johnson (Jo) also given in Fig. 3 may be used as a reference standard for relation to mobilities of the common phenotypes. See Table II for identification of the phenotypes. Reproduced by permission from Kirk (1968).

mined, and in some cases the chain involved has not been identified by subtyping (e.g., Hp 2-L, Hp 1-P, Hp 2-P, Hp 1-H). Robson *et al.* (1964) discovered a number of phenotypes that were detected as the Hp-Hb complex; some of these are observed on normal starch gel only when the haptoglobin is complexed with hemoglobin (Hp 1-P, Hp 2-P, Hp 2-L) and others whether complexed or not (Hp 1-H, Hp 2-H). In contrast, Hp 2-1D is not detectable when complexed with hemoglobin (Renwick and Marshall, 1966). These observations suggest that the hemoglobin-binding site in some cases is close to the locus of structural variation or that the binding of hemoglobin exposes the site in other cases.

Although most reported mutations affect the α chain, some of the best-studied structural variants of haptoglobin involve the hpβ chain; these are Hp Marburg (Hp 2-1 Mb and Hp 1-1 Mb) (Aly *et al.*, 1962; Cleve and Deicher, 1965; Weerts *et al.*, 1966) and Hp Bellevue (Hp 2-1 Bellevue) (Javid, 1967; Javid and Yingling, 1968b). As expected from the role of the hpβ chain in hemoglobin binding, these variants are less effective in binding Hb; furthermore a specific Hp antigenic site which is blocked in the Hp-Hb complex with the common phenotypes is not masked in the complex formed by these hpβ chain variants. In the case of Hp Marburg the structural change does not seem to be a single amino acid substitution, for comparison of the Marburg β chain (hpβ^{Mb}) with normal hpβ chains by the peptide map method showed several additional tryptic peptides to be present in the variant chain (Cleve *et al.*, 1969). Determination of the complete amino acid sequence of the normal hpβ chain should greatly facilitate identification of the type of mutation that has occurred in the hpβ^{Mb} chain.

C. Quantitative Variants

Aside from the changes in haptoglobin level that may occur in various diseases, there are several hereditary conditions that lead to a decrease in serum haptoglobin. These include (1) quantitative variants that cause a diminished expression of the gene for either α^1 or α^2, (2) hypohaptoglobinemia, and (3) an apparent anhaptoglobinemia.

A number of quantitative variants have been described; the most common of these are the Hp 2-1(mod) or Hp 2-1M phenotypes which represent modifications in the Hp 2-1 phenotype. In starch gel electrophoretic patterns of Hp 2-1(mod) phenotypes there is a diminution in the intensity of the slower moving polymeric bands attributable to the hpα^2 chain. The fast moving monomeric hpα^1 band, which is usually faint in Hp 2-1 patterns, becomes intense and several of the slowest moving bands may disappear (Fig. 3). A series of such Hp 2-1(mod) patterns has been described by several workers. They are all ascribed to a difference in the expression of the $Hp\alpha^1$ and $Hp\alpha^2$ genes. Because of an apparent deficiency in the production of the hpα^2 chain, the monomer tetrapolypeptide and the lower polymers become predominant. Several genetic theories to explain this phenomenon have been proposed (Parker and Bearn, 1963; Sutton and Karp, 1964), but none is completely satisfactory.

Although Hp 2-1(mod) phenotypes affecting the Hpα^2 gene occur in up to 10% of American Blacks and have a varying prevalence in African populations (Giblett and Steinberg, 1960; Sutton and Karp, 1964), quantitative variations affecting the $Hp\alpha^1$ gene product are quite rare. The first quantitative variant discovered was the Carlberg type (Hp 2-1 Carlberg) (Galatius-Jensen, 1958a). Other examples have since been reported. In normal starch gel Hp Carlberg resembles Hp 2-2, but closer examination shows that it is more like a mixture of Hp 2-2 and Hp 2-1 in that polymeric bands characteristic of both phenotypes appear. By use of the alkaline-urea subtyping technique Giblett (1964) has shown that the inheritance of Hp Carlberg is consistent with the existence of an allele at the $Hp\alpha$ locus which has a product indistinguishable from hpα^1 except for its diminished quantity. Giblett (1964) has described two other quantitative variants listed in Table II, Hp 2-1(Trans) and Hp 2-1 (Haw). Both of these result in reduced synthesis of the hpα^2 chain. Hp

2-1 (Trans), as its name implies, produces patterns transitional between Hp 2-1 and Hp 2-1(mod), whereas Hp 2-1(Haw) gives patterns intermediate between Hp 2-1 and Hp 1-1.

D. Hereditary Deficiencies and Genetic Control

A number of physiological and pathological conditions may cause the virtual absence of haptoglobin, resulting in hypohaptoglobinemia or anhaptoglobinemia. Anhaptoglobinemia is characteristic of the newborn infant up to 3 months (see Chapter 6 by Gitlin and Gitlin) and also results from severe liver disease or excessive intravascular hemolysis. In addition hereditary factors may result in deficient synthesis of haptoglobin causing hypo- or anhaptoglobinemia, designated Hp 0.

Generally in individuals of Hp type 1-1 the mean level of serum haptoglobin is higher than for Hp 2-2 (Nyman, 1959a). Hypohaptoglobinemia seldom occurs in persons of the Hp 1-1 phenotype but is not uncommon in the Hp 2-1(mod) phenotype which is thought to represent an inherited decrease in synthesis of the hpα^2 chain. Thus, there is a rather high frequency of anhaptoglobinemia in people of African ancestry—about 4% for adults and 12% for children among American Blacks (Giblett, 1975). The question has been raised whether Hp 0 is a "silent allele" that does not produce a recognizable gene product, i.e., a chain capable of combining with the hpβ chain to form haptoglobin (Harris *et al.*, 1958; Matsunaga, 1962). This would be difficult to prove by techniques of protein chemistry. Likewise because of the low frequency of anhaptoglobinemia and the presumed Hp° gene the probability of finding individuals homozygous for this gene is small. The frequency of the Hp° allele is estimated to be only 0.0005 (Pintera, 1971).

Anhaptoglobinemia rarely means the absolute absence of haptoglobin but rather that it is present in unusually low amount, more properly referred to as hypohaptoglobinemia. The riddle of anhaptoglobinemia, whether it is a qualitative or quantitative problem has puzzled many observers and has led to a great deal of speculation about the genetic control of haptoglobin synthesis. Kirk (1968), Giblett (1968), and Pintera (1971) all treat this subject at some length.

Although a series of papers by Gerald *et al.* (1964, 1967) gave a possible assignment of the haptoglobin locus $Hp\alpha$ to a D group chromosome, this assignment has been criticized by Robson *et al.* (1969). From study of a pedigree for a translocation between one arm of a No. 2 chromosome and one arm of a No. 16 chromosome that segregated in coupling with the $Hp\alpha^1$ allele, Robson *et al.* (1969) concluded that the data indicate a probability of 0.97 that Hp is on chromosome 16. No linkage between the hp locus and the ABO and Rh blood groups or serum antigenic markers has been established.

E. Population and Geographic Distribution

The presence of the three main types of haptoglobin (Hp 1-1, Hp 2-1, and Hp 2-2) in human populations throughout the world represents a true polymorphism. Many investigations of this polymorphism have been made in different ethnic groups in widely separated geographic areas; indeed, the number is far too numerous to attempt to list in this treatise. This subject is surveyed in depth by Kirk (1968) who gives a series of tables of gene frequencies and an extensive bibliography, as also does Giblett (1968).

Haptoglobin polymorphism is extremely old in human history, for it is present in all populations studied. Yet, the $hp\alpha^2$ mutation must have occurred within the human line, for the polymer pattern is not found in primates. However, the frequency of the $Hp\alpha^1$ and $Hp\alpha^2$ alleles varies widely among different populations. The highest incidence of the $Hp\alpha^1$ gene reported is about 0.89 in the Colorado Indians of Ecuador and the lowest is 0.07 among the Irulas of India. European populations have been extensively studied; their $Hp\alpha^1$ frequencies range from 0.31 to 0.45 with most of the values being within the narrow spread of 0.36 to 0.43 High $Hp\alpha^1$ frequencies occur among certain African populations (e.g., up to 0.77 in the Congo and 0.76 in Northern Nigeria), in some Central and South American Indian tribes (up to 0.80), and in Oceania (as high as 0.86). At the other extreme the three major ethnic groups in Ceylon have $Hp\alpha^1$ frequencies ranging from 0.14 to 0.19 and certain population groups in India have frequencies of only 0.10. This low incidence has led Smithies *et al.* (1962b) to suggest that India is the birthplace of the $Hp\alpha^2$ fusion gene. Isolated ethnic groups within the same region may have quite different frequencies of the $Hp\alpha^1$ gene. This is illustrated by Fig. 8 from Kirk (1968) showing the worldwide distribution of $Hp\alpha^1$ and $Hp\alpha^2$ genes for selected populations. For example, compare the Bushmen, Congolese and Nigerians in Africa. Indian populations in America show an especially wide range of frequency of the Hp genes as they do of other serum genetic markers. Among African populations with a higher incidence of Hp°, the gene frequency of $Hp\alpha^1$ may be overweighted and also in groups having decreased haptoglobin level because of an environmental disease such as malaria.

It is harder to estimate the gene frequencies of the Hp^{1F} and Hp^{1S} subtypes in populations because subtyping requires the more difficult procedure of electrophoresis in alkaline-urea gels after reductive cleavage

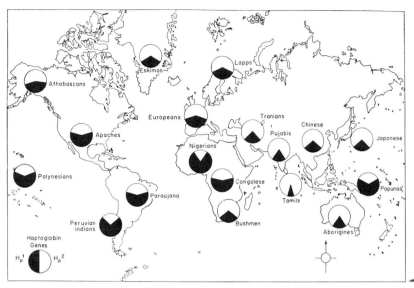

Fig. 8. World distribution of the Hp^1 and Hp^2 genes. Selected populations only. Reproduced by permission from Kirk (1968).

rather than the normal starch gel electrophoresis used for typing. Hence, fewer population groups have been studied, and the results are less reliable. The frequency of Hp^{1S} alleles is generally higher than that of Hp^{1F} alleles. The ratio of Hp^{1S}/Hp^{1F} ranges from 0.49 to 0.68 in European populations except for one aberrant value of 0.18 for Czechs. Quite discordant values have been published for Mongoloid populations, some authors reporting the absence of Hp^{1F} and others finding a significant incidence.

Kirk (1968) believes that the Hp^{1F} and Hp^{1S} subtypes could be valuable genetic markers in anthropological studies but that the results thus far have been too discrepant to be useful. On the other hand, the haptoglobin types Hp 1-1, Hp 2-1, and Hp 2-2 are important markers for the study of population genetics and almost 200 different population groups have already been typed. It is unknown to what extent the frequency of the $Hp\alpha^{1F}$ and $Hp\alpha^{1S}$ alleles reflects the action of selective factors; as described below, some authors think that there is an association with endemic diseases.

F. Applications in Forensic Medicine

As with other genetic markers in human blood, the haptoglobin types are potentially useful in forensic medicine. The applications include the proof of the presence of hemoglobin in blood stains and the exclusion of paternity in disputed cases. In the detection of blood by the peroxidase method the activity of hemoglobin is enhanced by the addition of haptoglobin. Hp typing may be done on both fresh and old dry blood samples by the immunoelectrophoretic method (Culliford and Wraxall, 1966). In cases of disputed paternity, Hp typing is done by the method of starch gel electrophoresis. The principles are obvious; for example, (1) If the mother and child are both of type Hp 1-1, the father cannot be of type Hp 2-2, (2) if the mother is Hp 1-1 and the child Hp 2-1, the father cannot be Hp 1-1, and so on. The theoretical exclusion rate depends on the Hp gene frequency in the population. Although the exclusion rate has been calculated to be 18% in Denmark (Galatius-Jensen, 1960), the value of Hp typing for paternity cases has been questioned by Harris *et al.* (1958) and others. Kirk (1968) has pointed out that the usefulness of haptoglobins in paternity cases would be greatly increased if subtyping were done. For example, if the mother and child are both of type Hp 1F-1F, paternity can be excluded if the father is of type Hp 1S-1S as well as Hp 2-2. Rare haptoglobin types found in both the supposed father and child greatly increase the probability of paternity. Since there is no genetic linkage of ABO and Rh blood groups with Hp types, the two methods can be used in conjunction to increase the percentage of exclusion.

V. Biosynthesis and Alterations in Disease

A. Normal Abundance

Nyman (1959a) defined the most commonly used concentration unit for haptoglobin as the hemoglobin-binding capacity, abbreviated HbBC, which is expressed as the amount of hemoglobin in mg that can be bound by the haptoglobin present in 100 ml of solution, usually serum. Haptoglobin levels are presented either as HbBC or as mg Hp/100 ml; the conversion factor is Hp = HbBC × 1.3 because 1 mg of Hb is bound per 1.3 mg Hp regardless of the type (Pintera, 1971). The HbBC normally varies between 30 and 180 mg/100 ml; haptoglobin thus represents about one-fourth of the normal α_2-globulin fraction. Individuals belonging to Hp type 2-2 have lower mean values than those belonging to type 1-1 (Nyman, 1959a; Laurell, 1960). The amount of haptoglobin normally present in the total plasma volume is enough to bind about 3 gm of Hb—the equivalent of about 10 ml of red cells or 12 mg of iron and about half the daily turnover of hemoglobin (Giblett, 1962). The affinity of haptoglobin for hemoglobin is so high, that no measureable quantities of free hemoglobin occur in plasma until all haptoglobin has been saturated with Hb. Thus, in the electrophoretic measurement of HbHC, Hb may be added in increments until free Hb appears (Bernier, 1967).

Although any given individual has a fairly constant HbBC while healthy, a wide range of normal values has been reported by different investigators and the mean values for various laboratories differ significantly (see Table XIII in Pintera, 1971). In part these variations are explained by the characteristic difference in levels of the three common Hp types mentioned above and also by the fact that men have a significantly higher average level than women (HbBC = 113 mg/100 ml, S.D. = 43 for men vs. 94 mg/100 ml, S.D. = 30 for women according to Nyman, 1959b). Obviously hormones influence the haptoglobin level.

Age also has a significant influence on haptoglobin level. Anhaptoglobinemia is common in the newborn being present in 80–90% of infants up to 3 months of age. This has been attributed both to the hemolysis of fetal red cells and to immaturity of the hepatic and reticuloendothelial system for forming haptoglobin. Although a number of authors have reported that haptoglobin could not be identified by starch gel electrophoresis in cord blood though present in the maternal serum (Engle and Woods, 1960), it has been detected immunochemically in fetal serum after the ninth week of gestation (Hirschfeld and Lunell, 1962; Gitlin and Biasucci, 1969). Moreover, by concentration of the serum or by use of special techniques haptoglobin can be identified in the serum of infants of only a few weeks of age. For more about the antenatal and postnatal development of haptoglobin see Chapter 6 by Gitlin and Gitlin.

Haptoglobin is present in low concentrations in many extravascular physiological fluids including cerebrospinal fluid, bile, lymph, synovial fluid, aqueous humor, saliva, gastric juice, seminal plasma, and milk, and is also present in small amounts in normal urine. The Hp concentration in most physiological fluids other than lymph is too low for typing. In pathological effusions the Hp content may be considerably elevated, for example, in pleural and ascitic fluids (Ng *et al.*, 1963). Synovial fluid normally has a low content of haptoglobin (Neuhaus and Sogoian, 1961), but the concentration may increase tenfold in rheumatoid arthritis (Niedermeier *et al.*, 1965) owing to damage to the synovial membrane.

In inflammatory exudates such as blister fluid considerable haptoglobin is often present. The Hp content in pathological fluids is usually sufficient for typing (Bundschuh *et al.*, 1962). Because of the lower molecular weight of the monomer Hp 1-1, it is more readily excreted in the urine than are the polymeric forms Hp 2-1 and Hp 2-2. Hap-toglobinuria as the result of nephrosis provides a source for preparation of Hp 1-1 (Marnay, 1961) as does ascites fluid (Barnett *et al.,* 1972).

B. Changes in Disease

Profound changes in serum haptoglobin level occur in disease making it a valuable indicator for diagnosis and prognosis (Owen *et al.,* 1964; Pintera, 1971). In general, serum haptoglobin is decreased or absent in hemolytic anemias and is increased in a variety of inflammatory condi-tions. Whereas the median normal value of HbBC was 125 mg/100 ml with a range of 75 to 175 mg/100 ml in one series, the sera of patients with inflammatory diseases had values as high as 650 mg/100 ml and sera of most patients with hemolytic diseases were below 75 mg/100 ml (Bernier, 1967). Low values of HbBC may have little clinical signifi-cance in the very young or in persons of African ancestry. Serial values of HbBC as a means of following hepatic or hemolytic disease are likely to be of more value than an isolated analysis.

A very extensive literature that has been well summarized by Pintera (1971) exists on the serum levels, diagnostic value, and prognostic sig-nificance of hyperhaptoglobinemia and hypohaptoglobinemia in a great variety of disease states, particularly in hemolytic diseases. Haptoglobin is one of the indicators of acute infections but may also rise in chronic infections such as tuberculosis, multiple sclerosis, and rheumatic dis-eases. In renal diseases, particularly the nephrotic syndrome (Marnay, 1961), values of HbBC as high as 700 mg/100 ml may be reached, and haptoglobin may be present in urine in concentrations sufficient to war-rant nephrotic urine as a source for preparation of Hp. Trauma and surgical injuries also induce an increase in HbBC. An increase in HbBC is often associated with malignancies and is said to be almost pathog-nomonic of Hodgkin's disease. In the latter case, the increase is at-tributed to increased Hp synthesis (Krauss *et al.,* 1966).

Low values of serum haptoglobin are most likely to be observed in severe liver disease, since liver is the chief site of Hp synthesis, and in hemolytic crises where the destruction of the Hp-Hb complex is much faster than the rate of Hp synthesis. In liver disease a decline in Hp is not uniform, for the level may rise in inflammations and obstructive jaundice but is uniformly low in severe chronic hepatocellular lesions. In a variety of hemolytic diseases, however, the serum HbBC is very low and continuing observation of the level is useful; the return to normal requires several days after the hemolytic episode. Low levels of HbBC are observed in a number of abnormal hemoglobin diseases such as sickle cell anemia, hemoglobin C disease, and the thalassemias; also after adverse transfusion reactions and autoimmune hemolysis as in acquired hemolytic anemia. In an acute hemolytic crisis all of the haptoglobin is usually depleted because of the one-way transit of the Hp-Hb complex to the reticuloendothelial system where it is catabolized primarily in the liver. In such cases some of the unbound Hb will spill over into the urine though much of it is catabolized in the liver.

The possible association of the haptoglobin types with various diseases has been examined by a number of workers without any clear conclusion. The greater frequency of Hp° phenotype in African populations has been noted. There has been some debate about the possible selective advantage of the $Hp\alpha^2$ allele because the polymer type is less readily excreted in the urine and is more rapidly catabolized as the Hp-Hb complex. The fact that some individuals with hereditary anhaptoglobinemia can exist in an apparently healthy state has taken some of the force out of this issue. There seems to be little effect of the Hp phenotype in most diseases.

C. Biosynthesis, Regulation, and Catabolism

As with most other plasma proteins, the liver is the main site of haptoglobin synthesis. This has been shown by several kinds of evidence; it was first indicated by the association of low haptoglobin levels with chronic liver disease and experimental liver poisoning and was then established by the incorporation of radioactive amino acids and galactose into Hp in isolated perfused rat liver (Krauss and Sarcione, 1964) and *in vivo* incorporation of ^{14}C-glycine in canine liver (Alper *et al.*, 1965), and by immunofluorescent studies (Peters and Alper, 1966). In the latter work specific fluorescence was found only in islands of hepatic parenchymal cells and Kupffer cells and in a few macrophage-like cells in the spleen. Immunofluorescent studies of human tissue in culture by Wada *et al.* (1970) confirmed that serum haptoglobin is produced largely in the liver but showed that it is also produced in such reticuloendothelial tissues as spleen, lymph nodes, and thymus. Neither the absence of amino acid and hormone supplementation nor even fasting for up to 6 days totally impairs the capacity of perfused rat liver to synthesize haptoglobin (Miller and John, 1970).

The serum level of haptoglobin is regulated largely by the amount of extracorpuscular hemoglobin in the blood. Because of the high affinity of haptoglobin for hemoglobin, any free hemoglobin is combined in the Hp-Hb complex until all the haptoglobin is saturated. In a classic experiment in which hemoglobin was administered to human volunteers,

Laurell and Nyman (1957) showed that the Hb-Hp complex is rapidly eliminated from the blood stream. The serum Hp concentration thus falls toward zero within 6 to 12 hr after injection of Hb intravenously in amounts sufficient to saturate all the Hp in the circulation. Once the Hp is all eliminated via the Hp-Hb complex, the serum level does not return to normal for a period of from 5 to 7 days. This indicates that rapid depletion of the serum Hp does not stimulate a reciprocal biosynthetic response. Experimentally, Hp biosynthesis can be stimulated by procedures inducing inflammation such as injection of turpentine to form a local abscess.

The liver also is the principal site for the clearance of the Hp-Hb complex and for ultimate catabolism of both haptoglobin and hemoglobin. If ^{14}C-labeled Hp-Hb complex is administered intravenously, a major portion of it is metabolized in the Kupffer cells in the liver (Wada *et al.,* 1970). Under normal conditions only about half of the haptoglobin is catabolized via the Hp-Hb complex (Pintera, 1971).

The turnover of haptoglobin in human and animal plasma has been studied by a number of laboratories since Nyman's first report (1959a) suggesting a maximum half-life time of 5 days. Lower values of from 1.4 to 4.4 days have been given, but the range is unaccountably large. For this reason no clear conclusion can be made as yet of the effect of hemolytic anemias, malignant tumors, or healing and injury on the normal rate of Hp turnover. The rate of normal biosynthesis is about 30–50% of the intravascular content per day (Noyes and Garby, 1967). For a compilation of metabolic data see Table XIX in Pintera (1971).

In metabolic studies account must be taken of differences in Hp phenotype and of the degree of saturation of serum Hp. Much of the Hp in normal serum is free or may be present in an intermediate complex. Although the metabolic fate of free and bound Hp is probably the same, the rate may differ significantly. Another factor is the distribution of haptoglobin between the intravascular and extravascular compartments. This depends on the phenotype; with the lower molecular weight Hp 1-1, the extravascular amount is about equal to the intravascular amount, whereas with Hp 2-2 the proportion in the extravascular compartment is considerably less (Pintera, 1971).

D. Physiological Function and Evolutionary Advantage

One would think that there should be no question about the physiological role and evolutionary advantage of a protein such as haptoglobin which has the specific biological property of forming the Hp-Hb complex. Yet, two factors have led to a questioning of physiological importance of haptoglobin; the first is the apparent lack of adverse effects in anhaptoglobinemic individuals, the second is the calculation that the Hp-Hb complex accounts for only a portion of the hemoglobin delivered to the reticuloendothelial system for catabolism (Nyman, 1959b).

When more hemoglobin enters the circulation than can be bound by haptoglobin, free Hb circulates in the plasma. This Hb is more rapidly eliminated from the plasma *in vivo* than is the Hp-Hb complex (Laurell, 1960). Most of the free Hb is taken up by the reticuloendothelial cells, but some 10% of it is excreted in the urine. Thus, in addition to transport and catabolism as the Hp-Hb complex, Hb in excess can be metabolized by the reticuloendothelial system without loss of the iron or amino acids as occurs in hemoglobinuria, i.e., hemoglobin is catabolized at the same site whether delivered as the Hp-Hb complex or as free Hb.

Because of the strength of the Hp-Hb complex and its relatively high molecular weight, free hemoglobin is not normally excreted in the urine in significant amounts. Haptoglobin is thus one of the group of components that act as a defense mechanism to prevent undue loss of iron; the other components are transferrin, which combines reversibly with iron, hemopexin which combines with heme, and to a lesser extent albumin which forms methemalbumin. Hemoglobin does not appear in the urine unless all haptoglobin in the circulation has been tied up in the Hp-Hb complex (Laurell and Nyman, 1957). The "renal threshold" of hemoglobin varies with the Hp concentration and is thus not dependent mainly on the functional capacity of the tubular cells to reabsorb Hb (Laurell and Nyman, 1957; Allison and ap Rees, 1957; Laurell, 1960).

How then is iron conserved in individuals who are anhaptoglobinemic? This question is especially pertinent to cases of inherited forms of hemolytic anemia such as in sickle cell anemia and other hemoglobinopathies. In these cases haptoglobin is removed from the circulation via the Hp-Hb complex as rapidly as the Hp is formed. This is a dead end for the haptoglobin for none of it returns to the circulation. In such patients tubular reabsorption of free Hb must play an important role in iron conservation.

VI. Comparative Biochemistry and Evolutionary Development

A. Comparative Biochemistry

Hemoglobin-binding proteins or haptoglobins have been found in the serum of many animals, including the horse, dog, cat, rabbit, ox, pig, duck, turtle, and frog (see Engle and Woods, 1960, for early references).

Because of the relative ease of identifying hemoglobin-binding proteins by the method of starch gel electrophoresis, the detection and qualitative study of haptoglobins in animal sera is easier than for most other plasma proteins. Although the great majority of the literature deals with human haptoglobin, structural studies have been made on canine Hp (Dobryszycka *et al.,* 1969), rabbit and rat Hp (Lombart *et al.,* 1965), horse Hp (Waks *et al.,* 1969), and porcine Hp (Lockhart *et al.,* 1972). Kurosky *et al.* (1975) have reported the N-terminal sequence for the first 30 residues of the β chain of rat, dog, and rabbit haptoglobins. However, no other sequence information is yet available on animal haptoglobins. The antigenic structure of haptoglobins in man and nonhuman primates has been compared (Javid and Fuhrman, 1971). The relative dearth of structural data on animal haptoglobins is very surprising since these proteins with their highly specific function and ready identification offer an excellent system for comparative structural study.

Few attempts have been made to identify haptoglobin allotypes and study their genetic control in animals. However, Chiao and Dray (1969) by the Ouchterlony immunodiffusion method distinguished two antigenically different genetic variants of haptoglobins in rabbit serum. Progeny data indicated that the two allotypes are controlled by allelic genes at an autosomal locus but that this locus is not closely linked to the loci for low density lipoproteins, α_2-macroglobulin, or immunoglobulin light or heavy chains.

B. Evolutionary Development

Extensive immunochemical studies of the phylogeny of haptoglobins have not been made comparable to those for serum albumin; however, a series of eight antigenic markers of haptoglobin in man and in five other primate species have been investigated by Javid and Fuhrman (1971). Like human Hp 1-1, all of the nonhuman primate haptoglobins lack a determinant that depends on the polymeric configuration of haptoglobin. This is consistent with the absence in animal sera of a component that resembles Hp 2-2 in gel electrophoretic media. All of the primates tested shared the determinants that are located near the binding site for hemoglobin. This suggests that the configuration at this site is preserved against selective pressures and that the ability to bind hemoglobin confers an evolutionary advantage as a biologically useful function. Of the eight antigenic determinants identified in human Hp 2-2 or Hp 2-1, seven are present in Hp 1-1. The nonhuman primates could be ranked in order by the number of determinants shared with man as follows: chimpanzee 6, gibbon 5, green monkey 3, rhesus 3, and baboon 2.

Since nonhuman primates do not have a polymeric haptoglobin component identifiable with Hp 2-2, the partial duplication of the *Hpα¹* gene to form the *Hpα²* gene must have occurred after the separation of man and the higher primates. Because both hpα^{1F} and hpα^{1S} are represented in the hpα² chain, the latter arose after the point mutation that produced the lysine-glutamic acid interchange at position 54 in the hpα^{1F} and hpα^{1S} chains. These events must have been relatively recent on an evolutionary scale because the duplicated sequence of hpα² has remained unchanged, yet long enough ago (perhaps 50,000 years) to permit the spread of the *Hpα²* gene to virtually all world populations.

An evolutionary relationship between haptoglobin and the immunoglobulins has been proposed by Black and Dixon (1968) because of a sequence homology between the Hp α chains and the light chains of immunoglobulins and because of the resemblance of Hp-Hb complex formation to the antibody—antigen reaction. However, unlike antibodies, which are a complex array of structurally related molecules that can be elicited in a wide spectrum of specificities by a multiplicity of antigens, haptoglobin has a single specificity. Also, the hereditary Hp allotype is produced early in neonatal development, and the three common types are under hereditary control and are almost universally distributed. Haptoglobin and antibodies also have different sites of biosynthesis.

There is a weak homology in certain regions between the sequence of the hpα chains and the κ and λ light chains of immunoglobulins and an even weaker homology to the heavy chains. This is illustrated in Fig. 9 taken from Wikler *et al.* (1969). However, there is no detectable homology between the hpβ chain and either the heavy or light chains of the immunoglobulins; on the contrary, the hpβ chain has a significant homology to the serine proteinases (Barnett *et al.*, 1972; Kurosky *et al.*,

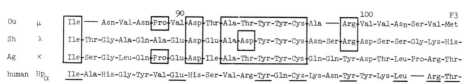

Fig. 9. Example of the weak sequence homology between the α chain of human haptoglobin and the light and heavy chains of human immunoglobulins. The immunoglobulin sequences begin at Ile-85 in the μ heavy chain Ou and in homologous positions for the λ light chain Sh and the κ light chain Ag. The haptoglobin α chain sequence begins at Ile-22. Residues that are identical with any of the immunoglobulin chains are underscored. Even though the variable regions of the immunoglobulin chains are being compared, it is obvious they have much more homology to each other than either of the light chains or the heavy chain has to the Hp α chain (from Wikler *et al.*, 1969).

1974, 1975). Although the hypothesis of an ancestral relationship between haptoglobin and the immunoglobulins is attractive, the homology between the hpβ chain and the serine proteinases requires a different line of descent between the two pairs of chains in haptoglobin whereas, as can be seen from Fig. 9 and is described more fully in a later chapter, the light and heavy chains of immunoglobulins have a common line of descent.

REFERENCES

Adams, E. C., and Weiss, M. R. (1969). *Biochem. J.* **115**, 441.
Alfsen, A., Chiancone, E., Wyman, J., and Antonini, E. (1970). *Biochim. Biophys. Acta* **200**, 76.
Allison, A. C. (1969). *Nature (London)* **183**, 1312.
Allison, A. C., and ap Rees, W. (1957). *Brit. Med. J.* **2**, 1137.
Alper, C. A., Peters, J. H., Birtch, A. G., and Gardner, F. H. (1965). *J. Clin. Invest.* **44**, 574.
Aly, F. W., Brinker, G., Deicher, H., Hartman, F., and Nix, W. (1962). *Nature (London)* **194**, 1091.
Barnett, D. R., Lee, T. H., and Bowman, B. H. (1970). *Nature (London)* **225**, 938.
Barnett, D. R., Lee, T. H., and Bowman, B. H. (1972). *Biochemistry* **11**, 1189.
Barnett, D. R., Kurosky, A., Fuller, G. M., Han-Hwa, K., Rasco, M. A., and Bowman, B. H. (1975). *Protides Biol. Fluids, Proc. Colloq.* **22**, 589.
Barnicot, N. A. (1961). *In* "Genetical Variation in Human Population" (G. A. Harrison, ed.), p. 41. Pergamon Press, Oxford.
Bearn, A. G., and Franklin, E. C. (1958). *Science* **128**, 596.
Bearn, A. G., and Franklin, E. C. (1959). *J. Exp. Med.* **109**, 55.
Berggård, I., and Bearn, A. G. (1962). *Nature (London)* **195**, 1311.
Bernier, G. M. (1967). *Clin. Chim. Acta* **18**, 309.
Bernini, L. F., and Borri-Voltattorni, C. (1970). *Biochim. Biophys. Acta* **200**, 203.
Black, J. A., and Dixon, G. H. (1968). *Nature (London)* **218**, 736.
Black, J. A., Chan, G. F. Q., Hew, C. L., and Dixon, G. H. (1970). *Can. J. Biochem.* **48**, 123.
Bundschuh, G., Menning, I., Handage, H., and Schubert, G. (1962). *Z. Aerztl. Fortbild.* **56**, 767.
Burrows, S., and Hosten, E. B. (1966). *Amer. J. Clin. Pathol.* **36**, 634.
Cheftel, R. I., and Moretti, J. (1966). *C. R. Acad. Sci.* **262**, 1982.
Cheftel, R. I., Cloarec, L., Moretti, J., Rafelson, M., and Jayle, M. F. (1960). *Bull. Soc. Chim. Biol.* **42**, 993.
Cheftel, R. I., Cloarec, L., Moretti, J., and Jayle, M. F. (1965). *Bull. Soc. Chim. Biol.* **47**, 385.
Cheftel, R. I., Parnaudeau, M. A., Bourrillon, R., and Moretti, J. (1969). *Eur. J. Biochem.* **9**, 585.
Chiancone, E. Wittenberg, J. B., Wittenberg, B. A., Antonini, E., and Wyman, J. (1966). *Biochim. Biophys. Acta* **117**, 379.
Chiao, J. W., and Dray, S. (1969). *Biochem. Genet.* **3**, 1.
Chiao, M. T., and Bezkorovainy, A. (1972). *Biochim. Biophys. Acta* **263**, 60.

Chung, J. H., and Shim, B.-S. (1973). *J. Catholic Medical College (Korea)* 25, 15.

Cleve, H., and Deicher, H. (1965). *Humangenetik* 1, 537.

Cleve, H., Gordon, S., Bowman, B. H., and Bearn, A. G. (1967). *Amer. J. Hum. Genet.* 19, 713.

Cleve, H., Bowman, B. H., and Gordon, S. (1969). *Humangenetik* 7, 337.

Cloarec, L., and Moretti, J. (1965). *Bull. Soc. Chim. Biol.* 47, 21.

Cohen-Dix, P., Noble, R. W., and Reichlin, M. (1973). *Biochemistry* 12, 3744.

Connell, G. E., and Shaw, R. W. (1961). *Can. J. Biochem.* 39, 1013.

Connell, G. E., and Smithies, O. (1959). *Biochem. J.* 72, 115.

Connell, G. E., Dixon, G. H., and Smithies, O. (1962). *Nature (London)* 103, 505.

Connell, G. E., Smithies, O., and Dixon, G. H. (1966). *J. Mol. Biol.* 21, 225.

Culliford, B. J., and Wraxall, B. G. D. (1966). *Nature (London)* 211, 872.

Dayhoff, M. O., ed. (1973). "The Atlas of Protein Sequence and Structure," Vol. 5, Suppl. I. Nat. Biomed. Res. Found., Washington, D.C.

Dobryszycka, W., Elwyn, D. H., and Kukral, J. C. (1969). *Biochim. Biophys. Acta* 175, 220.

Ehnholm, C. (1968). *Scand. J. Clin. Lab. Invest.* 21, Suppl. 101, 39.

Engle, R. L., Jr., and Woods, K. R. (1960). *In* "The Plasma Proteins" (F. W. Putnam, ed.), Vol. 2, pp. 183–265. Academic Press, New York.

Fagerhol, M. K., and Jacobsen, J. H. (1969). *Vox Sang.* 17, 143.

Ferris, T. G., Easterling, R. E., Nelson, K. J., and Budd, R. E. (1966). *Amer. J. Clin. Pathol.* 46, 385.

Fuller, G. M., Rasco, M. A., McCombs, M. L., Barnett, D. R., and Bowman, B. H. (1973). *Biochemistry* 12, 253.

Galatius-Jensen, F. (1958a). *Acta Genet. Med. Gemellol.* 8, 232.

Galatius-Jensen, F. (1958b). *Acta Genet. Med. Gemellol.* 8, 248.

Galatius-Jensen, F. (1960). Dansk Videnskabs Forlag, Copenhagen.

Galatius-Jensen, F. (1962). *Methods Forensic Sci.* 1, 497.

Gerald, P. S., Warner, S., Singer, J. D., Corcoran, P. A., and Umansky, I. (1964). *J. Clin. Invest.* 43, 1297.

Gerald, P. S., Warner, S., Singer, J. D., Corcoran, P. A., and Umansky, I. (1967). *J. Pediat.* 70, 172.

Gerbeck, C. M., Bezkorovainy, A., and Rafelson, M. E. (1967). *Biochemistry* 6, 403.

Giblett, E. R. (1962). *Progr. Med. Genet.* 2, 34.

Giblett, E. R. (1964). *Cold Spring Harbor Symp. Quant. Biol.* 29, 321.

Giblett, E. R. (1968). *Ser. Haematol.* [N.S.] 1, 1.

Giblett, E. R. (1969). "Genetic Markers in Human Blood." Blackwell, Oxford.

Giblett, E. R. (1975). *In* "Structure and Function of the Plasma Proteins" (A. C. Allison, ed.). Plenum, New York (in press).

Giblett, E. R., and Brooks, L. E. (1963). *Nature (London)* 197, 576.

Giblett, E. R., and Steinberg, A. G. (1960). *Amer. J. Hum. Genet.* 12, 160.

Gitlin, D., and Biasucci, A. (1969). *J. Clin. Invest.* 48, 1433.

Gordon, S., Cleve, H., and Bearn, A. G. (1968). *Proc. Soc. Exp. Biol. Med.* 127, 52.

Guinand, S., Tonnelat, J., Boussier, G., and Jayle, M. F. (1956). *Bull. Soc. Chim. Biol.* 38, 329.

Hamaguchi, H. (1969). *Amer. J. Hum. Genet.* 21, 440.

Hamaguchi, H., and Sasazuki, T. (1967). *Proc. Jap. Acad.* 43, 332.

Hamaguchi, H., Isomoto, A., Miyake, Y., and Nakajima, H. (1971). *Biochemistry* 10, 1741.

Harris, H., Robson, E. B., and Siniscalco, M. (1958). *Nature (London)* 182, 1324.

Harris, H., Robson, E. B., and Siniscalco, M. (1959). *Biochem. Hum. Genet., Ciba Found. Symp., 1959* p. 151.
Haupt, H., and Heide, K. (1970). *Blut* **20**, 1.
Heimburger, N., Heide, K., Haupt, H., and Schultze, H. E. (1964). *Clin. Chim. Acta* **10**, 293.
Herman-Boussier, G. (1960). "Prêparation et Propriétés Physiques et Chimiques des Haptoglobines Humaines." Foulon, Paris (cited by Schultze and Heremans, 1966).
Herman-Boussier, G., Moretti, J., and Jayle, M. F. (1960a). *Bull. Soc. Chim. Biol.* **42**, 817.
Herman-Boussier, G., Moretti, J., and Jayle, M. F. (1960b). *Bull. Soc. Chim. Biol.* **42**, 837.
Herman-Boussier, G., Cloarec, L., and Cheftel, R. I. (1962). *Nouv. Rev. Fr. Hematol.* **2**, 455.
Hew, C. L., and Dixon, G. H. (1971). Quoted in Dayhoff (1973, p. 579).
Hirschfeld, J. (1959). *Acta Pathol. Microbiol. Scand.* **47**, 160.
Hirschfeld, J. (1960). *Sci. Tools* **7**, 18.
Hirschfeld, J., and Lunell, N. O. (1962). *Nature (London)* **196**, 1220.
Hodgson, R., and Sewell, P. (1965). *J. Med. Lab. Technol.* **22**, 130.
Hommes, F. A. (1959). *Clin. Chim. Acta* **4**, 707.
Javid, J. (1964). *Proc. Nat. Acad. Sci. U.S.* **52**, 663.
Javid, J. (1965). *Vox Sang.* **10**, 330.
Javid, J. (1967). *Proc. Nat. Acad. Sci. U.S.* **57**, 920.
Javid, J., and Fuhrman, M. H. (1971). *Amer. J. Hum. Genet.* **23**, 496.
Javid, J., and Horowitz, H. I. (1960). *Amer. J. Clin. Pathol.* **34**, 35.
Javid, J., and Yingling, W. (1968a). *J. Clin. Invest.* **47**, 2290.
Javid, J., and Yingling, W. (1968b). *J. Clin. Invest.* **47**, 2297.
Javid, J., Fischer, D. S., and Spaet, T. H. (1959). *Blood* **14**, 683.
Jayle, M. F. (1951). *Bull. Soc. Chim. Biol.* **33**, 876.
Jayle, M. F. (1962). "Les Haptoglobines." Masson, Paris.
Jayle, M. F., and Boussier, G. (1954). *Bull. Soc. Chim. Biol.* **36**, 959.
Jayle, M. F., and Moretti, J. (1962). *Progr. Hematol.* **3**, 342.
Kawamura, K., Kagiyama, S., Ogawa, A., and Yanese, T. (1972a). *Biochim. Biophys. Acta* **285**, 15.
Kawamura, K., Kagiyama, S., Ogawa, A., and Yanese, T. (1972b). *Biochim. Biophys. Acta* **285**, 22.
Killander, J. (1964). *Biochim. Biophys. Acta* **93**, 1.
Kirk, R. L. (1968). "The Haptoglobin Groups in Man," Monogr. Hum. Genet., Vol. 4. Karger, Basel.
Kluthe, R., Faul, J., and Heimpel, H. (1965). *Nature (London)* **205**, 93.
Korngold, L. (1963). *Int. Arch. Allergy Appl. Immunol.* **23**, 268.
Korngold, L. (1965). *Immunochemistry* **2**, 103.
Krauss, S., and Sarcione, E. J. (1964). *Biochim. Biophys. Acta* **90**, 301.
Krauss, S., Schrott, M., and Sarcione, E. J. (1966). *Amer. J. Med. Sci.* **252**, 184.
Kurosky, A., Barnett, D. R., Rasco, M. A., Lee, T.-H., and Bowman, B. H. (1974). *Biochem. Genet.* **11**, 279.
Kurosky, A., Han-Hwa, K., Barnett, D. R., Rasco, M., Touchstone, B., and Bowman, B. H. (1975). *Protides Biol. Fluids, Proc. Colloq.* **22**, 597.
Laurell, C.-B. (1959). *Clin. Chim. Acta* **4**, 79.
Laurell, C.-B. (1960). *In* "The Plasma Proteins" (F. W. Putnam, ed.), Vol. 1, p. 459. Academic Press, New York.
Laurell, C.-B., and Grönvall, C. (1962). *Advan. Clin. Chem.* **5**, 135.
Laurell, C.-B., and Nyman, M. (1957). *Blood* **12**, 493.

Lockhart, W. L., Chung, W. P., and Smith, D. B. (1972). *Can. J. Biochem.* **50,** 775.

Lombart, C., Dautrevaux, M., and Moretti, J. (1965). *Biochim. Biophys. Acta* **97,** 270.

Makinen, M. W., and Kon, H. (1971). *Biochemistry* **10,** 43.

Makinen, M. W., Milstien, J. B., and Kon, H. (1972). *Biochemistry* **11,** 3851.

Malchy, B., and Dixon, C. H. (1970). *Can. J. Biochem.* **48,** 192.

Malchy, B., and Dixon, C. H. (1973a). *Can. J. Biochem.* **51,** 249.

Malchy, B., and Dixon, C. H. (1973b). *Can. J. Biochem.* **51,** 321.

Malchy, B., Rorstad, O., and Dixon, C. H. (1973). *Can. J. Biochem.* **51,** 265.

Malin, S. F., Baker, R. P., Jr., and Edward, J. R. (1972). *Biochem. Med.* **6,** 205.

Marnay, A. (1961). *Nature (London)* **191,** 74.

Matsunaga, E. (1962). *Jap. J. Hum. Genet.* **7,** 133.

Miller, L. L., and John, D. W. (1970). *In* "Plasma Protein Metabolism: Regulation of Synthesis, Distribution and Degradation" (M. A. Rothschild and T. Waldmann, eds.), pp. 199–222. Academic Press, New York.

Moretti, J., Cheftal, R. I., and Cloarec, L. (1966). *Bull. Soc. Chim. Biol.* **48,** 843.

Nagel, R. L., and Gibson, Q. H. (1967). *J. Biol. Chem.* **242,** 3428.

Nagel, R. L., and Gibson, Q. H. (1971). *J. Biol. Chem.* **246,** 69.

Nagel, R. L., and Gibson, Q. H. (1972). *Biochem. Biophys. Res. Commun.* **48,** 959.

Nagel, R. L., and Ranney, H. M. (1964). *Science* **144,** 1014.

Nagel, R. L., Wittenberg, J. B., and Ranney, H. M. (1965). *Biochim. Biophys. Acta* **100,** 286.

Nance, W. E., and Smithies, O. (1963). *Nature (London)* **198,** 869.

Neuhaus, O. W., and Sogoian, V. P. (1961). *Nature (London)* **192,** 558.

Ng, A., Owen, J. A., and Padanyi, R. (1963). *Clin. Chim. Acta* **8,** 145.

Niedermeier, W., Cross, R., and Beetham, W. P., Jr. (1965). *Arthritis Rheum.* **8,** 55.

Noyes, W. D., and Garby, L. (1967). *Scand. J. Clin. Lab. Invest.* **20,** 33.

Nyman, M. (1959a). *Scand. J. Clin. Lab. Invest.* **11,** Suppl. 39.

Nyman, M. (1959b). *Scand. J. Clin. Lab. Invest.* **12,** 121.

Ogawa, A., Kagiyama, S., and Kawamura, K. (1968). *Proc. Jap. Acad.* **44,** 1054.

Owen, J. A., Smith, H., Padanyi, R., and Martin, J. (1964). *Clin. Sci.* **26,** 1.

Parker, W. C., and Bearn, A. G. (1963). *Nature (London)* **198,** 107.

Pastewka, J. V., Reed, R. A., Ness, A. T., and Peacock, A. C. (1973). *Anal. Biochem.* **51,** 152.

Pavliček, Z., and Kalous, V. (1964). *Collect. Czech. Chem. Commun.* **29,** 1851.

Peacock, A. C., Pastewka, J. V., Reed, R. A., and Nees, A. T. (1970). *Biochemistry* **9,** 2275.

Perutz, M. F. (1970). *Nature (London)* **228,** 726.

Peters, J. H., and Alper, C. A. (1966). *J. Clin. Invest.* **45,** 314.

Pintera, J. (1971). *Ser. Haematol.* **4,** No. 2, 1–183.

Polonovski, M., and Jayle, M. F. (1938). *C. R. Soc. Biol.* **129,** 457.

Polonovski, M., and Jayle, M. F. (1939). *Bull. Soc. Chim. Biol.* **21,** 66.

Polonovski, M., and Jayle, M. F. (1940). *C. R. Acad. Sci.* **211,** 517.

Poulik, M. D. (1957). *Nature (London)* **180,** 1477.

Prokop, O., and Bundschuh, G. (1963). "Die Technik und die Bedeutung der Haptoglobine und Gm-gruppen in Klinik und Gerichtsmedizin." de Gruyter, Berlin.

Putnam, F. W. (1972). *J. Hum. Evol.* **1,** 591.

Rafelson, M. E., Cloarec, L., Moretti, J., and Jayle, M. F. (1961). *Nature (London)* **191,** 279.

Ramot, B., Kende, G., and Arnon, A. (1962). *Nature (London)* **196,** 176.

Ratcliff, A. P., and Hardwicke, J. (1964). *J. Clin. Pathol.* **17,** 676.

Renwick, J. H., and Marshall, H. (1966). *Ann. Hum. Genet.* **29,** 389.

Robson, E. B., Glen-Bott, A. M., Cleghorn, L. E., and Harris, H. (1964). *Ann. Human Genet.* **28,** 77.

Robson, E. B., Polani, P. E., Dart, S. J., Jacobs, P. A., and Renwick, J. H. (1969). *Nature (London)* **223,** 1163.

Rowe, D. S. (1961). *J. Clin. Pathol.* **14,** 205.

Roy, R. B., Shaw, R. W., and Connell, G. E. (1969). *J. Lab. Clin. Med.* **74,** 698.

Russo, S. F., and Chen, W. W.-C. (1974). *Biochemistry* **13,** 5300.

Sass, M. D., and Spear, P. W. (1962). *Nature (London)* **193,** 285.

Schultze, H. E., and Heremans, J. F. (1966). "Molecular Biology of Human Proteins. I. Nature and Metabolism of Extracellular Proteins," p. 200. Elsevier, Amsterdam.

Schultze, H. E., Haupt, H. Heide, K., and Heimburger, N. (1963). *Clin. Chim. Acta* **8,** 207.

Shim, B. S., and Bearn, A. G. (1964). *J. Exp. Med.* **120,** 611.

Shim, B. S., and Lee, T. H., and Kang, Y. S. (1965). *Nature (London)* **207,** 1264.

Shim, B. S., Jin, K. S., and Cleve, H. (1967). *Proc. Soc. Exp. Biol. Med.* **126,** 221.

Shinoda, T. (1965). *J. Biochem. (Tokyo)* **57,** 100.

Smith, H., and Owen, J. A. (1961). *Biochem. J.* **78,** 723.

Smith, H., Edman, P., and Owen, J. A. (1962). *Nature (London)* **193,** 286.

Smithies, O. (1955). *Biochem. J.* **61,** 629.

Smithies, O. (1959a). *Advan. Protein Chem.* **14,** 65.

Smithies, O. (1959b). *Biochem. J.* **71,** 585.

Smithies, O. (1964). *Cold Spring Harbor Symp. Quant. Biol.* **29,** 309.

Smithies, O., and Walker, N. F. (1956). *Nature (London)* **178,** 694.

Smithies, O., Connell, G. E., and Dixon, G. H. (1962a). *Amer. J. Hum. Genet.* **14,** 14.

Smithies, O., Connell, G. E., and Dixon, G. H. (1962b). *Nature (London)* **196,** 232.

Smithies, O., Connell, G. E., and Dixon, G. H. (1966). *J. Mol. Biol.* **21,** 213.

Steinbuch, M., and Quentin, M. (1961). *Nature (London)* **190,** 1121.

Sutton, H. E. (1970). *Progr. Med. Genet.* **7,** 163.

Sutton, H. E., and Karp, G. W., Jr. (1964). *Amer. J. Hum. Genet.* **16,** 419.

Tarukoski, P. H. (1966). *Scand. J. Clin. Lab. Invest.* **18,** 80.

Tsunoo, H., Sasazuki, T., Sato, H., and Nakajima, H. (1974). *Immunochemistry* **11,** 673.

Wada, T., Ohara, H., Watanabe, K., Kinoshita, H., and Nishio, H. (1970). *J. Reticuloendothel. Soc.* **8,** 195.

Waks, M., and Alfsen, A. (1966). *Arch. Biochem. Biophys.* **113,** 304.

Waks, M., and Alfsen, A. (1968). *Arch. Biochem. Biophys.* **123,** 133.

Waks, M., and Beychok, S. (1974). *Biochemistry* **13,** 15.

Waks, M., Alfsen, A., and Cittanova, N. (1967). *Biochem. Biophys. Res. Commun.* **27,** 693.

Waks, M., Alfsen, A., Beuzard, Y., Rosa, J., Lessin, L. S., Mayer, A., and Trautwein, A. (1968). *Biochem. Biophys. Res. Commun.* **32,** 215.

Waks, M., Alfsen, A., Schwaiger, S., and Mayer, A. (1969). *Arch. Biochem. Biophys.* **132,** 268.

Weerts, G., Nix, W., and Deicher, H. (1966). *Blut* **12,** 65.

Wheby, M. S., Barrett, O., and Crosby, W. H. (1960). *Blood* **16,** 1579.

Wikler, M., Köhler, H., Shinoda, T., and Putnam, F. W. (1969). *Science* **163,** 75.

2 / Ceruloplasmin

M. D. Poulik and M. L. Weiss

I. Introduction

Copper was probably the first metal known to man. Copper instruments were found in Egyptian tombs dating back as far as 5000 BC. The ancient copper mines were located on the island of Cyprus and the word copper was derived originally from *cyprium* and altered later to cuprum. Thus, the knowledge of this metal goes as far back as 5000 BC. The identification of copper in living organisms goes back only 150 years. That copper may be an essential body constituent was recognized when the respiratory pigment of cold-blooded animals, hemocyanin, was discovered and when a copper-containing pigment, turacin, was found in the feathers of touraco birds (Sass-Kortsak, 1965).

Progress in the elucidation of the role of copper for the sustenance of health was made when naturally occurring deficiency states in a number of domestic animals were discovered in cattle, sheep, and pigs feeding on plants grown on copper-deficient soil in North America (Neal *et al.,* 1931), Europe (Sjollema, 1933, 1938), and Australia (Bennetts and Chapman, 1937). Copper has been recognized as an essential constituent in a number of enzymes and in many of them it is indeed indispensable for the function of their active sites. Some of these enzymes are widespread in living tissues, e.g., cytochrome *c* oxidase, and involved *sine qua non* in basic life processes. Elaborate physiological mechanisms must be operational to insure that copper is made available in sufficient amounts, in the right place, in proper form and at the right time.

While trace amounts of copper are essential for life, an excess is toxic. Warburg and Krebs (1927) have shown that blood serum has a fairly constant copper content of about 100 μg/dl. Krebs (1928) found that there is a rise in serum copper during pregnancy and Heilmeyer *et al.* (1941) showed a similar rise during infection. Abderhalden and Moller (1928) showed that the copper in serum is nondialyzable and Boyden and Potter (1937) have demonstrated that low pH is able to dissociate copper from the constituents of serum. Similar findings were also made previously by Warburg and Krebs (1927) and Locke *et al.* (1932). Eisler *et al.* (1936) demonstrated binding of copper to albumin. Mann and Keilin (1938) prepared a crystalline copper–protein, hemocuprein, which contained about 0.34% copper. A similar protein was prepared from horse serum and the same investigators identified hepatocuprein from human liver. Later, a somewhat similar protein was isolated from human brain by Porter and Folch (1957) and nearly 10 years later Carrico and Deutsch (1969b) were able to prove that all three proteins are identical.

Luetscher (1940), and later Pedersen (1945) described a blue globulin in pig serum and Holmberg and Laurell (1947, 1948) found that 90% of serum copper is firmly bound to an α_2-globulin, ceruloplasmin, which exhibits oxidase properties. The molecular weight of this protein was estimated to be 151,000 (Holmberg and Laurell, 1951), and from the copper content of 0.35% it was calculated that there must be 8 atoms of copper per molecule of ceruloplasmin.

Since then a vast amount of work concerned with biophysical, biochemical, and immunological properties has been carried out (see reviews of Laurell, 1960; Peisach *et al.*, 1966; Malkin and Malmström, 1970). Ceruloplasmin has been shown to contain about 8% covalently bound carbohydrate (Schultze, 1957). A possible polymorphism was found by Broman (1958). New techniques for investigating the submolecular structure of proteins stimulated new interest in ceruloplasmin. Poulik (1962) first reported on the presence of several polypeptide chains in ceruloplasmin as analyzed by urea-starch gel electrophoresis and other investigators followed suit. The controversy still rages whether ceruloplasmin is a single or multichain protein. The content of sugar was reinvestigated by Jamieson (1965) and several glycopeptides were prepared and isolated by him. Electron paramagnetic resonance studies were conducted to learn more about the kinds of copper present in ceruloplasmin (Vänngård, 1967; Andrèasson and Vänngård, 1970). Similar studies were performed on a number of ceruloplasmins of different species. Genetically controlled polymorphic forms were demonstrated by Shreffler *et al.* (1967b). The catabolism of desialylated ceruloplasmin was studied extensively by the Scheinberg group and copper-free ceruloplasmin, apoceruloplasmin, was suggested as a therapeutic agent.

All these and other studies to be discussed in this review tried to answer the major question about ceruloplasmin, namely: What is the function of this protein? The answer to this question would be particularly helpful to our understanding of a rare, inherited disorder known as hepatolenticular degeneration or Wilson's disease or Wilson-Konovalov disease. The disease was described for the first time in 1912 by Wilson and until 1959 not more than 650 cases were recorded (Boudin and Pepin, 1959). This malady appears to be the only instance of primarily deranged copper metabolism in man. The condition is characterized by greatly reduced or undetectable ceruloplasmin and these low levels are associated with abnormal copper balance and copper deposits in various tissues, particularly in liver and brain (Scheinberg, 1966; Walshe, 1966; Walshe and Cumings, 1961). The argument exists that the role of ceruloplasmin is to bind absorbed copper and maintain zero copper balance (Scheinberg, 1966). If this hypothesis is correct, then the enzymatic property of this protein, namely, oxidase, would be only incidental.

Experimental data show that ceruloplasmin is a very inefficient catalyst of all its known substrates with the possible exception of ferrous ions as shown by Osaki et al. (1966b) and Osaki and Walaas (1967). Osaki et al. (1966a, 1971) demonstrated that ceruloplasmin is involved in iron mobilization and that ferrous iron is the physiological substrate of the protein. These authors suggested a new name for the protein, ferroxidase. Yet patients with undetectable ceruloplasmin do not show any symptoms of anemia except for the consequences of abnormal copper balance. None of the current theories of the function of ceruloplasmin account for all the physiological and clinical facts.

We hope to elucidate and review the present knowledge of this fascinating metalloprotein in the following pages. While an attempt is made to cover all subjects dealing with ceruloplasmin in an equitable fashion, it is painfully obvious that this ideal is prevented by the inequitable knowledge on the part of the authors for all the subjects covered.

II. Purification and Physical Properties

A. Purification

There are many methods of preparation and purification of ceruloplasmin. These can be divided into two major groups, (a) small-scale and (b) large-scale methods. The source of the starting material is usually serum or fractions thereof. Holmberg and Laurell (1948) have shown that most of the copper present in the serum is precipitable by 50% saturation with neutralized ammonium sulfate. They used the method of Cohn et al. (1940) to prepare an α-globulin fraction, of sky-blue color, which had a copper content of about 0.03%. If treated with alcohol and chloroform as Mann and Keilin (1938) did when preparing a copper-containing protein of red cells (haemocuprein) the supernatant could be further fractionated with ammonium sulfate (50–65% saturation) to prepare a copper protein with a copper content of 0.35%. Several investigators prepared ceruloplasmin directly from serum (Broman, 1958, 1964) by hydroxyapatite or from plasma (Deutsch, 1960) by ammonium sulfate fractionation and by calcium phosphate gel (Curzon and Vallet, 1960).

Sanders et al. (1959) described a procedure for isolation of ceruloplasmin from Cohn Fraction IV-1 prepared by Method 6 using ion-exchange chromatography. This material became by far the favorite starting material for preparation of ceruloplasmin. Škvařil et al. (1965) on the other hand used Cohn Fraction III as the starting material as did Péjaudier et al. (1970). Since normal serum is relatively expensive, still other sources were utilized for similar purposes, namely, placental serum by Broman and Kjellin (1964), placenta by Clausen *et al.* (1962), and ascitic fluid by Laurell (1960). It would be impractical to comment on all the methods used and consequently only a few will be described and two of them in considerable detail. Deutsch and his group (1962) provided the best physicochemical characterization of ceruloplasmin and Sgouris and his group (1962) prepared most of the ceruloplasmin for the American National Red Cross which subsequently released this material to a large number of workers in this field. Consequently the methods of these two groups are given below.

The method of Deutsch *et al.* (1962) is relatively rapid and gives high yields of ceruloplasmin. They have used 100 gm of Fraction IV-1 which was suspended in 500 ml of 0.05 M sodium acetate. This suspension was stirred for 30–60 min. The insoluble protein was spun down at 0°C. The residue was then reextracted with 200 ml of 0.05 M sodium acetate if an additional 10–15% higher yield was desired. Ion-exchange chromatography on DEAE-cellulose was then performed. The ion exchanger was equilibrated with 0.05 M sodium acetate, pH 5.5, and the supernatant added. The suspension was allowed to settle, the supernatant decanted, and the slurry poured into a column. The column was then washed with 0.05 M sodium acetate, pH 5.5, containing 0.05 M NaCl until the A_{280} value of the effluent was below 0.200. The ceruloplasmin was then eluted with the same acetate buffer, pH 5.5 containing 0.5 M NaCl. The eluted ceruloplasmin was then dialyzed against 0.05 M sodium acetate, pH 5.5, and then rechromatographed on DEAE-cellulose equilibrated in the same buffer. A constant volume continuous gradient was used (0.05 M sodium acetate, pH 5.5, 0.3 M NaCl). Fractions having $A_{280}:A_{610}$ ratios less than 50 were pooled, adjusted to pH 7.4 ($\pm$ 0.2) and dialyzed against 0.05 M sodium acetate. This fraction was now rechromatographed on DEAE-cellulose which had been adjusted to pH 7.4 and then equilibrated against 0.05 M sodium acetate. Again a constant volume continuous gradient elution technique was employed in which the higher salt concentration is 0.05 M sodium acetate containing 0.3 M NaCl. Fractions having an $A_{280}:A_{610}$ ratio less than 40 were pooled. The ceruloplasmin solution was then precipitated at 40% saturation of ammonium sulfate and diluted with water to give a ceruloplasmin concentration of 3–5%. The sample was dialyzed against 0.025 M sodium acetate pH 5.25 ($\pm$0.05) for 2–3 days. The ceruloplasmin crystallized within 24 hr. The crystals were removed by centrifugation in the cold and washed two times at 0°C with the 0.025 M sodium acetate buffer, pH 5.25, by centrifugation. The ceruloplasmin was then reconstituted to the desired working solution. The amounts of the Fraction IV-1 used were equivalent to 5-25 liters of plasma. The yield of the crystalline ceruloplasmin ranged from 30 to 55% of the amount of ceruloplasmin present in this plasma fraction. The copper content of the crystalline ceruloplasmin was 7.9–8.1 moles/160,000 gm protein. The copper–nitrogen ratio was 0.0216 and the nitrogen content was 15.0%. The A values at 280 nm and 610 nm were 14.9 and 0.68, respectively, when the protein was dissolved in 0.1–0.2 M solution of sodium chloride or sodium acetate at pH 6–8.

Škvařil *et al.* (1965) prepared ceruloplasmin from placental Cohn Fraction III of high purity using DEAE-Sephadex, precipitation with ammonium sulfate at 60% saturation and Sephadex G-200 gel filtration. Their A_{280} value was 16.3, A_{610} value 0.672, and the ratio of $A_{610}:A_{280}$ obtained was 0.041. Péjaudier *et al.* (1970) used caprylic acid as a precipitating agent to remove most of the nonceruloplasmin protein. The supernatant contained α_1-acid glycoprotein and prealbumin in addition to ceruloplasmin. After readsorption on DEAE-cellulose (Whatman) the ceruloplasmin was eluted with 0.25 M acetate buffer, pH 5.7, and upon dialysis against 0.015 M acetate buffer, pH 5.4, ceruloplasmin crystallized within hours at 4°C. The copper content of this preparation was 0.28–0.29% and the $A_{610}:A_{280}$ absorbance ratio 0.044–0.047.

Large-scale methods of preparations (up to several hundred grams) were also developed. Sgouris *et al.* (1962) started with 10 kg of Fraction IV-1 (preferably one having a bluish-green coloration) and suspended this amount of paste in 100 liters of cold distilled water. The flow diagram of the method is given in Fig. 1.

The overall yield averaged 56% based on copper analysis. The absorbance values were A_{610}, 0.68 and A_{280}, 14.4. One of the authors (M.D.P.) had at one time, while being associated with the American National Red Cross, nearly 2 kg of ceruloplasmin prepared by this method.

Björling (1963) described a method to obtain ceruloplasmin from several human blood fractions adaptable to small- and large-scale batch production. Twenty kilograms of Fraction III or IV as derived from 300 liters of retroplacental serum (stored at 5°C up to 1 week) were used in a routine batch. The flow sheet of this scheme is given in Fig. 2.

The author does not give any indication of purity as determined by spectral analysis. However, the material was relatively pure by electrophoretic methods. A number of possible subfractionation methods using ethanol, isoelectric precipitation, ammonium sulfate fractionation, DEAE-Sephadex chromatography, and combinations of these methods are also discussed. It should be noted that most of the large-scale methods utilized outdated plasma as collected from blood banks and few used fresh or relatively fresh serum or plasma for their preparation of

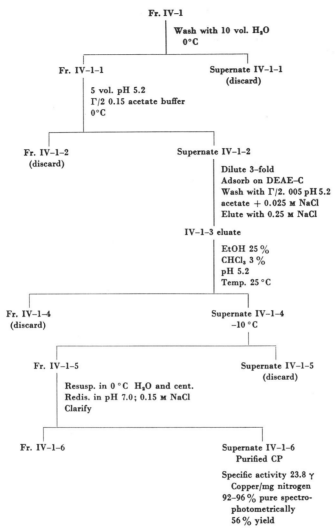

Fig. 1. The purification of ceruloplasmin from Fraction IV-1. From Sgouris *et al.* (1962).

ceruloplasmin. Rydén (1971a) questioned the integrity of ceruloplasmin prepared by large-scale methods. He provided some evidence that proteolytic degradation during the preparation might have occurred.

The preparation of apoceruloplasmin should be also mentioned. The possibility that the apoenzyme might be clinically effective in Wilson's disease led to preparation of such material by Morell and Scheinberg

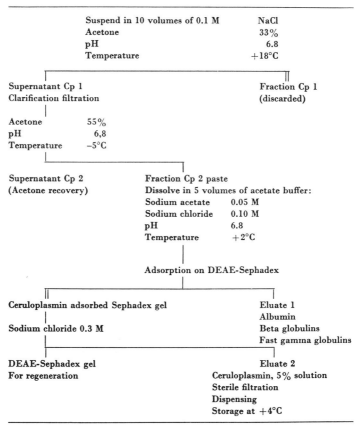

Fig. 2. The purification of ceruloplasmin from Fractions III and IV. From Björling (1963).

(1958). Previously, Scheinberg and Morell (1957) had shown that the copper–protein bond can be dissociated under certain conditions. Their results suggested that it might be possible to remove copper from ceruloplasmin and thus prepare an apoprotein capable of recombining with copper to reconstitute active ceruloplasmin. The procedure was carried out in acetate buffer and in the presence of a sufficient concentration of ascorbic acid to keep the ceruloplasmin copper in a monovalent state throughout its removal from the protein. Diethyldithiocarbamate ion was added also to form a colloidal suspension as this compound combines tightly with copper ions. The tightly bound copper was then removed by centrifugation. The apoprotein so prepared contained only 1.46 μg/ml of copper as compared to 30.7 μg/ml of the original solution. In other words, about 93% of the copper was removed by this process. The enzymatic activity was spectrophotometrically monitored by its effect on the rate of oxidation of paraphenylenediamine (Scheinberg and Morell, 1957). Only 57% of the original activity of the ceruloplasmin was regenerated with an ascorbic acid and cupric sulfate solution followed by passage through a column of acetate resin (IRA-400) and sodium resin (IR-120) which had been equilibrated with 0.2 *M* acetate buffer, pH 5.25. A clear blue solution of ceruloplasmin was obtained which contained 58.4% of ceruloplasmin copper of the original solution. The enzymatic activity was 86% of the original 100%. Addition of cupric ion without ascorbic acid to a solution of apoprotein did not result in formation of blue ceruloplasmin. However, considerable enzymatic activity was regenerated if the substrate paraphenylenediamine dichloride was added after the addition of the cupric ions. Sgouris *et al.* (1962) heated ceruloplasmin (10 hr, 60°C) and dialyzed it against 1.2 *M* sodium acetate buffer at pH 5.2. Then crystalline ascorbic acid was added with 0.4% sodium diethyldithiocarbamate and the copper complex removed by centrifugation (26,000 *g* for 2 hr). The excess of ascorbic acid and carbamate was removed by mixed bed resin (IR-120 sodium form and IRA-acetate form). The effluent was colorless and the apoenzyme was then precipitated by adding pH 4.0 acetate buffer to pH 5.2 acetate buffer and 95% ethanol to a concentration of 25% and lowering the temperature to −10°C. The preparation contained one major component and two minor components by electrophoresis. The copper content of this preparation was 0.12 μg copper/mg nitrogen. The efficacy of such preparations where used for treatment of Wilson's disease patients is questionable.

B. Electrophoretic Identification

The electrophoretic mobility of ceruloplasmin was measured by Holmberg and Laurell (1948) with the aid of free boundary electrophoresis at pH 7.4 in 0.2 ionic strength buffer. It migrated under these conditions close to the α-globulin fraction. Deutsch *et al.* (1962) showed that their crystalline ceruloplasmin is pure in a phosphate buffer at pH 7.0 and 0.1 ionic strength. Škvařil *et al.* (1965) determined the mobility of their preparation as 5.0×10^5 cm^2 V^{-1} sec^{-1} in a descending boundary, also in a phosphate buffer at pH 7.0. They found veronal (barbituric acid) buffers unsuitable for classic electrophoresis since during dialysis the blue color of the solution had a tendency to fade. In such a buffer three slowly migrating components were usually detected. Kasper and Deutsch (1963a) conducted free boundary electrophoresis in 0.1

ionic strength buffers, (a) acetate pH 5.48, (b) phosphate pH 7.01, and (c) barbiturate pH 8.6, on a preparation of ceruloplasmin obtained by the method of Deutsch *et al.* (1962). A single component was detected at pH 7.0 and 5.5. A faster migrating shoulder was seen at pH 8.6 which could be due to modification produced by losses or changes in the valency of copper. They have also prepared apoceruloplasmin by a cyanide method, by dialyzing a 1% solution of ceruloplasmin against changes of 0.05 M NaCN in 0.2 ionic strength potassium phosphate buffer, pH 7.4, and by the method of Morell and Scheinberg (1958). Apoceruloplasmin prepared by either method migrated with greater mobility to the anode. A smaller component of still higher anodal mobility was found in the ascorbic acid–diethyldithiocarbamate (DDC)-treated apoceruloplasmin but not in the apoceruloplasmin prepared by the cyanide method. Poulik (1962) has noticed that dialysis of pure ceruloplasmin against 0.1 M acetate buffer (pH 4.0) or against ascorbic acid or ethylenediaminetetraacetic acid (EDTA) in the presence of acetate buffer caused profound changes of the electrophoretic mobility of ceruloplasmin. On filter paper or agar gel electrophoresis two components instead of the usual one could be separated. Deutsch (1960) has demonstrated an electrophoretic component of higher anodic mobility after treatment with ascorbic acid. Kasper and Deutsch (1963a) have studied electrophoretic mobilities of ceruloplasmin and some of its derivatives by free boundary electrophoresis. The results are given in Table I.

Uriel *et al.* (1957) introduced a new method of detection of ceruloplasmin by exploiting its oxidase activity. With *p*-phenylenediamine as a substrate, two components were demonstrated after electrophoresis of purified ceruloplasmin in agar gel. Both components also contained copper. This method was later modified by Owen and Smith (1961) who used 0.1% orthodianisidine as a substrate. The enzymatic method of detection proved extremely useful especially in conjunction with electrophoresis in supporting media, e.g., filter paper, agar gel, and in particular starch gel. The advent of starch gel electrophoresis (Smithies, 1955) aided enormously the studies on ceruloplasmin heterogeneity, genetic polymorphic forms, and submolecular structure. Uriel (1957), Broman (1958), Richterich *et al.* (1960), as well as Rydén (1971b) and Sass-Kortsak *et al.* (1960) drew attention to the possibility that ceruloplasmin may exist in several molecular forms. Subsequently, Morell and Scheinberg (1960) applied starch gel electrophoresis to the analysis of a ceruloplasmin which was chromatographed on a hydroxyapatite gel. They found the presence of at least four ceruloplasmins which appeared to differ in histidine content. The authors thought that such differences might be genetic in origin.

TABLE I

Electrophoretic Mobilities of Ceruloplasmin and Some of Its Derivatives[a]

Protein	Buffer at 0.1 ionic strength	Mobility[b]
Native ceruloplasmin	Barbital, pH 8.60	5.20
	Barbital, pH 8.24[c]	5.24
	Tris, pH 8.41[c]	5.26
	Phosphate, pH 7.01	4.72
	Acetate, pH 5.48	2.74
DDC apoprotein		
Fast component	Phosphate, pH 7.01	6.39
Slow component	Phosphate, pH 7.01	~5
Cyanoapoprotein	Phosphate, pH 7.01	6.25
Colorless components from		
Ascorbic acid reduction	Phosphate, pH 7.01	6.10
Ascorbic acid reduction	Acetate, pH 5.48	3.97
Treatment with Tris	Phosphate, pH 7.01	6.14
Versene at pH 5.15		
Intermediate form	Phosphate, pH 7.01	6.11
Fast	Phosphate, pH 7.01	6.95

[a] Reproduced from Kasper and Deutsch (1963a) with permission.
[b] In cm^2 $volt^{-1}$ $sec^{-1} \times 10^5$.
[c] KCl contributed 80% of ionic strength.

In evaluating the significance of polymorphic systems it is important to decide whether the variants occur *in vivo* or whether the heterogeneity is induced by the method of preparation or storage. Poulik and Bearn (1962) provided evidence that ceruloplasmin prepared by large-scale methods consists of multiple components, as demonstrated by starch gel electrophoresis in borate buffer pH 8.6. Both protein stain (Amido Black 10B) and oxidase stain (0.5% solution of *p*-phenylenediamine hydrochloride in 0.1 *M* acetate buffer pH 5.7) were used to demonstrate the enzymatically active and inactive "ceruloplasmins." By use of two-dimensional zone electrophoresis (Poulik and Smithies, 1958), two of the ceruloplasmin preparations were separated into two zones on filter paper electrophoresis and into several zones by the subsequent starch gel electrophoresis. Major oxidase activity was localized mainly in one of the bands. However, all of the protein-stained zones reacted with a specific anticeruloplasmin antiserum. These results provided clear evidence that ceruloplasmin is a labile protein which can be easily denatured or/and polymerized during preparation and storage. Similar studies by Poulik (1963a) on well-defined batches of ceruloplasmin and apoceruloplasmin prepared by the method of Sgouris *et al.* (1962) mentioned above have shown that ceruloplasmin stored under liquid nitrogen was relatively intact (one major and one minor band on two-dimensional zone electrophoresis both stainable by protein and oxidase stains). Less carefully handled ceruloplasmins were separated into a faster migrating zone and a slower migrating zone by filter paper electrophoresis. The faster migrating zone was separated further into a number of zones by starch gel electrophoresis as demonstrated by staining for protein. Only a few of the slower migrating starch gel zones were still enzymatically active. The apoceruloplasmin migrated as a single zone on paper electrophoresis and separated into multiple zones on the subsequent starch gel electrophoresis. None of the zones were oxidase-positive. Screening of fresh sera of pregnant women has revealed that two oxidase-positive zones can be separated by vertical starch gel electrophoresis. Screening of such sera with the aid of the two-dimensional technique has shown that this minor oxidase-positive zone migrates with slightly faster electrophoretic mobility on the filter paper. In a significantly high proportion of pathological sera (lymphomas, myelomas), two oxidase-positive zones could be demonstrated. Both zones migrated with the same mobility on filter paper.

Kasper and Deutsch (1963a) found several slower migrating zones on vertical starch gel electrophoresis in borate buffer, pH 8.6, even in their crystalline ceruloplasmin. When screened in Tris-borate-EDTA gel at pH 8.5, the main ceruloplasmin resolved into two discrete bands. The authors attributed the lability of ceruloplasmin to various reagents and to storage to be due to changes in the valency and of amounts of copper or both. Indeed they produced change of crystalline ceruloplasmin by chromatography in DEAE-cellulose by elution with constant volume gradient technique ($0.05 \, M$ sodium acetate, pH $7.2 - 0.05 \, M$ acetate containing $0.3 \, M$ sodium chloride). They found that (a) some of the cupric copper was reduced to cuprous copper, (b) some of the cupric copper was no longer bound to groups in the molecule as complexes which have an intense absorption at 610 nm, or (c) both (a) and (b) had occurred. All these experiments indicate that ceruloplasmin is indeed a labile protein. Buffers containing barbital, Tris, EDTA, and other chelating substances or reducing agents are able to change the molecule and this modification is readily detectable by electrophoresis (Marriott and Perkins, 1966a,b). A typical example of such change is apoceruloplasmin. Yet, true genetic variants were discovered by Shreffler *et al.* (1967b) and will be discussed in detail in Section V.

C. Molecular Weight and Molecular Kinetic Properties

Determination of the molecular weight of ceruloplasmin was undertaken by several investigators. Ceruloplasmin prepared by Holmberg and Laurell (1948) was investigated by Pedersen (1953) and the molecular weight was estimated to be 151,000 daltons, sedimentation coefficient $s_{20,w}$ 6.8–7.3 S, diffusion coefficient $D^{\circ}_{20,w} = 4.5 \times 10^{-7}$ cm^2 sec^{-1}. Kasper and Deutsch (1963a) reinvestigated the molecular weight of ceruloplasmin and found their crystalline preparation to sediment as a single component ($s_{20,w}$ was 7.08 S at zero protein concentration). This value agrees with that obtained by Schultze and Schwick (1959). The results of the physicochemical studies done on native ceruloplasmin and two apoceruloplasmins prepared by two different methods are given in Table II.

Magdoff-Fairchild et al. (1969) have reported the molecular weight to be only 132,000 daltons. Since this value is derived from crystallographic data, these authors consider some of the sources of the errors and give a final molecular weight of 132,000 ± 4100. This value is outside the range of values determined by ultracentrifugal methods. The lowest value obtained by ultracentrifugal methods (Archibald's approach to equilibrium) was 153,000 daltons by Poillon and Bearn (1966b). The ceruloplasmin studied was prepared by a large-scale method of preparation (American National Red Cross, batch 1967) and was used previously by Poulik (1963a) for electrophoretic and structural characterization. This preparation contained 18.9 mg/ml of protein, 75 units of oxidase activity per milligram, 55.6 μg of copper per milliliter. A_{610}/A_{280}

TABLE II

Physicochemical Parameters of Ceruloplasmin and Apoceruloplasmin[a]

		Apoceruloplasmin	
Parameter	Native ceruloplasmin	Cyanide	DDC
Sedimentation coefficient (S)	7.08	6.01	6.15
Diffusion coefficient (D) (cm^2 sec^{-1} × 10^7)	3.76	3.22	2.96
Partial specific volume (v)	0.713[b]	0.728	0.728
Axial ratio ($a:b$)	11	16	18
Molecular weight (daltons)	160,000 155,000[c]	167,000	186,000

[a] Adapted from Kasper and Deutsch (1963a) with permission.
[b] Determined on DDC apoceruloplasmin.
[c] Approach to equilibrium.

was 0.041 and the percentage of copper 0.30%; consequently, it was 93% pure based on $A_{610}/A_{280} = 0.044$ for ceruloplasmin of 100% purity (Hirschman *et al.*, 1961). Nevertheless, two components were seen, 6.9 S and 10.8 S, respectively. The major component was estimated to be 90% of the sedimenting material. The faster sedimenting component appeared to be a dimer.

In view of these discrepancies, Rydén (1972a,c) prepared ceruloplasmin from fresh blood drawn directly into centrifuge bottles containing ϵ-aminocaproic acid (final concentration 0.02 M). Using a three-step method, a preparation was obtained which had an $A_{610}:A_{280}$ ratio as high as 0.049 and was homogeneous by electrophoresis in polyacrylamide gel (Rydén, 1971a). The sedimentation equilibrium technique was applied to a 0.05% solution of the reactive ceruloplasmin. The rotor speed was 11,000 rpm. Under these conditions, the material appeared homogeneous and had a molecular weight of 134,000 daltons. Rydén (1972a) argues that the value obtained from crystallographic data by Magdoff-Fairchild *et al.* (1969) might be more reliable since it is not dependent upon extrapolation procedures or possible association behavior. Taking into account the carbohydrate content (10%), the peptide moiety has a molecular weight of 120,000. From his work on commercial preparations of ceruloplasmin, degradation can be expected (Rydén, 1971a) which can hamper meaningful interpretation of the polypeptide structure of ceruloplasmin. In the most recent report by Freeman and Daniel (1973), the molecular weight of a ceruloplasmin prepared by affinity chromatography was reported as 126,000 (6000 rpm, interference optics), 122,000 (9000 rpm, absorption optics), and 123,000 (20,000 rpm, interference optics). The authors consider the value of 124,000 daltons most reliable and attribute the higher molecular weight values given by previous workers to errors in determining diffusion coefficients in the sedimentation-diffusion method and to difficulties in extracting the data necessary for the calculation of molecular weight by the Archibald method of approach to sedimentation equilibrium. Rydén (1972a) assumed that ceruloplasmin is a single chain protein and Freeman and Daniel (1973) that it is a multichain protein. This controversial question will be considered in detail in Section III.

Rydén (1972b) deduced the molecular weights of four mammalian ceruloplasmins by gel chromatography. Human, rabbit, horse, and pig ceruloplasmins were cyanoethylated and subjected to gel filtration on Sepharose 6B in 0.1 Tris-HCl, pH 8.5 and in 6 M guanidine · HCl. The minimum molecular weights reported were 110,000, 106,000, 106,000, and 102,000, respectively. These results will be discussed later in Section III in connection with the chain structure of ceruloplasmin. Osaki

(1960) prepared porcine ceruloplasmin and Kaya (1964) determined its molecular weight as 160,000. Optical properties of ceruloplasmin are summarized in Table III.

The copper content of ceruloplasmin ranges from 0.275 to 0.340% (Morell *et al.*, 1969; McKee and Frieden, 1971; Huber and Frieden, 1970a). McKee and Frieden (1971) have shown that the content of their ceruloplasmin sample decreased from 7 to 6 copper atoms/132,000 molecular weight by passing the sample over a chelating resin without any reduction of blue color or enzymatic activity. The presence of both cuprous and cupric atoms in ceruloplasmin has been shown by spectrophotometric titration with reducing agents (Laurell, 1960), electron paramagnetic resonance (Broman *et al.*, 1962; Blumberg *et al.*, 1963; Kasper *et al.*, 1963), and magnetic susceptibility (Ehrenberg *et al.*, 1962). Scheinberg and Morell (1957) have found that four of the eight copper atoms were exchangeable with free cuprous ions in the presence of reducing agents and Curzon (1958) could remove only four copper atoms after digestion with chymotrypsin. Kasper and Deutsch (1963a) found only four atoms of copper after dialysis against Tris-HCl, pH 8.0 buffer or ascorbic acid at pH 5.2. However, Marriott and Perkins (1966a) were able to exchange six of the eight copper atoms of reduced ceruloplasmin with free cuprous ions when oxygen was excluded. ^{64}Cu-labeled ceruloplasmin, if digested with chymotrypsin or dialyzed against 0.1 *M* Tris-HCl buffer, pH 8.0, seems to exchange only three atoms of copper. These authors suggest the presence of two groups of four atoms of copper. In group A all four copper atoms can be removed by either Tris or chymotrypsin, however, one of the copper atoms is not exchangeable with [64]Cu. Group B coppers are not attacked in either reaction and contain also one nonexchangeable copper atom. They suggest that the dif-

TABLE III

Optical Properties of Ceruloplasmin[a,b]

Wavelength (nm) of absorptive line centers	Gram atomic[c] absorption coefficient
794	850
610	4400
459	460
332	1600

[a] Adapted from Scheinberg (1966) with permission.
[b] A_{610} 0.680–0.740; A_{280} 14.9–16.2.
[c] Assuming that Cu^{2+} ions only contribute to all absorptions (Blumberg *et al.*, 1963).

ference between the two groups may be due to the folding of the molecule and not to differences in ligands or stereochemistry of the binding sites. In a subsequent report Marriott and Perkins (1966b) provided evidence that chelating agents are able to remove all eight copper atoms from the molecule. The rate of removal depends on the agent and no stable intermediates were found to be formed between the native ceruloplasmin and the final reaction product. The absence of copper-containing intermediates was demonstrated during irreversible decolorization by EDTA and urea. Aisen and Morell (1965) have shown the existence of a similar mechanism.

Several techniques are available for the study of protein-bound copper, but electron paramagnetic resonance (EPR) has been particularly valuable since it permits observation of the copper *in situ*. Malmström and Vänngård (1960) first observed that paramagnetic (cupric) copper ions were present in ceruloplasmin. Quantitative EPR and magnetic susceptibility measurements detect about 45% of the total copper (Broman *et al.*, 1962; Ehrenberg *et al.*, 1962; Carrico *et al.*, 1971). All these studies have indicated that the bonding of Cu^{2+} is unique among complexes of this ion (Malmström and Vänngård, 1960). The uniqueness is seen from the very narrow hyperfine splitting seen in the EPR and is responsible for the blue color (Type I or blue copper). The Type II nonblue copper has EPR parameters more like low molecular weight copper complexes and this diamagnetic copper was long believed to be cuprous. However, after the discovery that all copper ions in ceruloplasmin can accept electrons (Carrico *et al.*, 1971) it has been proposed to constitute tightly complexed pairs of cupric ions (Malkin and Malmström, 1970). While the chemical background of the unique bonding is not understood, it is established that it affects the reactivity of Cu^{2+} ceruloplasmin. Broman *et al.* (1963) have definitely established that the catalytic reaction involves reduction of Cu^{2+} by substrate and reoxidation of Cu^{1+} by oxygen. Morell *et al.* (1964) demonstrated that the intense blue color of ceruloplasmin does not depend on the presence of molecular oxygen in the ceruloplasmin molecule. The EPR spectra of native ceruloplasmin are the same in the presence of oxygen and helium.

D. Enzymatic Activity and Interaction with Other Metals

Ceruloplasmin in serum or in a purified form has a moderate oxidase activity as shown by Holmberg and Laurell (1951). They demonstrated activity toward a number of substrates [*p*-phenylenediamine (PPD), hydroquinone, catechol, pyrogallol, adrenaline, ascorbic acid, etc.].

Porter *et al.* (1957) demonstrated activity toward 5-hydroxytryptamine and 2-methyl-5-hydroxytryptamine, as did Curzon and Vallet (1960) toward hydroxyindole acetic acid and Blaschko and Levine (1960) toward 4-hydroxytryptamine and 6-hydroxytryptamine. An endless number of substrates were tested by Young and Curzon (1972). During the 20 years since the original report numerous modifications of the *p*-phenylenediamine-oxidase procedures have become widely adopted for routine use in clinical chemistry laboratories (Sunderman and Nomoto, 1970). Whether this protein may be also active as an oxidase toward ascorbic acid became a matter of a lively dispute (Morell *et al.*, 1962; Osaki, 1961; Humoller *et al.*, 1960; McDermott *et al.*, 1968; Curzon and Young, 1972). A similarly vigorous debate exists today as to whether diamine oxidase and histaminase are identical enzymes and whether these enzymes are not ceruloplasmin (Buffoni, 1966; Hampton *et al.*, 1971, 1972). Considerable work has also been done with regard to ceruloplasmin's substrates and inhibitors (Aprison *et al.*, 1959; Curzon and O'Reilly, 1960; Levine and Peisach, 1962; Walshe, 1963; Osaki *et al.*, 1964; Curzon and Cumings, 1966). Andrèasson and Vänngård (1970) have shown with the electron paramagnetic resonance method that a specific copper(II) in human ceruloplasmin acts as a binding site for inhibitory anions.

In spite of all these studies not too much was learned about the enzymatic structure of ceruloplasmin. According to Curzon and Cumings (1966) there are two main reasons for this: (a) many substances were selected as potential inhibitors of ceruloplasmin based on ceruloplasmin's implication in the regulation of mental health and (b) ceruloplasmin's oxidase activity is sensitive to iron. Nevertheless, the localization of the active center was sought by iodination procedures (Vasilets and Shavlovskii, 1972; Vasilets *et al.*, 1972b). These authors have shown that when 20 moles of iodine were added to ceruloplasmin dissolved in 0.2 *M* acetate buffer, pH 5.5, tyrosine residues were primarily iodinated, and when 60 moles were added per mole of protein, histidine was iodinated as well, and concomitantly, copper was lost as was oxidase activity. According to these authors tyrosines are involved in the maintenance of the conformation of the molecule and histidines participate directly in the catalytic center.

In a subsequent report Shavlovskii and Vasilets (1972) used methylene blue to photooxidize ceruloplasmin and determine the groups which bind copper. A study of peptide maps of tryptic hydrolysates of photooxidized ceruloplasmin showed that peptides containing histidine are located mainly in the region of neutral peptides. One of these peptides was isolated and it contained NH_2-terminal alanine, C-terminal lysine, and the following amino acids: histidine, aspartic acid, threonine, serine, glutamic acid, valine, tyrosine, and leucine.

Curzon and O'Reilly (1960) found that ferrous ions can reduce the cupric ion in ceruloplasmin via a ferrous–ferric couple. In accord with this they found that the ferrous ion enhanced the activity of ceruloplasmin toward DPD (dimethyl-p-phenylenediamine), although ferric ion, which should have the same stimulatory activity, is considerably less active. Levine and Peisach (1963) using PPD (p-phenylenediamine) as a substrate found that ferrous ions enhanced ceruloplasmin's oxidase activity, but found no enhancement whatever with ferric ions. However, they observed considerable stimulation in the absence of oxygen and attributed this to ferrous impurities in the ferric salts.

It is generally believed that the interconversion of ferrous to ferric ion is the function of hemoproteins, e.g., cytochromes, and other non-heme enzymes. The reaction of interconversion is assumed to proceed spontaneously, but recent evidence points to an enzymatically controlled mechanism(s). The ability of ferrous ion to reduce the cupric ion in ceruloplasmin was observed by Curzon and O'Reilly (1960) as mentioned above. The appreciation that ceruloplasmin is responsible for this ferroxidase activity came from the work of Osaki et al. (1966a). These authors have demonstrated that the spontaneous oxidation of ferrous to ferric ions was inadequate to account for the need for iron in the form of ferritransferrin. Consequently, this reaction needs a ferroxidase, a role supposedly filled by ceruloplasmin. This was confirmed in studies using perfused liver (Osaki et al., 1971) in which a specific and rapid mobilization of iron could be induced only by ceruloplasmin. The rate of maximum iron mobilization was reached at 0.2 μM of ceruloplasmin. Similar studies were conducted previously by Ragan et al. (1969) and Roeser et al. (1970) who showed that ceruloplasmin and not Cu(II) was responsible for the immediate mobilization of serum iron in copper-deficient pigs. More detailed discussion of this phase of copper and iron metabolism is given in Section IV.

Shaposhnikov and Derkachev (1971) demonstrated the interaction of ceruloplasmin with the electron transport systems of the cell. They observed a decrease in the concentration of ceruloplasmin upon incubation (under aerobic conditions) of heart mitochrondria with an oxidative substrate. Using inhibitors they showed that the electron transmitter which reacts with ceruloplasmin is situated in the region of cytochromes c_1–a_3. However, cytochromes of the microsomes did not interact with ceruloplasmin. Broman (1964) proposed that ceruloplasmin transports copper (or a copper-containing prosthetic group) for the synthesis of cytochrome oxidase in which copper is responsible for the catalytic activity (Nair and Mason, 1967).

Huber and Frieden (1970b) provided evidence that ferroxidase (ceruloplasmin EC 1.12.31) can be inhibited with trivalent ions. The cationic inhibitors were effective in the following order: In(III) > ZrO(II) > A1(III) > Sc(III) > Ga(III). Whanger and Weswig (1970) investigated the effect of copper antagonists on induction of ceruloplasmin levels in rats. The results showed that Ag is the strongest copper antagonist, followed by Cd, Mo, Zn, and SO_4 and evidence was given that Cu, as a Cu–Mo complex, was less available for ceruloplasmin synthesis than Cu or $CuSO_4$. The inhibitory action was explained by two mechanisms or a combination of both (a) prevention of copper from inducing the synthesis of apoceruloplasmin molecule, and (b) the elements could be incorporated into the ceruloplasmin molecule in the place of copper, resulting in reduced oxidase activity.

E. Immunological Properties

Specific antisera prepared against native ceruloplasmin were used mainly for quantitative estimation of the levels of ceruloplasmin (Goodman and Vulpe, 1961; Richterich *et al.*, 1962; Bickel *et al.*, 1956; Uriel *et al.*, 1957) and for studies of the possible enzymatically "silent" ceruloplasmin in various disease states, notably Wilson's disease (Scheinberg and Gitlin, 1952). The levels of this protein detected by the radial immunodiffusion technique (Mancini *et al.*, 1965) range from 7 to 15 mg/dl of serum at birth and from 20 to 35 mg/dl of serum in the adult. Specific antisera were prepared by Markowitz *et al.* (1955) by absorption with Wilson's disease serum and by Schultze and Schwick (1959) by immunization with 94% pure ceruloplasmin; however, Berggård (1960) demonstrated at least two different antibodies with their antisera by immunodiffusion.

Antisera against ceruloplasmin are not too difficult to prepare and in the author's laboratory (M.D.P.) numerous antisera were prepared against native ceruloplasmin, apoceruloplasmin, and ceruloplasmin which was reduced and alkylated in the presence of 8 *M* urea. With the aid of such antisera two precipitin lines were usually obtained even with crystalline ceruloplasmin stored under liquid nitrogen prior to use (Poulik, 1968). Apoceruloplasmin was always detected as a faster migrating component on immunoelectrophoresis with respect to "good" ceruloplasmin and both forms share some antigenic determinants. Similar observations were made previously by Uriel *et al.* (1957) and especially by Kasper and Deutsch (1963b) who prepared antisera against four different batches of crystalline ceruloplasmin. By using two-dimensional zone electrophoresis (Poulik and Smithies, 1958) in conjunction with starch gel immunoelectrophoresis (Poulik, 1959) evidence was obtained that oxidase-positive and oxidase-negative zones of ceruloplasmin gave lines of precipitation. A fast migrating fraction (filter paper) which was separated into several zones by the subsequent starch gel electrophoresis gave precipitation lines of immunological identity (Poulik and Bearn, 1962). Kasper and Deutsch (1963b) made a similar observation with aged DDC apoceruloplasmin. The same observation was made with ascorbic acid-treated ceruloplasmin and isolated fractions thereof. Poulik (1962) has shown by immunoelectrophoresis that treatment of ceruloplasmin with 0.1 M acetate buffer in the presence of 0.1 M EDTA changes the mobility of the protein with the appearance of new antigenic determinants.

Reductively cleaved (8 M urea) and alkylated ceruloplasmin was shown to contain several antigenic determinants by Poulik (1962) via immunodiffusion. These studies were extended with the aid of urea-starch gel immunoelectrophoresis (Poulik, 1963b, 1966). The structural subunits α, β, γ, and δ were shown to form precipitin lines with antisera prepared against the native ceruloplasmin. The α subunit afforded two precipitin lines which shared some of the antigenic determinants. The β subunit gave two independent ones while the γ and δ subunits yielded only one each. Similar results were obtained also with antiserum directed against apoceruloplasmin. All these results indicated that several antigenic determinants exist; however, the question still remains whether they are located on the same chain or several chains. Simons and Bearn (1969) studied the problem with antisera made against amino-ethylated ceruloplasmin. The results showed that these antisera reacted with their three fractions (α, β', and β'') on double diffusion. However, such antisera reacted poorly with native ceruloplasmin. They reached the conclusion that β' and β'' chains are partially antigenically identical and that the α chain is antigenically different.

Kasper and Deutsch (1963b) studied the immunological relationships of ceruloplasmins of various animal species. Rhesus monkey ceruloplasmin cross-reacted most strongly with rabbit antibody to human ceruloplasmin while the ceruloplasmins of ungulates cross-reacted to a lesser degree. They point out that in spite of the high degree of cross-reactivity the ceruloplasmins still may be different, while a portion of the ceruloplasmins may be quite similar immunologically.

Shreffler et al. (1967b) attempted to distinguish the various polymorphic forms of ceruloplasmin by immunological means. They used an antiserum which was obtained commercially and made against an unspecified ceruloplasmin. The results showed that the variant oxidase components on starch gel or agar gel electrophoresis are antigenically similar or even identical to the common form (Cp B) and thus the variants may be structurally altered ceruloplasmins due perhaps to differences in amino acid sequences.

Finally, Fisher and Deutsch (1970) addressed themselves to the question of possible anticomplementary activity of ceruloplasmin. Their results suggested that such an activity is a property of the protein and not the property of the accompanying impurities (immunoglobulins IgG and IgM). Removal of the loosely bound copper, accomplished with biscyclohexanoneoxalyldihydrazone (CHD) by the method of Peterson and Bollier (1955), increased the anticomplementary activity. Apoceruloplasmin showed considerably less activity than the native ceruloplasmin at low levels of protein, but at higher concentrations had more activity. Thus, the anticomplementary activity does not seem dependent on the copper content as shown by Audran and Steinbuch (1965).

III. Chemical Composition and Structure

A. Amino Acid Composition

The amino acid composition of ceruloplasmin was determined in at least three laboratories. The results are summarized in Table IV.

The results are quite similar in spite of the fact that the molecular weight of ceruloplasmin was taken as 160,000 by Heimburger *et al.* (1964) and Kasper and Deutsch (1963b) while Rydén (1972a) took it as 132,000.

Sulfhydryl groups of human ceruloplasmin were studied by Witwicki and Zakrzewski (1969). The authors used β-hydroxyethyl-2,4-dinitrophenyl disulfide which reacts with free sulfhydryl groups according to the reaction:

$$\text{Protein—SH} + \text{HOCH}_2\text{CH}_2\text{S—SC}_6\text{H}_3(\text{NO}_2)_2 \rightarrow$$
$$\text{protein—S—SCH}_2\text{CH}_2\text{OH} + \text{C}_6\text{H}_3(\text{NO}_2)_2\text{SH}$$

The amount of thiodinitrophenol liberated is a measure of the number of sulfhydryl groups in the protein (Bitny-Szlachto, 1965). In the native ceruloplasmin one sulfhydryl group was found. In urea solutions the number of sulfhydryl groups titrated depended on the concentration of urea and on the presence of EDTA. Two sulfhydryl groups were found in 7 M urea and a third one when EDTA was added to the solution. The unmasking of these groups is coincident with "bleaching" of the ceruloplasmin and with loss of its oxidase activity. These results contrast with those of Kasper and Deutsch (1963b) who detected only one sulfhydryl group after alkylation of the ceruloplasmin with iodoacetate according to

TABLE IV

Amino Acid Composition of Ceruloplasmin

| Amino acid | Moles per mole protein | | Residues/160,000 |
	Heimburger et al. (1964)	Rydén (1972c)[a]	Kasper and Deutsch (1963a)
Lys	73	68.4	68
His	46	44.1	43
Arg	45	41.5	46
Asp	132	120.6	135
Thr	85	73.0	86
Ser	67	61.5	69
Glu	135	116.7	130
Pro	53	48.0	57
Gly	84	76.1	57
Ala	55	49.9	56
½ Cys	11	14.7	14
Val	66	63.8	67
Met	24	17.6	26
Ile	58	53.8	56
Leu	78	72.1	76
Tyr	74	64.7	71
Phe	55	47.9	54
Trp	20	21.6	27
Cysteine plus cystine			
Reduction–alkylation			15.0–15.1
Performic acid oxidation			14.7–15.2
Cysteine			
S-Carboxymethylcysteine			1.0–1.2
p-Hydroxymercuribenzoate			1.1–2.1

[a] Based on a molecular weight of 132,000.

the method of Cole *et al.* (1958). This method also involves treatment of the protein with dodecyl sulfate. In order to clarify this discrepancy Witwicki and Zakrzewski (1969) carried out the reaction at pH 9 and in 0.17 *M* sodium dodecyl sulfate. Even after 90 min of reaction time only 1.5 SH/mole of ceruloplasmin were found. The explanation may be that Kasper and Deutsch (1963b) used relatively mild dissociating agents. The single SH group titrated in the absence of urea appears to be partially masked, since it could be reacted with β-hydroxyethyl-2,4-dinitrophenyl disulfide only in relatively concentrated Tris buffer. This buffer is known to alter the electrophoretic mobility of ceruloplasmin as shown by Kasper and Deutsch (1963b) and Marriott and Perkins (1966a). Furthermore, this easily accessible SH group is not bound to copper and does not appear to be involved in the chromophoric center of the active site of the protein. However, unmasking of the buried SH groups by urea is accompanied by destruction of both the chromophoric center and the active site. Erickson *et al.* (1970) found less than 0.5 —SH groups/molecule of ceruloplasmin and 4 —SH groups/molecule of apoceruloplasmin. These groups were necessary for reconstitution to an active ceruloplasmin.

The NH_2-terminal amino acids were also studied by several groups. Kasper and Deutsch (1963b) and Deutsch and Fisher (1964) found 0.9 residue of valine and 0.3 residue of lysine per 160,000 gm of ceruloplasmin. Schultze and Mahling (1961) found valine and lysine in less than 1 mole per mole of protein. However, the first step in the stepwise degradation according to Edman revealed four amino acids: phenylalanine, valine, aspartic acid, and threonine. The same authors determined also the C-terminal amino acids. The results obtained by hydrazinolysis showed that three amino acids are present: glycine, serine, and alanine. The total content of the latter three was about 4 moles per mole of protein. Simons and Bearn (1969) demonstrated valine and lysine as the terminal NH_2-amino acids and, in contrast, Rydén (1972a) found only valine. Kaya *et al.* (1961) studying porcine ceruloplasmin found phenylalanine as the NH_2-terminal and C-terminal amino acid. However, in a later report Mukasa *et al.* (1968a,b) give evidence that porcine ceruloplasmin contains 2 moles of NH_2-terminal tyrosine and 2 moles of NH_2-terminal serine.

B. Carbohydrate Composition and Saccharide Structure

Little attention has been given so far to the glycoprotein nature of ceruloplasmin. Schultze *et al.* (1955), Schultze (1957), and Heimburger *et al.* (1964) showed that ceruloplasmin contains 8% carbohydrate (3% hexose, 2.4% acetylhexosamine, 2.4% sialic acid, and 0.18% fucose). Classic studies were performed by Jamieson (1965) on ceruloplasmins prepared by the large-scale method and by column chromatography (Deutsch *et al.*, 1962). The summary of the carbohydrate analyses is given in Table V.

Extensive digestion with pronase at 37°C in phosphate buffer, 0.1 *M*, pH 7.2, containing $CaCl_2$ (0.01 *M*) in the presence of alcohol (approximately 10% w/v) for several days at room temperature followed by gel filtration on Sephadex G-25 resulted in a glycopeptide fraction containing approximately 65% of carbohydrate. The individual carbohydrates were present in molar ratios identical with those in intact ceruloplasmin. Aspartic acid was the principal amino acid (with small amounts of glutamic acid). Ammonia was released in stoichiometric amounts by hydrolysis with 2 *N* hydrochloric acid at 100°C. The average molecular

TABLE V

Carbohydrate Analyses of Ceruloplasmin[a]

	Large-scale method			Column chromatography[b]		
Carbohydrate	Percent	Moles	Molar ratio	Percent	Moles	Molar ratio
Sialic acid	1.8	10	1	1.6	9	1
N-Acetylglucosamine	2.7	20	2	2.5	18	2
Hexose	4.4	39	4	4.0	36	4
Fucose	0.16	2	0.2	ND	ND	ND

[a] Adapted from Jamieson (1965) with permission.
[b] ND, not determined.

weight of this glycopeptide was 1300 daltons. The glycopeptide was subfractionated into several fractions on DEAE-cellulose. Each of the fractions contained between two and three residues of amino acids (aspartic and glutamic acid as well as threonine, proline, and glycine being the most frequent). The molar ratio of the carbohydrate constituents varied within narrow limits suggesting constitutive variations in the individual glycopeptide chains.

Rydén (1971c, 1975) studied in detail two different ceruloplasmin forms obtained by chromatography on hydroxyapatite gel. Human ceruloplasmin was prepared from fresh blood by the method of Rydén (1972c). The carbohydrate composition is given in Table VI.

Differences in carbohydrate composition of ceruloplasmin forms were suggested by Richterich et al. (1962) but not confirmed by Deutsch and Fischer (1964). The hexose contents reported from the two laboratories were widely different: 7% (form I) and 3.3% (form II) in the first case and 2.2% (form I) and 2.0% (form II) in the second.

C. Polypeptide Chain Structure

Curzon (1959) envisaged a submolecular structure of ceruloplasmin in which each copper provided a strong link between side chains of four parallel polypeptide chains which were further stabilized by disulfide bridges and hydrogen bonds. Poulik (1962) provided the first evidence that ceruloplasmin may be composed of several polypeptide chains after reductive cleavage and alkylation of a ceruloplasmin of high purity with mercaptoethanol in 8 M urea (Poulik, 1960; Edelman and Poulik, 1961). When the products were subjected to electrophoresis in starch gel pre-

TABLE VI

Carbohydrate Composition of Human Ceruloplasmin Forms[a,b]

Carbohydrate residue	Residues per mole of protein		Comment
	Form I	Form II	
Glucosamine	15.5	9.4	Amino acid analyzer. Hydrolysis in 6 M HCl, 24 hr, 110°C. Assumed recovery 68%
Glucosamine	18.9	10.1	Gas chromatography. Methanolysis in 1.25
Mannose	14.0	9.4	M HCl in dry methanol at 80°C for 24 hr.
Galactose	12.1	7.3	Duplicate analysis on two parallel samples
Fucose	1.6	1.0	
Sialic acid	8.5	5.7	Thiobarbituric acid method (Warren, 1959)
Total number of carbohydrate residues	51.7	32.9	

[a] Reproduced from Rydén (1975) with permission.

[b] The proteins were prepared as described in Rydén (1975). The results are normalized to the same number of amino acids, 1055, for both proteins.

pared in acid buffer (formate, pH 3.1) containing 8 M urea and 0.02 M mercaptoethanol, four protein zones were usually detected and essentially similar patterns were obtained with four different batches of ceruloplasmin prepared by a large-scale method (Sgouris *et al.*, 1962). However, when ceruloplasmins heterogeneous by starch gel electrophoresis were used, more complicated patterns were observed (Poulik and Bearn, 1962). These results suggested that native ceruloplasmin can be dissociated into several structural subunits nonidentical by electrophoresis and immunoelectrophoresis. These results were corroborated in subsequent experiments (Poulik, 1963a) with well-defined and pure ceruloplasmin batches (American National Red Cross, batch 1967 and 1972). These findings have been confirmed by Kasper and Deutsch (1963a) who subjected ceruloplasmin and apoceruloplasmin to reductive cleavage and electrophoresis in urea-starch gel (formate buffer, pH 3). They could detect only two well-defined zones with the native ceruloplasmin and six zones with apoceruloplasmin. Velocity sedimentation was performed in 6 M urea on reduced and alkylated apoceruloplasmin in 6 M urea at pH 7.4 and native ceruloplasmin in 6 M urea and 0.1 M mercaptoethanol (incubation at room temperature for 1–3 days) and the native ceruloplasmin showed fast and slow sedimenting shoulders. The main component sedimented with an $s^\circ_{20,w}$ of 4.55 S, and similar experiments performed in the absence of urea did not affect the native sedimentation properties. The authors concluded that the subunits may have a molecular weight of about 50,000 daltons. Molecular weight estimation of the possible subunits was performed by Poulik (1966) with a novel technique of molecular weight estimation by urea-starch gel devised by Smithies (1962). The four zones (Poulik, 1962) obtained with batch 1967 were clearly separated and designated as α, β, γ, and δ, where α is fastest migrating and δ is the slowest migrating subunit. The retardation coefficient for each subunit was established and the molecular weight estimated to be 18,500–20,000 for subunits α, β, and γ. The molecular weight of subunit δ could not be estimated with certainty. These results were supported by gel filtration experiments (Sephadex G-100, acetate buffer, 0.01 M pH 5.5, 6 M urea or 0.5 M propionic acid containing 0.2 M mercaptoethanol). On the basis of these experiments ceruloplasmin appeared to be an octamer composed of four nonidentical subunits each present as a dimer; α_2, β_2, γ_2, and δ_2. Immunological investigation of the subunits demonstrated that they may contain different antigenic determinants as well as those which are shared by some of the subunits. The nonidentity was questioned and the following reasons were considered: artifacts, population heterogeneity of the starting material, conformational changes, deamidation, carbohydrate content, solubility, and aggregative properties. In view of these possibilities a new method of starch gel-urea starch gel electrophoresis on fresh single samples of sera was devised (Poulik, 1968) to screen large numbers of individuals. The δ zone was found with ease, and there also was a slower migrating zone. The α and β zones were also reproducible, however, the γ zone migrated always slower than the γ zone of a control pure ceruloplasmin. Furthermore, the β zone was usually subfractionated into two zones. All in all the patterns were quite complex. Poillon and Bearn (1966a) used yet another approach. Using the same batch of ceruloplasmin (batch 1967) they succinylated the protein or disrupted the quaternary structure in alkali (pH 12.5) and reported on dissociation by either treatment and combination of both. Stable half-molecules were obtained by increasing the pH from 7.1 to 10.2 and quarter-molecules by increasing the pH from 7.1 to 12.5. Succinylation at pH 7–8 produced stable half-molecules. Raising the pH of the succinylated half-molecule system from 7.1 to 12.5 provided one-eighth molecules, and two zones were separated in polyacrylamide gel (borate buffer, pH 12.0) from the one-eighth molecule system. The molecular weight of the succinylated protein was $87,990 \pm 6150$ and that of alkali-treated succinylated protein was $17,190 \pm 1030$. They proposed an octameric structure for ceruloplasmin, each monomer having a molecular weight of 18,000. They also envisaged two kinds of subunits differing by "at least one charge unit." Similar experiments were corroborated recently by Vasilets *et al.* (1972a). Treating the ceruloplasmin with succinic anhydride or alkali buffer, pH 12.3, as well as with both reagents, resulted in dissociation of the protein into subunits having a molecular weight of approximately 85,000. They questioned the results obtained by Poillon and Bearn (1966a) especially with regard to the 18,000-dalton subunits obtained by prolonged dialysis (several days) against alkaline buffer, pH 12. They quote the work of Vasilets *et al.* (1968) who treated ceruloplasmin with 0.2 *M* sodium borate buffer, pH 12.4, for 88 hr or more and were able to determine new NH_2-terminal amino acids not characteristic of the native protein. Simons and Bearn (1969) also questioned the results of Poillon and Bearn (1966a) on similar grounds since they were able to detect new NH_2-terminal acids after dialysis at pH 12.5. However, the same authors provided evidence that ceruloplasmin is composed of two different polypeptide chains. They used reduced and aminoethylated ceruloplasmin (batch 1967) for gel filtration in 5.5 *M* guanidine · HCl in 0.05 *M* Tris buffer, pH 7.7, and preparative polyacrylamide column electrophoresis in Tris buffer and 8 *M* urea (Jovin *et al.*, 1964). They separated an α chain that was homogeneous, had a molecular weight of 15,900, and had valine as its NH_2-terminal amino acid. A second chain was also isolated (β chain) that was heterogeneous and usually present as two chains: β' and β''. Both of these chains had lysine as their NH_2-terminal acid and the same elution volume on gel filtration. The molecular weight of the β'' chains was 58,900 daltons. They concede that one of the chains may be the product of deamidation *in vitro* or *in vivo*. However, they could, presumably, be derived also from different types of ceruloplasmin molecules claimed to be present in human serum by Walaas *et al.* (1967). Simons and Bearn (1969), on the basis of their results, proposed a general formula $\alpha_2\beta_2$ for the quaternary structure of ceruloplasmin. From their molecular weight determinations and peptide mapping the presence of a repeating unit in the molecule is conceivable. The amount of α chains was estimated to be 25% of the β chain. However, the aggregates seen in both column electrophoresis and gel filtration experiments precluded accurate estimates. From their work no clear indication of the role of interchain disulfide bridges could be postulated.

The proposed $\alpha_2\beta_2$ formula was recently supported by Freeman and Daniel (1973). They have found that ceruloplasmin is dissociated into three small species, L, H, and H' by sodium dodecyl sulfate in the presence of 2-mercaptoethanol, *p*-hydroxymercuribenzoate, 6 *M* urea, or 6 *M* guanidine · HCl. The molecular weights of the L, H, and H' species were determined by sodium dodecyl sulfate (SDS) polyacrylamide gel electrophoresis. The respective molecular weights found were 16,000, 53,000, and 69,000. Recombination of the subunits was achieved after removal of the sodium dodecyl sulfate by dialysis and up to 80% of the original oxidase activity was recovered. These results are claimed as unequivocal evidence that ceruloplasmin is a multichain protein. They proposed that ceruloplasmin is an L_2H_2 tetramer. In this model the three major protein bands would be L (16,000), H (53,000), and LH (69,000). However, two minor bands were also observed on sodium dodecyl sulfate acrylamide electrophoresis and they should correspond to L_2H (83,000) and L_2 (30,000). Since these authors determined the molecular weight of the native ceruloplasmin as 124,000 daltons their tetramer would have a molecular weight about 11% higher than the native molecule. Part of the discrepancy may be in the unreliability of the SDS-acrylamide gel technique, especially when a protein contains carbohydrate, as ceruloplasmin does. The authors mention one major difficulty with this model, "The H′ species would be none but an HL dimer and should, in principle, be capable of dissociation into L and H species. We have never been able to obtain complete dissociation of the H′ species."

As can be seen, the structure of ceruloplasmin is quite elusive. To compound or simplify the problem, Rydén (1972a) proposed a single chain structure for human ceruloplasmin. He studied a reduced and cyanoethylated ceruloplasmin prepared by his method (Rydén, 1971a) followed by gel filtration in Sepharose 4B or 6B in 0.1 M Tris-HCl, pH 8.5 and 6 M guanidine · HCl according to the method of Fish *et al.* (1969). The protein was dissolved in the buffer and incubated under liquid nitrogen with 2-mercaptoethanol for 4 hr and with acrylonitrile for another 2 hr. Two components were found on the 6% agarose, a major one corresponding to a molecular weight of about 110,000 and a small one (1% of the total) of 17,000. The molecular weight of the cyanoethylated ceruloplasmin in 6 M guanidine in 0.1 M Tris-HCl, pH 8.5 by the sedimentation equilibrium method, was determined to be 92,000. In 6 M guanidine · HCl and 0.02 M Tris-HCl, pH 8.5 the molecular weight was determined by intrinsic viscosity, sedimentation velocity, and combination of both. The molecular weights were 144,000, 122,000, and 129,000, respectively. As discussed previously in Section II, Rydén (1972a) proposed a molecular weight of 120,000 for the peptide moiety of the native ceruloplasmin. Thus, the values obtained by the above-mentioned agree with the value obtained for the native ceruloplasmin. This low molecular weight value of 92,000 is explained by the presence of low molecular weight impurities (Yphantis, 1964) present in the preparation used. From these data the author concluded that ceruloplasmin does not dissociate into subunits under the experimental conditions used. He argues (Rydén, 1972c) that since Simons and Bearn (1969) found 50–55 ninhydrin-positive spots on peptide maps, and of these 22 gave positive Pauly reactions specific for histidine (nearly half the expected number), redundant sequences are present. This strongly suggests that the single chain ceruloplasmin evolved by duplication of its structural genes. However, from his data ceruloplasmin appears to be one of the longest chains found (approximately 1000 amino acid residues) in serum or plasma. Shavlovskii and Vasilets (1970) obtained 53 peptides by peptide mapping of reduced carboxymethylated ceruloplasmin after tryptic digestion. This number is practically equal to the number obtained from theoretical consideration and this indirectly supports the conviction that human ceruloplasmin consists of four subunits belonging to two different types. These results are also supported by determination of N- and C-terminal amino acids by Konnova *et al.* (1969).

One, two, four, eight — only the future will tell

D. Amino Acid Sequences of the Glycopeptides

Sequence data on ceruloplasmin are still lacking. Rydén and Eaker (1974) provided limited sequence data for three glycopeptides isolated from human ceruloplasmin. Matsunaga and Nosoh (1970) isolated three glycopeptides from porcine ceruloplasmin and determined their amino acid composition. Rydén and Eaker (1974) assigned the sequences of the latter three glycopeptides from the amino acid data and aligned them with the determined sequences of their three glycopeptides as shown in Fig. 3. Determination of the amino acid sequence of ceruloplasmin will be of the utmost importance for this field.

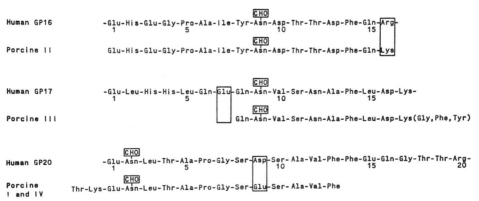

Fig. 3. Determined and assigned amino acid sequences of three human and porcine glycopeptides. Reproduced with permission from Rydén and Eaker (1974).

IV. Physiological Functions, Variation in Health and Disease, and Biosynthesis and Catabolism

A. Normal Levels and Determinations

The ceruloplasmin level in normal adult humans is roughly 30–35 mg% as shown by many researchers. However, sizable interindividual variation exists. Cox (1966) found that the average ceruloplasmin level in 163 adults was $30.4 \pm .5$ mg% with 95% confidence limits of 20.7–40.2 mg%. Carruthers *et al.* (1966) found a mean of 31.2 mg% ±5.7 while Ravin (1961) found a mean of 32.3 mg% in 100 adults.

Ontogenetic changes in serum ceruloplasmin do occur. (See Chapter 6.) At birth ceruloplasmin is present in very small amounts, averaging about 6.5 mg% (Scheinberg *et al.*, 1958; Shokeir, 1971b). These low ceruloplasmin levels, determined by ceruloplasmin's oxidase activity, probably reflect a deficiency in the incorporation of copper into apoceruloplasmin rather than a deficiency in the protein. Shokeir (1971b), using an immunochemical method to determine ceruloplasmin, found nearly normal concentrations of the protein moiety, most of which was devoid of copper and oxidase activity. Evans *et al.* (1970a) found age-dependent alterations of hepatic copper and serum ceruloplasmin in rats.

By the age of 2 the serum ceruloplasmin level ($\bar{X} \simeq 42.5$ mg%) has risen above the normal adult value and proceeds to decline until adult levels are reached in early adolescence. Except for the cases of pregnant women or women taking birth control pills (see below), there does not appear to be any effect of sex on ceruloplasmin levels, nor does the menstrual cycle appear to influence this parameter (Cox, 1966).

Ceruloplasmin levels in other human body fluids have been determined. The mean level in amniotic fluid is 2.6 mg% (Fischbacher and Quinlivan, 1970), 0.22 mg% in cerebrospinal fluid (Schuller *et al.*, (1971), about 3.3 mg% in human tears (Liotet, 1969), and 90 mg% and 120 mg% in liver and gallbladder bile, respectively (Lorentz *et al.*, 1969).

Recently Matsuda *et al.* (1974) developed a radioimmunoassay for apoceruloplasmin and measured its levels in nutritional and copper deficiency, Menkes' Kinky Hair syndrome, Wilson's disease, and umbilical cord blood. The levels determined in these conditions did not differ significantly from those of normal serum (3.3 ± 3.1 mg/dl). However, the concentration of apoceruloplasmin in umbilical cord blood of normal neonates was found to be lower (0.7 ± 0.5 mg/dl; $p < 0.01$). The concentration of "normal" ceruloplasmin (holoceruloplasmin) was also low in these sera.

Although ceruloplasmin's physiological function is still under debate, most determinations are based on its ability to act as a weak polyphenol and polyamine oxidase, the substrate most commonly used *in vitro* being *p*-phenylenediamine.

The most commonly used methods are those of Ravin (1961), Scheinberg and Morell (1957), or Cox's (1966) modification of the latter. Briefly, Cox's procedure utilizes recrystallized *p*-phenylenediamine dried over NaOH and stored in sealed vials. Ion-free water is used throughout to avoid contamination with copper and iron. Serum (1.15 ml), acetate buffer (2.0 ml, 1.0 M, pH 5.2) and 1 ml of a 9.4% solution of *p*-phenylenediamine are read in a 1-cm pathlength cuvette at 530 nm for 6–8 min at 37°C. The slope of the recorded line is measured to yield the change in optical density per minute. Under these conditions, ΔOD per minute $\times$ 790 gives the concentration of ceruloplasmin in mg%.

Because this enzymatic reaction can be affected by many factors, meticulous care must be taken to insure that the results reflect only variation in ceruloplasmin concentration. The pH must be maintained at the reaction's optimum. Trace contamination with iron and copper must be avoided. Temperature, too, must be carefully regulated. The ΔOD must be read after an initial 2-min lag period of unknown cause.

Quantitation can also be performed by an immunodiffusion technique (Preer, 1956). Antiserum to ceruloplasmin, usually made in rabbits, and the serum to be assayed are allowed to diffuse through an agar column. The ratio of the distance of the precipitin arc from the agar–antigen interface and from the agar–antibody interface is proportional to the initial ceruloplasmin concentration. This technique offers the advantage of permitting the study of apoceruloplasmin. Radial immunodiffusion (Mancini *et al.*, 1965) provides a more desirable method of quantification. The plates are commercially available.

A third technique, rarely used today, is a colorimetric method. Devised by Scheinberg and Morell (1957) it is based on the blue color of ceruloplasmin which disappears in the presence of cyanide or ascorbic acid. However, it requires large amounts of serum and is disturbed by any turbidity change.

B. Physiological Functions

The physiological function(s) of ceruloplasmin has been debated for some time without a final decision. At least three roles have thus far been suggested: (a) ceruloplasmin acts as a ferroxidase, (b) ceruloplasmin serves to transport copper, and (c) ceruloplasmin aids in the maintenance of hepatic copper homeostasis.

The ability of ceruloplasmin to increase the rate of oxidation of ferrous iron has been demonstrated (Curzon and O'Reilly, 1960; Osaki *et al.*, 1966a) resulting in the proposal that ceruloplasmin is important in the binding of iron by apotransferrin. Lee *et al.* (1968, 1969) have also shown that copper-deficient swine exhibited iron metabolism abnormalities; their mucosal, reticuloendothelial, and hepatic parenchymal cells showed impaired ability to release iron. This group later (Roeser *et al.*, 1970) reasoned that if ceruloplasmin functions as a ferroxidase and if the metabolic disturbances in copper-deficient swine result from ferroxidase deficiency, these animals (a) should be ceruloplasmin-deficient, (b) should show a reduced release of iron into plasma following a reduction in ceruloplasmin levels, (c) should show an increase in serum ceruloplasmin and then in serum iron after copper administration, (d) should exhibit lower levels of transferrin after injection of ferrous iron than after administration of ferric iron, and (e) should show increased plasma iron after administration of ceruloplasmin, but if given ceruloplasmin of low ferroxidase activity should show little increase in plasma iron.

Testing of all of these hypotheses indicated that ceruloplasmin is, in fact, a physiological ferroxidase. For instance, following intravenous administration of copper, ceruloplasmin levels rose within 15 min. Plasma iron, however, did not increase until the ceruloplasmin levels reached 1% of normal at which point the iron level increased rapidly. When ferric iron was administered to copper-deficient and control swine, both showed equal increases in plasma iron. When both received ferrous iron, the deficient animals showed a markedly lower plasma iron value, indicating the need for an enzyme with ferroxidase activity. Additionally, iron metabolism in eight patients with Wilson's disease was studied. Of the eight, five had ferroxidase levels less than 5% of normal and all of these, as well as one other patient, had iron deficiency as evidenced by absence of bone marrow iron stores and reduced transferrin saturation. *In vitro* experiments by Osaki *et al.* (1971) also point to the conclusion that ceruloplasmin is a ferroxidase; they found that ceruloplasmin, but not $CuSO_4$, HCO_3^-, citrate, apotransferrin, glucose, fructose, or serum albumin, caused an efflux of iron from perfused dog and pig livers. The scheme of ceruloplasmin action proposed by both groups (Osaki's and Roeser's) is shown in Fig. 4.

Shokeir is the primary opponent to the proposed physiological ferroxidase role for ceruloplasmin. In 1969, Shokeir and Shreffler suggested that ceruloplasmin acts to mediate enzymatically the transfer of copper

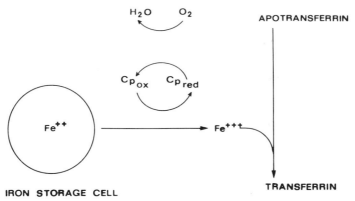

Fig. 4. Proposed scheme of ceruloplasmin's action as a ferroxidase. Ferrous iron is presented at the iron storage cell's surface and upon entering the blood is oxidized to the ferric form by ceruloplasmin. Fe^{3+} is then incorporated into transferrin. Adapted from Osaki *et al.* (1971) with permission.

to copper-containing enzymes such as cytochrome c oxidase and tyrosinase. Their data on Wilson's disease patients' leukocytes evidenced decreased cytochrome c oxidase activity.

Corroborating evidence for this view was provided by Marceau *et al.* (1970) who showed that ceruloplasmin labeled with ^{64}Cu could transfer the copper to cytochrome c oxidase, while similarly labeled albumin could not.

Subsequently, Shokeir (1972) investigated the ferroxidase activity in newborns, their mothers, and male and female control populations. While the newborns had the lowest serum ceruloplasmin levels (1.8 ± 1.1 mg/100 ml), they had the highest percent saturation of transferrin (73%). Their mothers had the highest serum ceruloplasmin activity (53.8 ± 5.1 mg%) and the lowest mean percent saturation of serum transferrin (20%). The controls had roughly 35 mg% ceruloplasmin and 37% saturation of serum transferrin. However, Roeser *et al.* (1970) did note that only 1% of normal ceruloplasmin levels were necessary for adequate ferroxidase activity. Also, infants have low absolute levels of serum transferrin.

If, indeed, ceruloplasmin is a ferroxidase, an intriguing physiological and evolutionary question is raised. Why does such a great redundancy exist in the adult? Possibly the seemingly excessive amounts of ceruloplasmin are required during periods of physiological stress.

A third possible function was advanced by Evans *et al.* (1970b). They noted that the major pathway for removal of hepatic copper, biliary excretion, is blocked by removal of the hypophysis and adrenals in rats. Subsequent to removal of either of these organs, a "compensatory" increase is observed in serum ceruloplasmin. Some evidence for such a case in man can be mustered. Patients with biliary cirrhosis have high hepatic copper and serum ceruloplasmin levels. Also, Holtzman *et al.* (1966) observed an increase in serum ceruloplasmin following copper intoxication. The conclusion drawn is that "the elevated ceruloplasmin accompanying increased hepatic copper is an indication of the body's attempt to maintain cellular homeostasis."

There is, however, no established reason to assume that any of these proposed functions are mutually exclusive.

C. Variation in Disease

Ceruloplasmin levels are markedly altered in many disease states as well as under several normal, physiologically altered circumstances (Table VII). For additional information, see Wolf *et al.* (1973).

1. Hyperceruloplasminemia

Being an acute phase reactant, serum ceruloplasmin is increased during acute and chronic infections resulting from a variety of viral, bac-

TABLE VII

Serum Ceruloplasmin Levels in Health and Disease[a]

Decreased	*Increased*
Wilson's disease	Leukemia
Malnutrition	Hodgkin's disease
Nephrosis	Neoplasia
Malabsorption	Myocardial infarction and tissue necrosis
	Rheumatoid arthritis
	Ataxia telangiectasia
	Pellagra
	Aplastic anemia
	Infections
	Postoperatively
	Biliary cirrhosis
	Schizophrenia
	Delirium tremens (?)
	Physical exercise
	Pregnancy
	Oral contraceptives

[a] Adapted from Wolf *et al.* (1973) with permission.

terial, and parasitic agents, but returns to normal as the inflammation subsides. Other inflammatory conditions such as rheumatoid arthritis and Reiter's syndrome also cause elevated serum ceruloplasmin levels (Roux *et al.,* 1971). Hyperceruloplasminemia is also noted in liver disorders which result in blockage of biliary excretion of copper.

It has been known for some time that serum ceruloplasmin levels are elevated in at least some forms of cancer (Goulien and Fahey, 1961). In a large-scale study involving more than 1000 cancer patients suffering from malignancies of a spectrum of organs, Hughes (1972) found high levels in virtually all groups; the average being about 93 mg%.

As ceruloplasmin will oxidize amines of the central nervous system, much research has been directed toward the role of ceruloplasmin in disorders of the nervous system. Akerfeldt (1957) found high serum ceruloplasmin levels in schizophrenics although others could not confirm this (Frohman *et al.,* 1958). In 1972, Alias *et al.* did show that ceruloplasmin activity is elevated in acute schizophrenias, but is not abnormal in chronic schizophrenia. Among the acute cases, patients in a catatonic stupor consistently gave the highest values.

Some have suggested that the apparently high ceruloplasmin values, in fact, reflect low ascorbic acid levels resulting from poor nutrition. Assay of plasma ascorbic acid in a sample of 19 normals, 22 acute schizophrenics, and 13 chronic schizophrenics found no significant differences between any of these groups. Neither is there any apparent correlation between ascorbic acid and ceruloplasmin levels in any of the groups (Alias *et al.,* 1972).

The elevated serum ceruloplasmin levels are presumed to be related to stress-induced alterations in pituitary regulation of adrenocortical activity. Along these lines, Cleghorn and McClure (1966) found that administration of ACTH can, at times, cause psychotic states indistinguishable from acute schizophrenia. Nevertheless, because ceruloplasmin is an acute phase reactant, and because of the high incidence of infections in the mentally ill, it is still necessary to find an explanation for the high ceruloplasmin levels.

There is further evidence to suggest the involvement of ceruloplasmin in proper functioning of the central nervous system. The centrally active drug LSD is known to elevate brain levels of 5-hydroxytryptamine and depress brain levels of catecholamines. As both are substrates for ceruloplasmin, Barrass and Coult (1972) sought to clarify the effect of LSD on ceruloplasmin activity. They found that LSD inhibited the oxidation of 5-hydroxytryptamine and enhanced that of noradrenaline and dopamine. They concluded that if proper functioning of the central nervous system depends on a balance among noradrenaline, dopamine, and 5-hydroxytryptamine, LSD could produce aberrant functioning by upsetting this balance through interaction with ceruloplasmin or a similar enzyme.

2. Hypoceruloplasminemia — Wilson's Disease

Decreased serum ceruloplasmin levels appear in several pathological states, the most noted of which is Wilson's disease or hepatolenticular degeneration, first described by Kinnier Wilson in 1912.

The clinical features of the disorder are variable; the only pathognomonic sign being Kayser-Fleischer rings at the limbus of the cornea. The ring consists of orange or green pigment granules and these are usually most marked in the superior or inferior aspects of the cornea; they are not always complete. Patients with neurological manifestations virtually always exhibit Kayser-Fleischer rings. In young patients, slit-lamp examination may be necessary to detect their presence or absence.

The neurological features of Wilson's disease are tremor, dysarthria, ataxia, and abnormal posture. Occasionally, epileptic seizures may develop, as may psychotic behavior. Some Wilson's disease patients have been erroneously diagnosed as schizophrenics.

Sass-Kortsak states, "The early hepatic signs are those of acute or chronic hepatitis, which then develops into a postnecrotic type of cirrhosis. There is nothing to distinguish the symptoms referable to involvement of the liver in the course of Wilson's disease from those of postnecrotic cirrhosis due to a number of other etiological factors. Liver function tests are generally abnormal, with mild to severe jaundice . . . , moderately elevated alkaline phosphatase, abnormal flocculation tests, low blood levels of albumin and elevated γ-globulin, low esterified cholesterol and prothrombin deficiency . . . (1965:40–41)." Often, portal hypertension can be demonstrated. Various other clinical signs can be detected at times. Hepatic coma occurs rarely as does severe hemolytic anemia. Osseous changes can result in spontaneous fractures. Kidney tubule damage, although not clinically obvious, often develops. Dent (1948) and Uzman and Denny-Brown (1948) found that the kidney tubule damage can result in amino aciduria. This increase in amino acid excretion is not a constant feature of the disease nor is the glycosuria reported by Bearn et al. (1957).

The foremost biochemical feature of Wilson's disease is the disruption of normal copper metabolism. Greatly increased copper deposits in brain, liver, kidney, and cornea undoubtedly account for many of the symptoms. In 1952, Bearn and Kunkel, Scheinberg, and Gitlin reported that the circulating protein-bound copper, primarily ceruloplasmin, is markedly reduced in most Wilson's disease patients, in some to the point of being undetectable. The nonceruloplasmin-bound serum copper is elevated, however. Although generally diminished, some patients do have normal serum ceruloplasmin levels.

It seems that the increased copper levels result from decreased biliary excretion, although increased copper absorption has been offered as an alternative explanation. ^{64}Cu injected intravenously remains in the blood for a longer period in patients than in controls, and reaches higher peak levels. A secondary peak occurs in controls, but not in patients, as radioactive copper is incorporated into ceruloplasmin. Gibbs and Walshe (1971) have found by the use of radioactive copper that the turnover time for liver copper was approximately 20–30 days in controls and more than 1800 days in patients.

Some have suggested that an abnormal ceruloplasmin is the root cause of Wilson's disease, hypothesizing that low levels of serum ceruloplasmin allow excess copper to be absorbed from the gastrointestinal tract, in turn leading to the accumulation of copper in the tissues. This does not appear to be correct for several reasons:

(a) Some patients have normal ceruloplasmin levels and, as shown below, "Wilsonian" ceruloplasmin has not been proved to be qualitatively abnormal.

(b) Treatment with chelating agents such as penicillamine may result in decreased ceruloplasmin levels as well as decreased tissue copper.

(c) Sternlieb *et al.* (1961) could not show an *in vivo* equilibrium between copper bound in ceruloplasmin and free copper, hence leading one to doubt that copper absorption is controlled by ceruloplasmin.

Further discussion of Wilson's disease is contained in Chapter 7, Section V of this chapter, as well as being covered more fully in Bearn (1972) and Sass-Kortsak (1965) and the *Mayo Clinic Proceedings* (1974).

D. Variation in Health

Ceruloplasmin levels are also altered by some nondisease states. Trained, high performance athletes exhibit elevated levels as do nonathletes who excercise for at least several hours (Haralambie, 1969). Ontogenetic changes have been previously discussed. Probably the best known causes of ceruloplasmin alterations are pregnancy and birth control pills.

It has been known for many years that serum ceruloplasmin is increased during pregnancy (Russ and Raymunt, 1956) and, predating this observation, was the knowledge that pregnancy also elevated serum copper levels (Thompson and Watson, 1949).

During pregnancy, there is a gradual rise in the levels of both serum copper and ceruloplasmin. At their peaks, both may reach values as high as three times normal, but the normal case is a doubling of the normal levels. Burrows and Pekala (1971) found that serum copper levels reached a peak at 25 weeks of gestation and then showed a slight decline until delivery, while serum ceruloplasmin peaked at 22 weeks, fell, and gradually rose to maximum levels near term.

Because of the intimate relationship between endogenous estrogens and serum ceruloplasmin and copper levels, it was hoped that monitoring of ceruloplasmin and copper levels might provide a method of assaying the welfare of the fetoplacental unit. Several studies have suggested that this approach is of little clinical value. In Burrows and Pekala's (1971) longitudinal study of 14 pregnancies, no irregularities in serum copper or ceruloplasmin levels were noted in 7 patients who suffered preeclampsia or in 4 patients who aborted. However, the determinations were not always performed shortly prior to the abortions. Willman *et al.* (1972) found that serum ceruloplasmin levels are not altered during saline-induced abortions. Theoretically, the increased ceruloplasmin levels during pregnancy may well be primarily a function of estradiol and not estriol. Thus, serum ceruloplasmin levels might be expected not to reflect the status of the fetoplacental unit.

The increased levels of serum ceruloplasmin and serum copper are mimicked by the administration of some oral contraceptives. O'Leary and Spellacy (1968) determined serum copper alterations by atomic absorption spectrophotometry on 14 healthy women before and after administration of 10 mg of norethynodrel with mestranol daily for 21 days. Prior to treatment, the mean serum copper level was 142 μg per 100 ml. After one cycle of the oral contraceptive, the average rose to 241 μg/100 ml, a highly significant difference.

Dealing with the effect of other estrogen-containing contraceptives on serum ceruloplasmin levels, researchers (Mendenhall, 1970; Briggs *et al.,* 1970; Laurell *et al.,* 1967; Halsted *et al.,* 1968) have found similar results. Carruthers *et al.* (1966), for instance, found a mean serum ceruloplasmin level of 80.3 mg/100 ml in 25 women taking one or another estrogen-containing contraceptive, as compared to a mean of 31.2 mg% in a control group of 23 healthy women of similar ages.

Oral contraceptives which contain progestogen alone, without added estrogen, do not appear to affect serum copper or ceruloplasmin in this fashion. Briggs *et al.* (1970) administered an estrogen-containing contraceptive (Minovlar) to one small group and norethisterone acetate ('SH−420C'; Schering) to another. As expected, Minovlar caused marked increases in serum copper and ceruloplasmin, but the progestogen alone had no significant effects on these serum components.

Although norethisterone acetate is known to produce estrogenic metabolites in humans, their data indicate that at dose levels no significant amount of estrogenic substances were formed. In an earlier study, Laurell *et al.* (1969) actually found a slight drop in ceruloplasmin levels after 6–9 months use of a progestogen — chloromadionone acetate — as a contraceptive. As chronically elevated ceruloplasmin levels have been implicated in the etiology of some side effects of estrogen-containing "pills" (migraine and chloasma), progestogen alone may obviate the problem.

The rate at which ceruloplasmin and other plasma protein levels returned to their original levels after pregnancy or discontinuance of oral contraceptives was investigated by Laurell *et al.* (1970). Ceruloplasmin decreased markedly for 3 weeks after cessation of the oral contraceptive and reached normal levels approximately 2 weeks later. This was the case even in patients who had been taking the "pill" for as long as 32 months. As the levels were somewhat higher in pregnant patients, serum ceruloplasmin did not reach normal levels until 6 weeks after delivery. Others (Friedman *et al.*, 1969) have found that the serum copper does not reach nonpregnant levels until 8 to 12 weeks postpartum.

In order to clarify the mechanism by which estrogen increased serum ceruloplasmin, Evans *et al.* (1970b) examined the incorporation of ^{64}Cu into ceruloplasmin. Female rats which had been treated with daily subcutaneous injections of 0.125 mg of estradiol were injected with 100 μCi of ^{64}Cu intraperitoneally after the tenth day of treatment. On the eleventh day, the rats were sacrificed and the blood collected. The specific activity of ceruloplasmin in the estrogen-treated rats was markedly higher than that of a control group not treated, indicating an increased synthesis of ceruloplasmin accompanying elevated estrogen levels. In contrast, oophorectomized rats did not show a decrease in serum ceruloplasmin in comparison to control rats. The explanation given for these results was that "estrogen may act as an inducer for the synthesis of ceruloplasmin RNA templates," resulting in a subsequent increase in ceruloplasmin.

E. Biosynthesis and Catabolism

Information on the biosynthesis, regulation, and catabolism of ceruloplasmin is still rather limited. The incorporation of copper into ceruloplasmin was shown to take place in the liver by Bush *et al.* (1955) and Bearn and Kunkel (1955), specifically at the microsomal level (Sternlieb *et al.*, 1962). Later, Holtzman and Gaumnitz (1970a) showed that ^{64}Cu is incapable of binding to circulating apoceruloplasmin in the rat.

Additional work by Holtzman and Gaumnitz (1970b) indicates that copper does not stimulate the release of newly synthesized ceruloplasmin. The rate of release of apoceruloplasmin in copper-deficient rats was equivalent to that for ceruloplasmin in nondeficient rats. However, the concentration of apoceruloplasmin in the copper-deficient animals is 25% of normal as judged by an immunological technique. This reduction appears to be a result of decreased stability of apoceruloplasmin rather than as a result of any influence of copper on ceruloplasmin release rates as judged by following the fate of radiolabeled ceruloplasmin. However, Evans *et al.* (1970c) found that incorporation of ^{14}C-L-lysine into plasma ceruloplasmin from copper-injected adult rats was higher than that of control animals.

The mechanism by which ceruloplasmin is catabolized has been elucidated in the past several years by a series of studies conducted at Albert Einstein College of Medicine and NIH.

Hickman *et al.* (1970) describe the preparation of rat asialoceruloplasmin by the use of several neuraminidase preparations. Sialyl transferase prepared from a rat liver homogenate, in the presence of cytidine monophosphate *N*-acetylneuraminic acid-1-^{14}C and completely desialylated ceruloplasmin, restored approximately 70% of the normal complement of sialic acid. When the partially reconstituted ceruloplasmin was injected into a rabbit the radioactivity was completely cleared from the circulation within 30 min. However, if the ceruloplasmin was only partially desialylated, the radioactive protein formed had about 85% of the *N*-acetylneuraminic acid content of the native protein. This material had a much longer survival time *in vivo;* 50% of this preparation survived in the serum with a normal half-life of 54 hr. The authors interpreted this to mean that the exposure of a very small number of galactosyl residues is sufficient to mark the ceruloplasmin molecule for removal by the liver.

Subsequently, the group (Morell *et al.,* 1966, 1968, 1971; van den Hamer *et al.,* 1970) fit the results to a Poisson distribution in order to quantify the number of galactosyl residues that must be exposed to result in the catabolism of a ceruloplasmin molecule. It appears that the removal of any two of the 10 sialic acid residues from one molecule will result in its destruction.

Gregoriadis *et al.* (1970) labeled asialoceruloplasmin with ^{64}Cu and its galactose residues with ^{3}H and followed its fate in the rat. By radioautography and by blockage of the reticuloendothelial system, they showed that the site of copper and galactose cleavage is primarily the hepatocytic lysosomes. This *in vivo* finding is consistent with Coffey and de Duve's (1968) finding that plasma proteins are degraded *in vitro* by lysosomal extracts. Gregoriadis *et al.* (1970) found that galactose is cleaved off of ceruloplasmin twice as rapidly as copper. Within 30 min of injection, the cleavage of copper is 80% complete.

In part based on these results, Winterburn and Phelps (1972) hypothc-
sized that the carbohydrate portion of glycoproteins serves to determine
the extracellular fate of the protein. The sugar may result either in the
recognition of a protein by its target cell or, as in the catabolism of
ceruloplasmin, the code may be hidden and recognized only after the
removal of terminal residues.

V. Genetic Variation

A. Genetic Polymorphism

For several years after Holmberg and Laurell first isolated ceruloplasmin, the protein was considered to be homogeneous. In 1958, however, Broman separated two human serum proteins with the characteristics of ceruloplasmin and subsequently other workers (Uriel, 1958;
Deutsch, 1960; Morell and Scheinberg, 1960) confirmed its heterogeneous nature. As many other serum proteins were being shown to
exhibit genetically caused variation, some ascribed genetic significance
to the heterogeneity of ceruloplasmin. Further studies (Poulik and
Bearn, 1962; Poulik, 1963a) indicated that the variability was of no
genetic significance, resulting rather from polymerization as well as
denaturation caused by the methods of preparation and/or storage.

In the early 1960's, a possible genetic variant was discovered by
McAlister *et al.* (1961) and later by Martin *et al.,* 1963. Detected by
vertical starch gel electrophoresis, the allelic product was found to
migrate ahead of normal ceruloplasmin and was named Cp 1F. Pedigree
studies showed that Cp 1F was transmitted through four generations of
one family as a dominant trait. During the ensuing years, ceruloplasmin
typing was carried out on a large scale in several laboratories, but this
allele was never reencountered.

A true genetic polymorphism was not repeated until Shreffler *et al.*
(1967a,b), surveying a series of American Black sera by alkaline starch
gel (electrode buffer 0.21 M boric acid, 0.085 M NaOH, pH 9.0; stained
with 0.1% *o*-dianisidine and 20% ethanol in 0.04 M acetate buffer, pH
5.5), found an individual heterozygous for two unusual ceruloplasmins.
As the variants have mobilities close to that of the common form, they
had previously escaped notice. Since 1966, several other variants have
been described (Shokeir and Shreffler, 1970), again primarily in Negroes, so that today there are five genetically determined forms of
ceruloplasmin encountered at, or near, polymorphic frequencies: the
common form found in all populations, Cp B; a more anodally migrating
form, Cp A; and two more cathodal types Cp C and Cp NH. Shokeir *et*

al. (1968) have also briefly described Cp Th from a Thai sample. Electrophoretically, Cp Th appears similar to Cp A. A very rare, fast variant, Cp Bpt, has been reported in only one family of American Blacks (Shokeir and Shreffler, 1970). Twin, family, and/or population studies support the contention that all these ceruloplasmin forms are the result of codominant alleles at a single autosomal locus (Fig. 5).

McCombs *et al.* (1970) have described another fast variant in a Negro female, Cp Galveston. Although they contend that it is of genetic significance, there is no evidence to support this view at the moment. Buettner-Janusch *et al.* (1973) typed 405 samples from Madagascar and found one with the mobility of Cp Galveston. But as McCombs *et al.* (1970) point out "a band with identical electrophoretic mobility (to Cp Galveston) is observed in aged serum which originally had only the Cp B types."

In addition to Cp Galveston, Buettner-Janusch *et al.* (1973) revealed two other variants which may be genetically determined. Cp Tan moves anodally to Cp A and Cp Galveston in acrylamide gels and was never phenotypically associated with the ubiquitous Cp B. If genetic in origin, Cp Tan may be dominant to Cp B. Another band, Cp X, appeared anodal to Cp A when samples which had previously been typed as ceruloplasmin zero were subjected to prolonged incubation in the staining solution. Assignment to allelic status for Cp Tan and Cp X must await pedigree studies.

Shokeir (1971a) biochemically and immunologically characterized ceruloplasmin of the following phenotypes: Cp A, Cp AB, Cp AC, Cp ANH, Cp BNH, and Cp BptB. As judged by gel filtration, all forms are of equal molecular size, about 150,000. The minor component of ceruloplasmin, considered to be a polymeric form, eluted in the first fractions on a Sephadex G-200 column, indicating that it has a molecular weight greater than 200,000.

Charge differences must account for the varying electrophoretic mobilities. However, as treatment with neuraminidase uniformly retarded

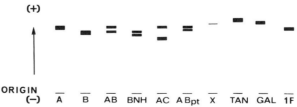

Fig. 5.   Electrophoretic mobilities of ceruloplasmin phenotypes.

the migration of all allelic products, the charge differences are not a function of sialic acid content.

Immunologically, antibodies to human ceruloplasmin were unable to differentiate between the variants when tested by Ouchterlony immunodiffusion. In addition, an anticeruloplasmin serum made by immunization with ceruloplasmin from a heterozygote could be rid of all immunological activity by absorption with ceruloplasmin from a homozygote.

Differences between forms were found in regards to inhibition of oxidase activity by either cyanide or azide. Compared to the normal form Cp B, Cp A is more resistant and Cp Bpt more susceptible to inhibition, while Cp NH and Cp C are inhibited to the same degree as Cp B. All forms are equally affected by inhibition with sodium citrate. Interestingly, Cp AB heterozygotes are not intermediate between Cp A and Cp B individuals in degree of inhibition. Rather, they are much closer to the Cp A homozygote.

The total level of ceruloplasmin in the serum of all phenotypic classes is the same except for Cp BptB (no Cp Bpt homozygotes were available for testing). Significantly higher levels (59.24 mg%) of ceruloplasmin were found in nine Cp BptB subjects.

Coupling the disparity in inhibition in Cp A, Cp AB, and Cp B with the equivalence of ceruloplasmin levels, Shokeir (1971a) concludes that the *Cp A* allele contributes twice the amount of ceruloplasmin in the Cp AB heterozygote as does the *Cp B* allele.

B. Population and Geographic Distribution

Table VIII lists the frequencies of the ceruloplasmin alleles in several populations. Because of the rather meager variability and the confusion surrounding the genetics of the protein, not many groups have been screened. At present, a polymorphism appears to be present only in Africans and American Blacks. In these groups, the frequency of *Cp NH* is underestimated because of the difficulty in distinguishing between the Cp BNH and Cp B phenotypes.

Of evolutionary interest is the fact that the frequency of *Cp A* in American Blacks is about one-third its frequency in West Africans. White admixture cannot account for this sizable reduction in frequency, as only 20% of the genes in the American Black gene pool are derived from White ancestors. The decline in *Cp A* frequency can tentatively be ascribed to a difference in selective forces in North America and Africa. Shokeir and Shreffler (1970) hypothesized that the Cp AB phenotype

TABLE VIII

Ceruloplasmin Allele Frequencies

Population/country	Number	Cp^A	Cp^B	Cp^C	Cp^{NH}	Reference
American Black	576	0.053	0.944	0.003		Shreffler *et al.*, 1967b
American Black	1126	0.0519	0.9392	0.0027	0.0062	Shokeir and Shreffler, 1970
Haiti, Black	323	0.1131	0.8735	0.0015	0.0119	Shokeir and Shreffler, 1970
Nigeria	520	0.1490	0.8365	0.0029	0.0115	Shokeir and Shreffler, 1970
West Africa	236	0.070	0.924	0.006		Kellermann and Walter, 1972
Angola	909	0.052	0.935	0.004	0.009	Kellermann and Walter, 1972
Mozambique	580	0.041	0.955	0.004		Kellermann and Walter, 1972
South Africa, Bantu	302	0.035	0.960		0.005	McDermid and Vos, 1971
India, Hindu	212	0.016	0.982	0.002		Walter *et al.*, 1972
India, Mahato	213	0.014	0.986			Walter *et al.*, 1972
India, Scheduled Castes	380	0.008	0.991	0.001		Walter *et al.*, 1972
India, Tribal	155	0.013	0.984	0.003		Walter *et al.*, 1972
India, Muslim	18	0.028	0.972			Walter *et al.*, 1972
India, Bombay	287		1.0			McDermid, 1971
India, West Bengal	978	0.012	0.986	0.002		Kellermann and Walter, 1972
Iran	198	0.003	0.990	0.007		Bajatzadeh and Walter, 1969
Pakistan	96	0.005	0.995			Bajatzadeh and Walter, 1969
Korea	115	0.009	0.978	0.013		Bajatzadeh and Walter, 1969
Australia, Aborigine	520	0.0019	0.9981			McDermid, 1971
New Guinea	560		1.0			McDermid, 1971
American White	334	0.006	0.994			Shreffler *et al.*, 1967b
Iceland	106	0.004	0.996			Bajatzadeh and Walter, 1969
Germany	224	0.013	0.985	0.002		Bajatzadeh and Walter, 1969
Ireland	240	0.010	0.988	0.002		Kellermann and Walter, 1972
Greece	210	0.036	0.960	0.004		Kellermann and Walter, 1972
Crete	155	0.068	0.932			Kellermann and Walter, 1972

might exhibit heterozygote advantage when faced with falciparum malaria.

Disregarding Wilson's disease for the moment, several studies have implicated genetic factors in ceruloplasmin quantitative variation. Hosenfeld and Schröter (1970) quantitated ceruloplasmin in 30 healthy subjects over a period of 9 months and found that the intraindividual fluctuation over time is relatively small compared with the interindividual variation of the whole group. They feel that the constancy in ceruloplasmin levels seems to indicate "an independence from exogenous effects." In a follow-up study, Hosenfeld and Drössler (1970) investigated the activity of ceruloplasmin in MZ and DZ twin pairs. They found that the intrapair variance in MZ twins is significantly lower than that of DZ twinships. At the 0.5% level, the intraclass correlation of MZ twins was significantly higher than that of DZ pairs. The heritability estimate for ceruloplasmin levels in this study was also quite high, 0.79. These results are in accord with Cox's (1966) report on two families in which low ceruloplasmin levels showed a regular pattern of inheritance. A particularly interesting test case for genetic influences on ceruloplasmin quantitative variation would be the analysis of the protein levels in MZ twins separated since birth.

Shokeir (1970) also has gathered data which would seem to indicate genetic factors are operating to produce quantitative variation between populations. Sera from five populations (American Black, American White, American Oriental, Orientals in the Far East, and a South American Indian tribe) were assayed for ceruloplasmin activity by both enzymatic and immunochemical techniques. Both data sets showed the Amerindians to have significantly higher ceruloplasmin levels than the Blacks and Caucasians. The two Oriental samples were significantly lower in activity than the Black and Caucasian groups. As he concludes, "Since Orientals living in America tend to have levels closer to Orientals living in the Far East than to American Caucasians, racial difference seems to play a more important role than the influence of environment. Inasmuch as diet, climate, and state of health are concerned, no major differences obtain between the Orientals and Caucasians in America who were investigated. These considerations may favor a genetic rather than an environmental basis for the reported variation" (Shokeir, 1970). The similarity of ceruloplasmin levels in American Blacks and Whites would tend to bolster this claim. On the other hand, Amerindians are known to be derived from a relatively recent Asian ancestor, yet the Amerindians and modern Asians are at opposite poles of ceruloplasmin quantitative variation, leading one to question a genetic explanation for the variation.

The high serum ceruloplasmin levels in the Amerindians are particularly intriguing in light of the fact that proteinuria is ubiquitous in the tribe studied (Neel *et al.*, 1964). Trip *et al.* (1970), among others, have shown that serum ceruloplasmin levels are decreased in proteinuria, implying that Indians without increased urinary protein excretion would have even higher serum ceruloplasmin levels. Nevertheless, further work must be done on the question of population differences in ceruloplasmin levels.

C. Genetics and Wilson's Disease

The most widely known cause of variation is Wilson's disease. Although the development of the syndrome of Wilson's disease has been greatly clarified during the past several years, the genetics of the disorder remains obscure. As Bearn (1972) notes, it has been tempting to assume that the primary defect is an inability to synthesize ceruloplasmin, for low serum levels are such a common feature in most patients. However, there are several previously mentioned observations which make this assumption untenable.

An alternative which has been suggested is that the structural gene for ceruloplasmin is abnormal in Wilson's disease. To date, the evidence on this point has been contradictory. Holtzman *et al.* (1967) reported that "Wilsonian" ceruloplasmin from a Negro male patient was not distinguishable from normal by starch gel or acrylamide electrophoresis, by tryptic peptide mapping, or by amino acid composition. Needleman *et al.* (1970), in a brief report, found the reverse for the ceruloplasmin of a Wilson's disease patient of unspecified race. In this case, both disc electrophoresis and tryptic peptide maps showed the "Wilsonian" ceruloplasmin to be more basic than the normal serum ceruloplasmin. Judging from their peptide maps, the major compositional differences in "Wilsonian" ceruloplasmin are (a) the increased basicity of three peptides, (b) the substitution of a basic peptide for a neutral one, and (c) a decrease in the number of acidic peptides.

Sahgal *et al.* (1970) provided evidence that the alteration in "Wilsonian" ceruloplasmin affects its antigenic sites. Rabbit antihuman ceruloplasmin produced a precipitation arc with normal ceruloplasmin in the Ouchterlony double diffusion test, yet at the same protein concentration and copper content ceruloplasmin from Wilson's disease homozygotes did not react with the antiserum. Neither could the "Wilsonian" ceruloplasmin inhibit the reaction of normal ceruloplasmin with the antiserum. However, "Wilsonian" ceruloplasmin could produce precipitin inhibition when highly concentrated. Carrico and Deutsch (1969a) however did not find "Wilsonian" ceruloplasmin to be distinct, physically, chemically, or immunologically from the protein of normal controls.

Alternatives other than a variant ceruloplasmin have been advanced. In one (Sass-Kortsak, 1965), the defect is thought to interfere with copper transport in the liver cells, leading to copper accumulation in the liver and a decreased availability of copper for incorporation into ceruloplasmin. Data gathered by Simons and Gahmberg (reported in Bearn, 1972) show that "Wilsonian" ceruloplasmin and ceruloplasmin from normal cord serum have a low K_m value for N,N'-dimethyl-p-phenylenediamine. These data suggest that the conversion from neonatal ceruloplasmin to the adult form with a higher K_m does not occur in individuals homozygous for Wilson's disease.

Research conducted by Bearn (1953, 1956, 1959, 1960) has provided much information on the population biology of Wilson's disease. The data on consanguinity rates in families of patients with Wilson's disease show that it is inherited as an autosomal, recessive trait. However, the possibility exists that the disease results from homozygosity for different genes in different populations. Bearn examined 22 patients of East European Jewish origin (14) or South Italian-Sicilian origin (8) and found several differences between the groups. The Jewish group, on the average, tended to show a greater degree of inbreeding, a later onset of the disease and, as a result, increased fertility. The Jews also had a greater variance for both serum copper and ceruloplasmin levels and all of the patients with normal serum ceruloplasmin levels were from the East European group. Thus, the possibility exists that Wilson's disease can result from different genetic causes; either different mutations at the "Wilson's disease locus" or as a result of different modifying genes. This conclusion is in agreement with the study of Cox *et al.* (1972) which presented evidence derived from pedigree analyses for at least three genetic types of Wilson's disease. If true, this could explain the apparent discrepancies between the work of Holtzman *et al.* (1967) and Needleman *et al.* (1970).

Estimates of the gene frequency for Wilson's disease are quite problematic, since the disease might not be one genetic entity. Another problem is that the gene frequencies are often calculated by a procedure which makes use of first cousin marriage estimates (Dahlberg, 1953), a parameter which often is poorly known. With this in mind Bearn (1972) estimates the gene frequency for the East European and Italian populations to be roughly 0.0006, with the disease incidence at 0.001 and heterozygous carriers 0.002. A study in Japan (Arima and Kurumada, 1963) yielded similar estimates.

D. Variation in Other Species

Very little information is available on the genetics of ceruloplasmin in other species. McCombs and Bowman (1970) examined sera from 11 primate species by acrylamide gel electrophoresis and found multiple bands in the spider monkey (*Ateles geoffryi*). However, there is only presumptive evidence that this is the result of a genetic polymorphism. As the sample sizes ranged between 1 and 6 animals per species, it is rather difficult to accept their concluding remark: "Of particular interest is that all members within one species had identical electrophoretic types."

From their typings, it tentatively appears, however, that the ceruloplasmins of the baboon, chimp, rhesus, and wooly monkey all have electrophoretic mobilities more anodal than the human Cp B; the patas and vervet monkeys are of the same mobility as Cp B while the capuchin and spider monkey ceruloplasmins are more basic. Poulik (1968) studied 250 chimpanzee sera by the method of Shreffler *et al.* (1967b) and found no polymorphism.

The one other species which is known to exhibit inherited ceruloplasmin variants is the pig (Imlah, 1964). By horizontal starch gel electrophoresis, he demonstrated 2 alleles *Cp a* and *Cp b* in the Landrace breed. *Cp b* had a frequency of 95% in this breed and was fixed at 100% in two other breeds tested. Imlah's segregation data fits a proposed 2-allele codominant model.

VI. Other Copper-Binding Proteins in Body Tissues and Fluids

Ceruloplasmin-bound copper accounts for 90–95% of the plasma copper. The remainder is loosely bound to albumin. As mentioned elsewhere, copper cannot bind to apoceruloplasmin except in the liver, and albumin appears to provide the vehicle necessary for copper transport. ^{64}Cu, administered orally or intravenously, first appears in the albumin fraction. Shortly later, as the ^{64}Cu-albumin disappears, the labeled ceruloplasmin appears. This rapid disappearance of the copper–albumin complex indicates that albumin bound copper easily exchanges with extravascular copper pools (Bearn and Kunkel, 1954; Earl *et al.* 1954; Jensen and Kamin, 1957; Scheinberg and Morell, 1957).

In other body tissues copper is also found complexed to protein, for free ionic copper probably does not exist in appreciable amounts in living organisms. In man, most of the liver copper, about 60–80% (Morell *et al.*, 1961) is contained in hepatocuprein. Erythrocyte and brain copper are primarily found in erythrocuprein and cerebrocuprein, respectively (Porter, 1966). These three proteins have been shown to be identical as mentioned previously.

High concentrations of a copper-containing protein are found in the liver mitochrondria of the neonate in neonatal hepatic mitochrondrocuprein. It has been suggested (Porter, 1966) as a corollary of its high copper content (3%) that neonatal hepatic mitochrondrocuprein is a copper storage protein.

As copper is a very effective catalytic agent, several metalloenzymes are known to incorporate this element. Uricase catalyzes the oxidation of uric acid to allantoin and CO_2. Found in the liver of nonprimate mammals, this copper flavoprotein contains 1 gm atom of copper per mole.

Tyrosinase, another copper protein, loses its enzymatic properties, as does uricase, upon the removal of copper. Tyrosinase has both catecholase and cresolase activities. Its molecular weight is 33,000.

The terminal electron acceptor in the mitochondrial oxidative pathway, cytochrome *c* oxidase, also is a copper metalloenzyme. Nair and Mason (1967) showed a reduction in its activity upon removal of copper, the activity being restored after the reincorporation of copper.

It has been known for some time that some mollusks and arthropods utilize a copper protein as an oxygen carrier in place of hemoglobin. This protein, hemocyanin, is extremely large, one form having a molecular weight of more than 6.5×10^6. The presence of hemocyanin in a limited number of invertebrates raises many fascinating evolutionary questions; most obviously, why did these creatures opt for a copper-based oxygen carrier in the blood while they depend on an iron protein — myoglobin — in their muscle tissues? It has been suggested that the ancestral oxygen carrier was copper based but that the ability to carry more oxygen provided a selective pressure favoring the transition to an iron protein. Why mollusks and arthropods nevertheless retained the ancestral form is still very much open to debate.

Further information on copper proteins is found in Table IX and in Vallee and Wacker (1970).

VII. Conclusions

The preceding pages of this review leave little doubt that ceruloplasmin is a fascinating plasma protein. It is also obvious that too little is known about most of its properties. Elucidation of its amino acid sequence and crystallographic data could provide new leads toward an

TABLE IX

Other Copper Proteins[a]

Protein	Molecular weight	Stoichi- ometry	Source	Physiological function	Enzymatic activity (cofactor)	Reference
Hemocyanin	25,000– 75,000	2	Blood of mollusks, cephalopods, gastropods	Respiratory protein	–	Polson and Wyckoff (1947) Ghiretti-Magaldi et al. (1966)
Erythrocuprein	~35,000	2	Mammalian erythrocytes		–	Porter (1966)
Hepatocuprein			Mammalian liver	?		Carrico and Deutsch (1969b)
Cerebrocuprein			Mammalian brain			Carrico and Deutsch (1969b)
Neonatal hepatic mitochondrocuprein	Insoluble	2.5– 4.4%	Human neonatal liver	Copper storage (?)	–	Porter (1966)
Cytochrome c oxidase	93,000	1 Cu/heme	Bovine heart	Electron transport	+(Heme)	Nair and Mason (1967)
Tyrosinase	33,000	4	Mushroom Mammalian tissue	Phenol oxidase	+	Kertesz (1954) Bouchilloux et al. (1963)
Uricase	100,000	4	Nonprimate mammalian tissue	Urate oxidation	+	Mahler (1963)
Monamine oxidase	170,000	1	Vertebrate tissue	Oxidative deami- nation of cat- echolamines	–(PLP)	Yamada and Yasunobu (1962) Achee et al. (1968)
β-Mercaptopyruvate transsulfurase	10,000	1	Rat liver	Transsulfuration of β-mercap- topyruvate	+	Fanshier and Kun (1962)

[a] Adapted from Sass-Kortsak (1965) and Vallee and Wacker (1970) with permission.

understanding of the various possible biological functions of this metalloenzyme.

ACKNOWLEDGMENTS

The authors wish to express their gratitude to Dr. Harold Civin and Dr. Emmanuel Epstein for their help. Ms. K. Wesley was of great aid in tracking down references. Our secretaries, Mrs. Tami Satow and Mrs. Colleen Collier, deserve much credit and gratitude for deciphering and preparing the manuscript.

The writing of this review was supported, in part, by United States Public Health Service Grant AI-11335 from National Institutes of Health, Children's Leukemia Foundation, and William Beaumont Hospital Research Institute.

REFERENCES

Abderhalden, E., and Moller, P. (1928). *Hoppe-Seyler's Z. Physiol. Chem.* **176,** 95.
Achee, F. M., Chervenka, C. H., Smith, R. A., and Yasunobu, K. T. (1968). *Biochemistry* **7,** 4329.
Aisen, P., and Morell, A. G. (1965). *J. Biol. Chem.* **240,** 1974.
Akerfeldt, S. (1957). *Science* **125,** 117.
Alias, A. G., Vijayan, N., Nair, D. S., and Sukumaran, M. (1972). *Biol. Psychiat.* **4,** 231.
Andrèasson, L. E., and Vänngård, T. (1970). *Biochim. Biophys. Acta* **200,** 247.
Aprison, M. H., Hanson, K. M., and Austin, D. C. (1959). *J. Nerv. Ment. Dis.* **128,** 249.
Arima, M., and Kurumada, T. (1963). *Paediat. Univ. Tokyo* **7,** 7.
Audran, R., and Steinbuch, M. (1965). *Protides Biol. Fluids, Proc. Colloq.* **13,** 463.
Bajatzadeh, M., and Walter, H. (1969). *Humangenetik* **8,** 134.
Barrass, B. C., and Coult, D. B. (1972). *Biochem. Pharmacol.* **21,** 677.
Bearn, A. G. (1953). *Amer. J. Med. Sci.* **15,** 442.
Bearn, A. G. (1956). *Postgrad. Med. J.* **32,** 477.
Bearn, A. G. (1959). *Proc. Roy. Soc. Med.* **52,** 61.
Bearn, A. G. (1960). *Ann. Hum. Genet.* **24,** 33.
Bearn, A. G. (1972). *In* "The Metabolic Basis of Inherited Disease" (J. B. Stanbury, J. B. Wyngaarden, and D. S. Fredrickson, eds.), 3rd ed., pp. 1033–1050. McGraw-Hill, New York.
Bearn, A. G., and Kunkel, H. G. (1952). *J. Clin. Invest.* **31,** 616.
Bearn, A. G., and Kunkel, H. G. (1954). *Proc. Soc. Exp. Biol. Med.* **85,** 44.
Bearn, A. G., and Kunkel, H. G. (1955). *J. Lab. Clin. Med.* **45,** 623.
Bearn, A. G., Yu, T. F., and Gutman, A. B. (1957). *J. Clin. Invest.* **36,** 1107.
Bennetts, H. W., and Chapman, F. E. (1937). *Aust. Vet. J.* **13,** 138.
Berggård, I. (1960). *Clin. Chim. Acta* **6,** 413.
Bickel, M., Schultze, H. E., Gruter, W., and Golner, I. (1956). *Klin. Wochenschr.* **34,** 361.
Bitny-Szlachto, S. (1965). *Progr. Biochem. Pharmacol.* **1,** 112.
Björling, H. (1963). *Vox Sang.* **8,** 641.
Blaschko, H., and Levine, W. G. (1960). *Brit. J. Pharmacol. Chemother.* **15,** 625.
Blumberg, W. E., Eisinger, J., Aisen, P., Morell, A. G., and Scheinberg, I. H. (1963). *J. Biol. Chem.* **238,** 1675.

Bouchilloux, S., McMahill, P., and Mason, H. S. (1963). *J. Biol. Chem.* **238,** 1699.
Boudin, G., and Pepin, B. (1959). "Degénérescence hépatolenticulaire." Masson, Paris.
Boyden, R., and Potter, V. R. (1937). *J. Biol. Chem.* **122,** 285.
Briggs, M., Austin, J., and Staniford, M. (1970). *Nature (London)* **225,** 81.
Broman, L. (1958). *Nature (London)* **182,** 1655.
Broman, L. (1964). *Acta Soc. Med. Upsal.* **69,** Suppl. 7, 75.
Broman, L., and Kjellin, K. (1964). *Biochim. Biophys. Acta* **82,** 101.
Broman, L., Malmström, B. G., and Vänngård, T. (1962). *J. Mol. Biol.* **5,** 301.
Broman, L., Malmström, B. G., Aasa, R., and Vänngård, T. (1963). *Biochim. Biophys. Acta* **75,** 365.
Buettner-Janusch, J., Reisman, R., Coppenhaver, D., Mason, G. A., and Buettner-Janusch, V. (1973). *Amer. J. Phys. Anthropol.* **38,** 661.
Buffoni, F. (1966). *Pharmacol. Rev.* **18,** 1163.
Burrows, S., and Pekala, B. (1971). *Amer. J. Obstet. Gynecol.* **109,** 907.
Bush, J. A., Mahoney, J. P., Markowitz, H., Gubler, C. J., Cartwright, G. E., and Wintrobe, M. M. (1955). *J. Clin. Invest.* **34,** 1766.
Carrico, R. J., and Deutsch, H. F. (1969a). *Biochem. Med.* **3,** 117.
Carrico, R. J., and Deutsch, H. F. (1969b). *J. Biol. Chem.* **244,** 6087.
Carrico, R. J., Malmström, B. G., and Vänngård, T. (1971). *Eur. J. Biochem.* **20,** 518.
Carruthers, M. E., Hobbs, C. B., and Warren, R. L. (1966). *J. Clin. Pathol.* **19,** 498.
Clausen, J., Hansen, A., and Jensen, R. (1962). *Protides Biol. Fluids, Proc. Colloq.* **9,** 269.
Cleghorn, R. A., and McClure, D. J. (1966). *In* "Comprehensive Textbook of Psychiatry" (A. M. Freedman and H. I. Kaplan, eds.), pp. 1085–1093. Williams & Wilkins, Baltimore, Maryland.
Coffey, J. W., and de Duve, C. (1968). *J. Biol. Chem.* **243,** 3255.
Cohn, E. J., McMeekin, T. L., Oncley, J. L., Newell, J. M., and Hughes, W. L. (1940). *J. Amer. Chem. Soc.* **62,** 3386.
Cole, R. D., Stein, D. W., and Moore, S. (1958). *J. Biol. Chem.* **233,** 1359.
Cox, D. W. (1966). *J. Lab. Clin. Med.* **68,** 893.
Cox, D. W., Fraser, F. C., and Sass-Kortsak, A. (1972). *Amer. J. Hum. Genet.* **24,** 646.
Curzon, G. (1958). *Nature (London)* **181,** 115.
Curzon, G. (1959). *Proc. Roy. Soc. Med.* **52,** 64.
Curzon, G., and Cumings, J. N. (1966). *In* "Biochemistry of Copper" (J. Peisach, P. Aisen, and W. E. Blumberg, eds.), pp. 545–557. Academic Press, New York.
Curzon, G., and O'Reilly, S. (1960). *Biochem. J.* **74,** 279.
Curzon, G., and Vallet, L. (1960). *Biochem. J.* **74,** 279.
Curzon, G., and Young, S. N. (1972). *Biochim. Biophys. Acta* **268,** 41.
Dahlberg, G. (1953). *In* "Clinical Genetics" (A. Sorsby, ed.), pp. 83–100. Butterworth, London.
Dent, C. E. (1948). *Trans. Conf. Liver Injury, 6th, 1947,* p. 53.
Deutsch, H. F. (1960). *Arch. Biochem. Biophys.* **89,** 225.
Deutsch, H. F., and Fisher, G. B. (1964). *J. Biol. Chem.* **239,** 3325.
Deutsch, H. F., Kasper, C. B., and Walsh, D. A. (1962). *Arch. Biochem. Biophys.* **99,** 132.
Earl, C. J., Moulton, M. J., and Selverstone, B. (1954). *Amer. J. Med.* **17,** 205.
Edelman, G. M., and Poulik, M. D. (1961). *J. Exp. Med.* **113,** 861.
Ehrenberg, A., Malmström, B. G., Broman, L., and Mosbach, R. (1962). *J. Mol. Biol.* **5,** 450.
Eisler, B., Rosdahl, K. G., and Theorell, H. (1936). *Biochem. Z.* **286,** 435.
Erickson, J. O., Gray, R. D., and Frieden, E. (1970). *Proc. Soc. Exp. Biol. Med.* **134,** 117.

Evans, G. W., Myron, D. R., Cornatzer, N. F., and Cornatzer, W. E. (1970a). *Amer. J. Physiol.* **218**, 298.

Evans, G. W., Cornatzer, N. F., and Cornatzer, W. E. (1970b). *Amer. J. Physiol.* **218**, 613.

Evans, G. W., Majors, P. F., and Cornatzer, W. E. (1970c). *Biochem. Biophys. Res. Commun.* **41**, 1120.

Fanshier, D. W., and Kun, E. (1962). *Biochim. Biophys. Acta* **58**, 266.

Fischbacher, P. H., and Quinlivan, W. L. (1970). *Amer. J. Obstet. Gynecol.* **108**, 1051.

Fish, W. W., Mann, K. G., and Tanford, C. (1969). *J. Biol. Chem.* **244**, 4989.

Fisher, G. B., and Deutsch, H. F. (1970). *Vox Sang.* **18**, 349.

Freeman, S., and Daniel, E. (1973). *Biochemistry* **12**, 4806.

Friedman, S., Bahary, C., Eckerling, B., and Gans, B. (1969). *Obstet. Gynecol.* **33**, 189.

Frohman, C. E., Goodman, M., Luby, M., Beckett, P. G. S., and Senf, R. (1958). *AMA Arch. Neurol. Psychiat.* **79**, 730.

Ghiretti-Magaldi, A., Nuzzulo, C., and Ghiretti, F. (1966). *Biochemistry* **5**, 1943.

Gibbs, K., and Walshe, J. M. (1971). *Clin. Sci.* **41**, 189.

Goodman, M., and Vulpe, M. (1961). *World Neurol.* **2**, 589.

Goulien, M., and Fahey, J. L. (1961). *J. Lab. Clin. Med.* **57**, 408.

Gregoriadis, G., Morell, A. G., Sternlieb, I., and Scheinberg, I. H. (1970). *J. Biol. Chem.* **245**, 5833.

Halsted, J. A., Hackley, B. M., and Smith, J. C., Jr. (1968). *Lancet* **2**, 278.

Hampton, J. K., Jr., Rider, L. J., and Parmelee, M. L. (1971). *Proc. Int. Cong. Primatol. 3rd, 1970* Vol. 2, p. 95.

Hampton, J. K., Jr., Rider, L. J., Goka, T. J., and Preslock, J. P. (1972). *Proc. Soc. Exp. Biol. Med.* **141**, 974.

Haralambie, G. (1969). *Z. Klin. Chem.* **7**, 352.

Heilmeyer, L., Kinderling, W., and Stuwe, G. (1941). "Kupfer und Eisen als Körpereigene Wirkstoffe und ihre Bedeutung beim Krankheitsgeschehen." Fisher, Jena.

Heimburger, M., Heide, K., Haupt, H., and Schultze, H. E. (1964). *Clin. Chim. Acta* **10**, 293.

Hickman, J., Ashwell, G., Morell, A. G., van den Hamer, C. J. A., and Scheinberg, I. H. (1970). *J. Biol. Chem.* **245**, 759.

Hirschman, S. Z., Morell, A. G., and Scheinberg, I. H. (1961). *Ann. N.Y. Acad. Sci.* **94**, 960.

Holmberg, C. G., and Laurell, C.-B. (1947). *Acta Chem. Scand.* **1**, 944.

Holmberg, C. G., and Laurell, C.-B. (1948). *Acta Chem. Scand.* **2**, 550.

Holmberg, C. G., and Laurell, C.-B. (1951). *Acta Chem. Scand.* **5**, 476.

Holtzman, N. A., and Gaumnitz, B. M. (1970a). *J. Biol. Chem.* **245**, 2350.

Holtzman, N. A., and Gaumnitz, B. M. (1970b). *J. Biol. Chem.* **245**, 2354.

Holtzman, N. A., Elliot, D. A., and Heller, R. H. (1966). *N. Engl. J. Med.* **275**, 347.

Holtzman, N. A., Naughton, M. A., Iber, F. L., and Gaumnitz, B. M. (1967). *J. Clin. Invest.* **46**, 993.

Hosenfeld, D., and Drössler, E. (1970). *Acta Genet. Med. Gemellol.* **19**, 122.

Hosenfeld, D., and Schröter, E. (1970). *Humangenetik* **9**, 38.

Huber, C. T., and Frieden, E. (1970a). *J. Biol. Chem.* **245**, 3973.

Huber, C. T., and Frieden, E. (1970b). *J. Biol. Chem.* **245**, 3979.

Hughes, N. R. (1972). *Aust. J. Exp. Biol. Med. Sci.* **50**, 97.

Humoller, F. L., Mockler, M., Halthaus, J. M., and Mahler, D. I. (1960). *J. Lab. Clin. Med.* **222**, 56.

Imlah, P. (1964). *Nature (London)* **203**, 658.

Jamieson, G. A. (1965). *J. Biol. Chem.* **240**, 2019.

Jensen, W. N., and Kamin, H. (1957). *J. Lab. Clin. Med.* **49**, 200.
Jovin, T., Krambach, A., and Naughton, M. A. (1964). *Anal. Biochem.* **11**, 219.
Kasper, C. B., and Deutsch, H. F. (1963a). *J. Biol. Chem.* **238**, 2325.
Kasper, C. B., and Deutsch, H. F. (1963b). *J. Biol. Chem.* **238**, 2343.
Kasper, C. B., Deutsch, H. F., and Beinert, H. (1963). *J. Biol. Chem.* **238**, 2338.
Kaya, T. (1964). *J. Biochem.* (*Tokyo*) **56**, 122.
Kaya, T., Osaki, S., and Sato, T. (1961). *J. Biochem.* (*Tokyo*) **50**, 24.
Kellermann, G., and Walter, H. (1972). *Humangenetik* **15**, 84.
Kertesz, D. (1954). *J. Nat. Cancer Inst.* **14**, 1081.
Konnova, L. A., Vasilets, I. M., and Shavlovskii, M. M. (1969). *Biokhimiya* **34**, 816.
Krebs, H. A. (1928). *Klin. Wochenschr.* **7**, 584.
Laurell, C.-B. (1960). *In* "The Plasma Proteins" (F. W. Putnam, ed.), Vol. 1, pp. 349–378. Academic Press, New York.
Laurell, C.-B., Kullander, S., and Thorell, J. (1967). *Scand. J. Clin. Lab. Invest.* **21**, 337.
Laurell, C.-B., Kullander, S., and Thorell, J. (1969). *Scand. J. Clin. Lab. Invest.* **24**, 387.
Laurell, C.-B., Kullander, S., and Thorell, J. (1970). *Scand. J. Clin. Lab. Invest.* **26**, 345.
Lee, G. R., Nacht, S., Lukens, J. N., and Cartwright, G. E. (1968). *J. Clin. Invest.* **47**, 2058.
Lee, G. R., Nacht, S., Christensen, D., Hansen, S. P., and Cartwright, G. E. (1969). *Proc. Soc. Exp. Biol. Med.* **131**, 918.
Levine, W. G., and Peisach, J. (1962). *Biochim. Biophys. Acta* **63**, 528.
Levine, W. G., and Peisach, J. (1963). *Biochim. Biophys. Acta* **77**, 602.
Liotet, S. (1969). *Ann. Ocul.* **202**, 629.
Locke, A., Main, E. R., and Rosbash, D. O. (1932). *J. Clin. Invest.* **11**, 527.
Lorentz, K., Niemann, E., Jaspers, G., and Oltsmanns, D. (1969). *Enzymol. Biol. Clin.* **10**, 528.
Luetscher, J. A. (1940). *J. Clin. Invest.* **19**, 313.
McAlister, R., Martin, G. M., and Benditt, E. P. (1961). *Nature* (*London*) **190**, 927.
McCombs, M. L., and Bowman, B. H. (1970). *Tex. Rep. Biol. Med.* **28**, 69.
McCombs, M. L., Bowman, B. H., and Alperin, J. B. (1970). *Clin. Genet.* **1**, 30.
McDermid, E. M. (1971). *Aust. J. Biol. Med. Sci.* **49**, 309.
McDermid, E. M., and Vos, G. H. (1971). *S. Afr. J. Med. Sci.* **36**, 63.
McDermott, J. A., Huber, C. T., Osaki, S., and Frieden, E. (1968). *Biochim. Biophys. Acta* **151**, 541.
McKee, D. J., and Frieden, E. (1971). *Biochemistry* **10**, 3880.
Magdoff-Fairchild, B., Lovell, F. M., and Low, B. W. (1969). *J. Biol. Chem.* **244**, 3497.
Mahler, H. R. (1963). *In* "The Enzymes" (P. D. Boyer, H. Lardy, and K. Myrbäck, eds.), 2nd ed., Vol. 8, Part B, pp. 285–296. Academic Press, New York.
Malkin, R., and Malmström, B. G. (1970). *Advan. Enzymol.* **33**, 177.
Malmström, B. G., and Vänngård, T. (1960). *J. Mol. Biol.* **2**, 118.
Mancini, G., Carbonara, A., and Heremans, J. F. (1965). *Immunochemistry* **2**, 84.
Mann, T., and Keilin, D. (1938). *Proc. Roy. Soc., Ser. B* **126**, 303.
Marceau, N., Aspin, N., and Sass-Kortsak, A. (1970). *Can. Fed. Biol. Soc. Abstr.* **13**, 127.
Markowitz, H., Gubler, C. J., Mahoney, J. P., Cartwright, G. E., and Wintrobe, M. M. (1955). *J. Clin. Invest.* **34**, 1498.
Marriott, J., and Perkins, D. J. (1966a). *Biochim. Biophys. Acta* **117**, 387.
Marriott, J., and Perkins, D. J. (1966b). *Biochim. Biophys. Acta* **117**, 395.
Martin, G. M., McAlister, R., Pelter, W., and Benditt, E. P. (1963). *Proc. Int. Congr.*

Hum. Genet., 2nd, 1961 Vol. 2, p. 752.

Matsuda, I., Pearson, T., and Holtzmann, N. A. (1974). *Pediat. Res.* **8**, 821.

Matsunaga, A., and Nosoh, Y. (1970). *Biochim. Biophys. Acta* **215**, 280.

Mayo Clinic Proceedings. (1974). "Symposium on Copper Metabolism and Wilson's Disease," Vol. 49, No. 6, pp. 361–411. Mayo Found., Rochester, Minnesota.

Mendenhall, H. W. (1970). *Amer. J. Obstet. Gynecol.* **106**, 750.

Morell, A. G., and Scheinberg, I. H. (1958). *Science* **127**, 588.

Morell, A. G., and Scheinberg, I. H. (1960). *Science* **131**, 930.

Morell, A. G., Shapiro, J. R., and Scheinberg, I. H. (1961). *In* "Wilson's Disease, Some Current Concepts" (J. M. Walshe and J. N. Cumings, eds.), pp. 36–41. Thomas, Springfield, Illinois.

Morell, A. G., Aisen, P., and Scheinberg, I. H. (1962). *J. Biol. Chem.* **237**, 3455.

Morell, A. G., Aisen, P., Blumberg, W. E., and Scheinberg, I. H. (1964). *J. Biol. Chem.* **239**, 1042.

Morell, A. G., van den Hamer, C. J. A., Scheinberg, I. H., and Ashwell, G. (1966). *J. Biol. Chem.* **241**, 3745.

Morell, A. G., Irvine, R. A., Sternlieb, I., Scheinberg, I. H., and Ashwell, G. (1968). *J. Biol. Chem.* **243**, 155.

Morell, A. G., van den Hamer, C. J. A., and Scheinberg, I. H. (1969). *J. Biol. Chem.* **244**, 3494.

Morell, A. G., Gregoriadis, G., Scheinberg, I. H., Hickman, J., and Ashwell, G. (1971). *J. Biol. Chem.* **246**, 1461.

Mukasa, H., Kajiyama, S., Sugiyama, K., Funakubo, K., Itoh, M., Nosoh, Y., and Sato, T. (1968a). *Biochim. Biophys. Acta* **168**, 132.

Mukasa, H., Nosoh, Y., and Sato, T. (1968b). *Biochim. Biophys. Acta* **168**, 483.

Nair, P. M., and Mason, H. S. (1967). *J. Biol. Chem.* **242**, 1406.

Neal, W. M., Becker, R. B., and Shealy, A. L. (1931). *Science* **74**, 418.

Needleman, S. B., Sahgal, V., and Boshes, B. (1970). *Experientia* **26**, 495.

Neel, J. V., Salzano, F. M., Junqueira, P., Keiter, C., and Maybury-Lewis, D. (1964). *Amer. J. Hum. Genet.* **16**, 52.

O'Leary, J. A., and Spellacy, W. N. (1968). *Science* **162**, 682.

Osaki, S. (1960). *J. Biochem. (Tokyo)* **48**, 190.

Osaki, S. (1961). *J. Biochem. (Tokyo)* **50**, 29.

Osaki, S., and Walaas, O. J. (1967). *J. Biol. Chem.* **242**, 2653.

Osaki, S., McDermott, J. A., and Frieden, E. (1964). *J. Biol. Chem.* **239**, 364.

Osaki, S., Johnson, D. A., and Frieden, E. (1966a). *J. Biol. Chem.* **241**, 2746.

Osaki, S., McDermott, J. A., Johnson, D. A., and Frieden, E. (1966b). *In* "Biochemistry of Copper" (J. Peisach, P. Aisen, and W. E. Blumberg, eds.), pp. 559–569. Academic Press, New York.

Osaki, S., Johnson, D. A., and Frieden, E. (1971). *J. Biol. Chem.* **246**, 3018.

Owen, J. A., and Smith, M. (1961). *Clin. Chim. Acta* **6**, 441.

Pedersen, K. O. (1945). "Ultracentrifugal Studies on Serum and Serum Fractions." Almqvist & Wiksell, Uppsala.

Pedersen, K. O. (1953). *In* "Les Protéines: Rapport et Discussions" (R. Stoops, ed.), pp. 19–50. Institutes Solvay Brussels, Institut International de Chimie, Brussels.

Peisach, J., Aisen, P., and Blumberg, W. E., eds. (1966). "Biochemistry of Copper." Academic Press, New York.

Péjaudier, L., Audras, R., and Steinbuch, M. (1970). *Clin. Chim. Acta* **30**, 387.

Peterson, R., and Bollier, M. (1955). *Anal. Chem.* **27**, 1195.

Poillon, W. N., and Bearn, A. G. (1966a). *Biochim. Biophys. Acta* **127**, 407.

Poillon, W. N., and Bearn, A. G. (1966b). *In* "Biochemistry of Copper" (J. Peisach, P. Aisen, and W. E. Blumberg, eds.), pp. 525–536. Academic Press, New York.

Polson, A., and Wyckoff, R. W. G. (1947). *Nature (London)* **160**, 153.

Porter, C. C., Titus, D. C., Sanders, B. E., and Smith, E. V. C. (1957). *Science* **126**, 1014.

Porter, H. (1966). *In* "Biochemistry of Copper" (J. Peisach, P. Aisen, and W. E. Blumberg, eds.), pp. 159–172. Academic Press, New York.

Porter, H., and Folch, J. (1957). *AMA Arch. Neurol. Psychiat.* **77**, 8.

Poulik, M. D. (1959). *J. Immunol.* **82**, 636.

Poulik, M. D. (1960). *Biochim. Biophys. Acta* **44**, 390.

Poulik, M. D. (1962). *Nature (London)* **194**, 842.

Poulik, M. D. (1963a). *Protides Biol. Fluids, Proc. Colloq.* **10**, 170.

Poulik, M. D. (1963b). *Protides Biol. Fluids, Proc. Colloq.* **11**, 385.

Poulik, M. D. (1966). *Methods Biochem. Anal.* **14**, 455.

Poulik, M. D. (1968) *Ann. N.Y. Acad. Sci.* **151**, 476.

Poulik, M. D., and Bearn, A. G. (1962). *Clin. Chim. Acta* **7**, 374.

Poulik, M. D., and Smithies, O. (1958). *Biochem. J.* **68**, 636.

Preer, J. R., Jr. (1956). *J. Immunol.* **77**, 52.

Ragan, H. A., Nacht, S., Lee, G. R., Bishop, C. R., and Cartwright, G. E. (1969). *Amer. J. Physiol.* **217**, 1320.

Ravin, H. A. (1961). *J. Lab. Clin. Med.* **58**, 161.

Richterich, R., Gautier, E., Stillhart, H., and Rossi, E. (1960). *Helv. Paediat. Acta* **15**, 424.

Richterich, R., Temperli, A., and Aebi, H. (1962). *Biochim. Biophys. Acta* **56**, 240.

Roeser, H. P., Lee, G. R., Nacht, S., and Cartwright, G. E. (1970). *J. Clin. Invest.* **49**, 2408.

Roux, H., Aquaron, R., Bergeaud, F., Grangier, J., and Recordier, A. M. (1971). *Rev. Rhum. Mal. Osteo-Articulaires* **38**, 99.

Russ, E. M., and Raymunt, J. (1956). *Proc. Soc. Exp. Biol. Med.* **92**, 465.

Rydén, L. (1971a). *FEBS (Fed. Eur. Biochem. Soc.) Lett.* **18**, 321.

Rydén, L. (1971b). *Int. J. Protein Res.* **3**, 131.

Rydén, L. (1971c). *Int. J. Protein Res.* **3**, 191.

Rydén, L. (1972a). *Eur. J. Biochem.* **26**, 380.

Rydén, L. (1972b). *Eur. J. Biochem.* **28**, 46.

Rydén, L. (1972c). *Acta Univ. Upsal.* **222**, 10.

Rydén, L. (1975). *Protides Fluids, Proc. Colloq.* **22** (in press).

Rydén, L., and Eaker, D. (1974). *Eur. J. Biochem.* **44**, 171.

Sahgal, V., Needleman, S. B., McKelvey, E. M., and Boshes, B. (1970). *Neurology* **20**, 402.

Sanders, B. E., Miller, O. P., and Richard, M. N. (1959). *Arch. Biochem. Biophys.* **84**, 60.

Sass-Kortsak, A. (1965). *Advan. Clin. Chem.* **8**, 1.

Sass-Kortsak, A., Jackson, S. J., and Charles, A. F. (1960). *Vox Sang.* **5**, 87.

Scheinberg, I. H. (1966). *In* "Biochemistry of Copper" (J. Peisach, P. Aisen, and W. E. Blumberg, eds.), pp. 513–524. Academic Press, New York.

Scheinberg, I. H., and Gitlin, D. (1952). *Science* **116**, 484.

Scheinberg, I. H., and Morell, A. G. (1957). *J. Clin. Invest.* **36**, 1193.

Scheinberg, I. H., Harris, R. S., Morell, A. G., and Dubin, D. (1958). *Neurology* **8**, Suppl. 1, 44.

Schuller, E., Allinquant, B., Garcia, M., Lefèvre, M., Moreno, P., and Tompe, L. (1971). *Clin. Chim. Acta* **33**, 5.

Schultze, H. E. (1957). *Scand. J. Clin. Lab. Invest.* **10**, Suppl. 31, 135.

Schultze, H. E., and Mahling, A. (1961). *Bibl. Haemotol. (Basel)* **12**, 197.

Schultze, H. E., and Schwick, G. (1959). *Clin. Chim. Acta* **4**, 15.

Schultze, H. E., Gollner, I., Heide, K., Schoenenberger, M., and Schwick, G. (1955). *Z. Naturforsch. B* **10**, 463.

Sgouris, J. T., Coryell, F. C., Gallick, M., Storey, R. W., McCall, K. B., and Anderson, H. D. (1962). *Vox Sang.* **7**, 394.

Shaposhnikov, A. M., and Derkachev, È. F. (1971). *Biokhimiya* **36**, 3.

Shavlovskii, M. M., and Vasilets, I. M. (1970). *Biokhimiya* **35**, 1031.

Shavlovskii, M. M., and Vasilets, I. M. (1972). *Biokhimiya* **37**, 507.

Shokeir, M. H. K. (1970). *Clin. Genet.* **1**, 166.

Shokeir, M. H. K. (1971a). *Clin. Genet.* **2**, 41.

Shokeir, M. H. K. (1971b). *Clin. Genet.* **2**, 223.

Shokeir, M. H. K. (1972). *Clin. Biochem.* **5**, 115.

Shokeir, M. H. K., and Shreffler, D. C. (1969). *Proc. Nat. Acad. Sci. U.S.* **62**, 867.

Shokeir, M. H. K., and Shreffler, D. C. (1970). *Biochem. Genet.* **4**, 517.

Shokeir, M. H. K., Rucknagel, D. L., Shreffler, D. C., Na-Nakorn, S., and Wasi, P. (1968). *Amer. Soc. Hum. Genet. Abstr.* **21**, 68.

Shreffler, D. C., Brewer, G. J., Gall, J. C., and Honeyman, M. S. (1967a). *Abstr. Contrib. Pap., Int. Congr. Hum. Genet., 3rd, 1966* p. 91.

Shreffler, D. C., Brewer, G. J., Gall, J. C., and Honeyman, M. S. (1967b). *Biochem. Genet.* **1**, 101.

Simons, K., and Bearn, A. G. (1969). *Biochim. Biophys. Acta* **175**, 200.

Sjollema, B. (1933). *Biochem. Z.* **267**, 151.

Sjollema, B. (1938). *Biochem. Z.* **295**, 372.

Škvařil, F., Hobzová, J., Kalous, V., and Sigmundová, V. (1965). *Collect. Czech. Chem. Commun.* **30**, 1713.

Smithies, O. (1955). *Biochem. J.* **61**, 629.

Smithies, O. (1962). *Arch. Biochem. Biophys., Suppl.* **1**, 125.

Sternlieb, I., Morell, A. G., Tucker, W. D., Greene, M. W., and Scheinberg, I. H. (1961). *J. Clin. Invest.* **40**, 1834.

Sternlieb, I., Morell, A. G., and Scheinberg, I. H. (1962). *Trans. Ass. Amer. Physicians* **75**, 228.

Sunderman, F. W., and Nomoto, S. (1970). *Clin. Chem.* **16**, 903.

Thompson, R. H. S., and Watson, D. (1949). *J. Clin. Pathol.* **2**, 193.

Trip, J. A., Que, G. S., van der Hem, G. K., and Mandema, E. (1970). *J. Lab. Clin. Med.* **75**, 403.

Uriel, J. (1957). *Bull. Soc. Chim. Biol., Suppl.* **1**, 105.

Uriel, J. (1958). *Nature (London)* **181**, 999.

Uriel, J., Gotz, H., and Grabar, P. (1957). *Schweiz. Med. Wochenschr.* **87**, 431.

Uzman, L. L., and Denny-Brown, D. (1948). *Amer. J. Med. Sci.* **215**, 599.

Vallee, B. L., and Wacker, W. E. C. (1970). "The Proteins" (H. Neurath, ed.), 2nd ed., Vol. 5, p. 45. Academic Press, New York.

van den Hamer, C. J. A., Morell, A. G., Scheinberg, I. H., Hickman, J., and Ashwell, G. (1970). *J. Biol. Chem.* **245**, 4397.

Vänngård, T. (1967). *In* "Magnetic Resonance in Biological Systems" (A. Ehrenberg, B. C. Malmström, and T. Vänngård, eds.), Wenner-Gren Center, Int. Symp. Ser., Vol. 9, pp. 213–219. Pergamon, Oxford.

Vasilets, I. M., and Shavlovskii, M. M. (1972). *Biokhimiya* **37**, 258.

Vasilets, I. M., Konnova, L. A., Kushner, V. P., Boshkov, V. M., Zdrodovskaya, E. P., and Mukma, G. V. (1968). *Biokhimiya* **33**, 1285.

Vasilets, I. M., Moshkov, K. A., and Kushner, V. P. (1972a). *Mol. Biol.* **6**, 246.

Vasilets, I. M., Shavlovskii, M. M., and Neifakh, S. A. (1972b). *Eur. J. Biochem.* **25,** 498.

Walaas, E., Løvstad, R. A., and Walaas, O. (1967). *Arch. Biochem. Biophys.* **121,** 480.

Walshe, J. M. (1963). *J. Clin. Invest.* **42,** 1048.

Walshe, J. M. (1966). *In* "Biochemistry of Copper" (J. Peisach, P. Aisen, and W. E. Blumberg, eds.), pp. 475–498. Academic Press, New York.

Walshe, J. M., and Cumings, J. N., eds. (1961). "Wilson's Disease, Some Current Concepts." Thomas, Springfield, Illinois.

Walter, H., Kellermann, G., Bajatzadeh, M., Krüger, J., and Chakravartti, M. R. (1972). *Humangenetik* **14,** 314.

Warburg, O., and Krebs, H. A. (1927). *Biochem. Z.* **187,** 255.

Whanger, P. D., and Weswig, P. H. (1970). *J. Nutr.* **100,** 341.

Willman, K., Salmi, T. T., Vanharanta, H., and Pulkkinen, M. O. (1972). *Acta Obstet. Gynecol. Scand.* **51,** 161.

Wilson, S. A. K. (1912). *Brain* **34,** 295.

Winterburn, P. J., and Phelps, C. F. (1972). *Nature (London)* **236,** 147.

Witwicki, J., and Zakrzewski, K. (1969). *Eur. J. Biochem.* **10,** 284.

Wolf, P. L., Williams, D., and von der Muehll, E. (1973). "Practical Clinical Enzymology. I. Techniques and Interactions. II. Biochemical Profiling." Wiley, New York.

Yamada, H., and Yasunobu, K. T. (1962). *J. Biol. Chem.* **237,** 3077.

Young, S. N., and Curzon, G. (1972). *Biochem. J.* **129,** 273.

Yphantis, D. A. (1964). *Biochemistry* **3,** 297.

3 / Fibrinogen and Fibrin

Russell F. Doolittle

I. Introduction

The blood plasma of vertebrate animals contains a soluble protein, *fibrinogen,* which can be transformed under suitable provocation into an insoluble polymeric gel called *fibrin.* This gelation is the central event in blood coagulation and, as such, protects the individual against excessive blood loss in many traumatic situations. The molecular basis of fibrin formation is primarily attributable to the thrombin-catalyzed[1] release of some small polar peptides (fibrinopeptides). The result of this "trimming" is the spontaneous polymerization of the individual parent molecules, which at this stage are called, somewhat inappropriately, "fibrin monomers." After the self-assembly of the individual fibrin units into a gel network, another enzyme, Factor XIII, catalyzes the introduction of a small number of covalent bonds between certain side chains of adjacent molecules in the polymer, thereby stabilizing the fibrin clot.

$$\text{Fibrinogen} \xrightarrow[\text{H}_2\text{O}]{\text{thrombin}} \text{"fibrin monomers"} + \text{fibrinopeptides} \tag{1}$$

$$\text{"Fibrin monomers"} \xrightarrow{\text{(spontaneous)}} \text{fibrin polymer} \tag{2}$$

$$\text{Fibrin polymer} \xrightarrow[\text{Ca}^{2+}]{\text{Factor XIII}} \text{cross-linked fibrin} \tag{3}$$

Although this simple scheme of events has been appreciated for the better part of a generation, the molecular details of the process remain shrouded in mystery on a number of fronts, and the fibrinogen–fibrin area continues to be a very popular and exciting field of research. From the point of view of the protein chemist, the fibrinogen molecule is fascinating not only because its structure has so far defied analysis, but also because it has seemed to flaunt some of the traditional physicochemical rules for protein structure. And while crystallographers patiently wait for suitable fibrinogen crystals, scores of workers around the world are pecking away at its enormous primary structure, and hundreds more are trying to reconstruct the natural arrangement of variously derived subunit fragments. For only when the structure of the parent molecule is better known can there be any reasonable understanding of the transition leading to fibrin, including the packing arrangement of the individual units and the various forces holding them together in the polymeric fibers.

Over and beyond the intrinsic interest of structure–function relationships, there are a number of related questions about fibrinogen and

---

[1] The complicated series of events surrounding the generation of thrombin is discussed in Chapter 7, Volume III by Davie and Hanahan (1976).

fibrin whose answers are currently being sought. For example, where did the system come from? In keeping with the general dictum that new proteins evolve from older, previously existing proteins, it ought to be possible to identify other proteins which have descended from a common ancestor with fibrinogen. If we could reconstruct some primitive form of the system, perhaps some insight could be gained into the mystery of its action.

From the metabolic point of view, there is considerable interest in the circumstances which regulate the amounts of fibrinogen in the blood plasma. Like all plasma proteins, fibrinogen is constantly being synthesized and destroyed or removed; in fact, fibrinogen probably has the shortest half-life of the major plasma proteins, not only because of being consumed in any clotting which may occur, but also because the parent molecule seems particularly vulnerable to abuse by proteolytic enzymes other than thrombin. Moreover, the degradation products resulting from these attacks may be involved in the stimulation of fibrinogen biosynthesis. As for the latter, the big question to be answered is, how is this complicated molecule assembled? Is there, as has been suggested, a more prosaic precursor molecule which is artfully dissected and snipped to yield the exquisitely delicate fibrinogen molecule?

Finally, the clinical importance of the fibrinogen–fibrin conversion cannot be overstated, there being a wide variety of ills involving thrombosis and hemorrhage. The hope is, of course, that with an emerging appreciation of the molecular events will come a rational approach for regulating the coagulability of the blood. For all of these reasons, the fibrinogen-fibrin field has become one of the most competitive in biomedical research. In this article I could not possibly do justice to all the persons, past and present, contributing to the state of the art. What I will attempt is to bring the reader abreast of what seems to be most clearly established, as well as making some comments on those aspects most feverishly under study at the present time.

II. Preparation and Purification of Fibrinogen

Fibrinogen occurs in the blood plasma of most vertebrates at concentrations in the range of 2–4 gm per liter. Because it is one of the least soluble of the proteins in plasma, it is particularly amenable to simple precipitation procedures, and a century ago Hammarsten (1879) prepared high purity fibrinogen by repeated precipitation with half-saturated sodium chloride solutions. Not long thereafter, ammonium sulfate was introduced as a protein precipitant, and many early twentieth century investigators utilized one-fourth saturation of ammonium sulfate to pre-

TABLE I

Preparation of Human Fibrinogen by a Cold Ethanol-Glycine Extraction Procedure[a]

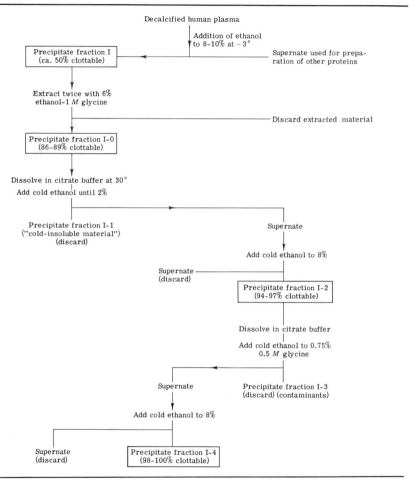

[a] From Blombäck and Blombäck, 1956.

pare fibrinogen from plasma. Fibrinogen is a euglobulin and can therefore be precipitated at low ionic strength also. Accordingly, the simple
dilution of plasma has been used as an initial step in some instances,
although it is not a recommended procedure.

A. Cold Alcohol Methods

During the 1940's the Harvard group of E. J. Cohn pioneered the use
of ethanol at low temperatures for the systematic fractionation of blood

plasma proteins. A major advantage to these methods using volatile organic liquids was that simple sterile techniques could be maintained throughout, permitting clinical administration of the fractions (Pennell, 1960). Cohn Fraction I—which is the material that precipitates upon the addition to plasma of a cold ethanol solution to a final alcohol concentration of 8–10 vols% (pH 7.2, temperature $= -3°C$, ionic strength $= 0.14$)—still serves as the starting material for the most widely used fibrinogen preparations today. Many variations have been tried over the years, including the substitution of other organic liquids (methanol, ether, acetone, etc.), but none has proved more convenient than the now classic method (Cohn *et al.,* 1946).

The observation that glycine lowered the solubility of fibrinogen, whereas other proteins actually became more soluble in its presence (Edsall and Lever, 1951), was put to use by Blombäck and Blombäck (1956), who undertook a painstaking investigation of the factors involved in the precipitation and extraction of fibrinogen by the Cohn procedures. Their method, which combines the glycine effect with the cold ethanol approach, results in a series of precipitated fibrinogen preparations of progressively higher clottability (Table I). Similar extractive procedures omitting glycine have been devised which are especially useful for chemical characterization purposes where glycine contamination ought to be minimized (Doolittle *et al.,* 1967). Another very popular procedure (Laki, 1951) for the purification of bovine fibrinogen starts with commercially available freeze-dried Cohn Fraction I, involves a cold settling step to remove cold-insoluble material, and then goes over to a classic precipitation with ammonium sulfate (final concentration $= 25\%$ of saturation). The product is highly clottable and has been widely used in physicochemical experiments.

B. Miscellaneous Precipitation Methods

A variety of procedures involving other precipitants has appeared over the years. Glycine alone (i.e., without ethanol) has been successfully used (Kazal *et al.,* 1963; Walker and Catlin, 1971) as has β-alanine (Jakobsen and Kierulf, 1973). A simple method employing a heavy metal coordination complex [potassium tetrathiocyanato-(*S*)-mercurate II] yields a product of high chemical and biological purity and reportedly has the advantage that the precipitated material is much more readily reintroduced into solution than most fibrinogen precipitates (Brown and Rothstein, 1967). Fibrinogen, by virtue of its low solubility at low temperatures, can also be prepared simply by thawing frozen plasma and collecting the most slowly dissolving material (Ware *et al.,* 1947).

C. Chromatography

Although precipitation methods can yield products which are, for all practical purposes, completely coagulable by thrombin, this is not to say that the preparations are chemically homogeneous. Moreover, these fibrinogen preparations usually contain biologically detectable amounts of various plasma enzymes and other activities, plasminogen and Factor XIII being particularly nuisancesome under many experimental circumstances (although their presence can be conveniently utilized under others). A major advance in the purification of fibrinogen was accomplished by Finlayson and Mosesson (1963) who showed that highly purified human fibrinogen exhibited two peaks when chromatographed on DEAE-cellulose, both of which were completely clottable. This same chromatographic procedure was found to be more or less suitable for the purification of many vertebrate fibrinogens (Finlayson and Mosesson, 1964), although recently Mosher and Blout (1973) have demonstrated that bovine fibrinogen, which gives a single peak on DEAE-cellulose, can be resolved into several fractions when chromatographed on DEAE-Sephadex A-50.

The heterogeneity of native fibrinogen is due in large part to proteolysis of the molecule *in vivo.* In this regard, Mosesson and Sherry (1966) have isolated high solubility fibrinogen derivatives from plasma which they have designated Fractions I-8 and I-9. These preparations are fully clottable by thrombin, albeit at a reduced rate compared with the less soluble Fraction I-4, which is generally regarded as material closely corresponding to "native fibrinogen" (Table I). *In vitro,* some heterogeneity attributable to contaminating plasmin or plasminogen can be held in check by the presence of ϵ-aminocaproic acid (EACA) in the buffers used during purification.

Not all of the heterogeneity observed among fibrinogen preparations is necessarily the result of proteolysis, of course. Some of it may derive from incomplete biosynthetic operations whereby a full complement of carbohydrate, phosphate, sulfate, etc., is not completely attached or other posttranscriptional modifications are not made. Alternatively, the heterogeneity may come from the hydrolytic removal of some of these moieties. Finally, there may be a genetic basis for some of the observed differences (Section VIII,B).

III. The Size and Shape of Fibrinogen

During the past 30 years virtually every known physical method has been brought to bear in an effort to determine the size and shape of the fibrinogen molecule. In the cases of the human and bovine molecules — which have been the targets for most of these studies — there is general agreement that the native molecular weight is 340,000 ± 20,000, a value based both on sedimentation-diffusion data and on light scattering measurements. Physical characterization of the subunits produced upon cleavage of all disulfide bonds is in agreement with this value when taken together with quantitative end group data which clearly show that the native molecule is a dimer (Blombäck and Yamashina, 1958). The molecular weights of fibrinogens from most other mammals examined are in this range also, although occasionally higher values are found (Doolittle, 1973).

A. Physical Properties

The generally accepted values of various physicochemical parameters as determined for human and bovine fibrinogens are listed in Table II. Although there may be widespread agreement on the molecular weight, the general shape of the molecule is another matter. Clearly the molecule does not behave hydrodynamically like a perfect compact sphere, its frictional ratio (f/f_0) being a relatively high 2.34 (Table II). The

TABLE II

Accepted Values of Physicochemical Parameters of Human and Bovine Fibrinogen[a]

Molecular weight (MW)	340,000 ± 20,000
Sedimentation coefficient ($S_{20,w}$)	7.9 S
Translational diffusion coefficient[b] ($D_{20,w}$)	2.0×10^{-7} cm^2 sec^{-1}
Rotary diffusion coefficient[b] ($\theta_{20,w}$)	40,000 sec^{-1}
Intrinsic viscosity ($|\eta|$)	0.25 dl/gm
Partial specific volume ($\bar{v}$)	0.71–0.72
Frictional ratio (f/f_0)	2.34
Molecular volume (calculated, unhydrated)	3.9×10^5 Å^3
Extinction coefficient[c] ($E^{1\%}_{1\,cm,280}$)	15–16
Isoelectric point[d] (IEP)	5.5
Percent α-helix[e]	33

[a] Although most of these values have been determined rigorously only for human and bovine fibrinogens (Scheraga and Laskowski, 1957), the physical properties of most vertebrate fibrinogens follow the same general pattern.

[b] A recent report using a laser-dependent viscoelastic scattering approach suggests that the translational diffusion coefficient might be as low as 1.5×10^{-7} cm^2 sec^{-1} (Birnboim and Lederer, 1972).

[c] At neutral pH.

[d] Seegers *et al.* (1945).

[e] Mihalyi (1965).

problem lies in determining whether this departure from the idealized minimum-volume sphere is the result of a very elongated molecule or a highly water-swollen structure—the effective volume of which is more than the simple sum of the volumes of the constituent amino acids and sugars—or some combination of the two. At one extreme, if the molecule is not in the least hydrated, then the hydrodynamic data are most consistent with a prolate ellipsoid of revolution with an axial ratio of about 30, and the approximate dimensions of the molecule would be 30×900 Å. At the other extreme, if the frictional ratio had to be attributed exclusively to hydration effects, then the structure would have to involve about 8 gm of water associated for every gram of protein; in this case a sphere of diameter about 200 Å would not be far removed from accounting for the data. There are ancillary data which indicate that a situation nearer the truth would be a compromise structure resembling a prolate ellipsoid with an axial ratio of about 5, the dimensions of which might be roughly 90×450 Å, and for which there would still have to be a larger than usual amount of associated water.

1. Nodular Structures

Spheres and prolate ellipsoids are not the only shapes proteins can assume of course, and one must be careful of accepting "equivalent" interpretations too literally. It was obvious to many of the physical chemists doing early studies on fibrinogen that the data could be accommodated by a variety of shapes, and the suggestion was made from the start that a chain of linked spheres, each of which was compact in itself, could also account for their observations (Fig. 1). Consistent with this depiction, Siegel *et al.* (1953) observed a molecule with the electron microscope which was comprised of four linked globules and measured $60–80 \times 500$ Å. The first electron microscope study of fibrinogen to meet with wide acceptance, however, was that of Hall and Slayter (1959), who published striking electron micrographs showing three linearly attached globules. The overall length of these triads was about 475 Å (Fig. 2). The terminal spheres were somewhat larger than the central one, the diameters being 65 and 50 Å, respectively, and the calculated volumes of the spheres added up to something very close to the unhydrated volume of the molecule.

Over the years there has been significant support for a three-ball structure of this sort from enzymatic degradation studies (Section III,C). Furthermore, some of these studies combined with physicochemical approaches, including fluorescence depolarization, have indicated that

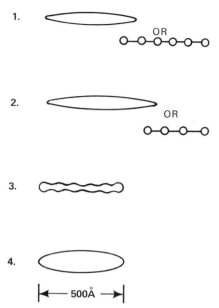

Fig. 1. Some schematic depictions of fibrinogen which can accommodate the hydrody-namic data. (1) Ellipsoid and string of beads consistent with intrinsic viscosity and sedi-mentation data; (2) ellipsoid and string of beads from sedimentation and diffusion data; (3) compromise of ellipsoid and string of beads for sedimentation and diffusion data; (4) equiv-alent hydrodynamic ellipsoid for a full hydrated molecule. (Redrawn from Shulman, 1953.)

the nodules are flexibly linked and independent (Johnson and Mihalyi, 1965).

2. Other Electron Microscope Results

Not all electron microscopists have found nodular-looking fibrinogen molecules. In particular, Köppel (1966, 1967) published electron micro-graphs of negatively stained fibrinogen preparations which indicated that fibrinogen has a cagelike geometry approximating the shape of a pentag-onal dodecahedron (Fig. 2). The edges of this isotropic structure were hypothesized to be helically interwoven polypeptide chains, and the overall width of the molecule was set at 240 Å. Since more than 90% of the effective volume would be water, the unusual hydrodynamic data alluded to above could be accounted for, and indeed, occasionally physi-cal evidence has been reported which seems most consistent with a structure of this sort (Lederer and Finkelstein, 1970; Lederer, 1972; Birnboim and Lederer, 1972). Recently some other electron micro-scopists have reported similar polygonal structures (Pouit *et al.,* 1972;

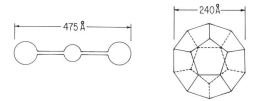

Fig. 2. Schematic comparison of two different models of fibrinogen derived from electron microscope studies. The nodular structure on the left is from Hall and Slayter (1959) and the open isotropic structure on the right from Köppel (1967).

Belitser *et al.*, 1973). On the other hand, the fact that fibrinogen can exhibit both flow and electric birefringence under appropriate circumstances is usually taken as evidence of an elongated structure, and these phenomena are not readily accounted for by the isotropic Köppel model. Nor, as indicated below, are the plethora of chemical data emerging from enzymatic degradation studies (Section III,C).

Recently Tooney and Cohen (1972) reported the electron microscopy of microcrystals obtained from a fibrinogen preparation that had been partially degraded by treatment with a bacterial enzyme preparation. The removal of a relatively small portion of the molecule (apparently from the carboxy terminal section of the α chain) was evidently sufficient modification that limited crystallization at low ionic strength was possible. The pictures exhibit a high degree of order, and a packing unit of dimensions 90×450 Å has been detected. It should be noted that a cylinder of these dimensions has a volume of 2.9×10^6 Å^3, and, depending on the disposition of the peptide chains in that volume, can obviously accommodate either a compact structure or the highly swollen molecule suggested by some of the hydrodynamic data (Table II). Optical superposition of these plates yields a characteristic fibrin pattern, emphasizing how much like the native structure these preparations are. Utilization of three-dimensional image reconstruction techniques may ultimately result in the refinement necessary to yield an approximate shape for these molecules.

Fibrinogen is an unusually delicate, easily denatured molecule, and it obviously exhibits different structural personalities under different conditions of pH, ionic strength, etc. Observations made under many conditions may have no bearing on the true (native) molecular structure at all. For example, it is entirely possible that the observed birefringence of fibrinogen is the result of the molecule being distorted by the high shearing forces or electric fields involved, and that the native molecule is not at all elongated. On the other hand, there are some investigators who feel that all the diverse shapes reported are a part of the molecule's natural countenance. It seems more likely, however, that the only ones which have any significance are those that are determined under a very narrow set of conditions approximating the physiological. What the geometry of that particular molecule is remains undetermined.

B. Chemical Characterization

1. Amino Acid and Carbohydrate Composition

The amino acid compositions of the four mammalian fibrinogens which have been analyzed are similar and undistinguished, all the usual amino acids being present in reasonable amounts (Fig. 3). A few unusual amino acids do occur in fibrinogen, including a tyrosine-O-sulfate which is present in most fibrinopeptides B (Bettelheim, 1954). This unusual derivative—found elsewhere in only a few polypeptide hormones and vasoactive factors—has been identified in a wide variety of fibrinopeptides B, including a fish (Doolittle, 1965b), the frog (Gladner, 1968), and a large number of mammals. It is not present in higher primates and the

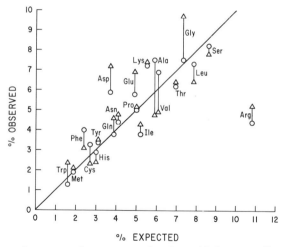

Fig. 3. Average frequency of occurrence of amino acids in mammalian fibrinogen (four species: human, pig, sheep, ox) compared with theoretical distribution (solid line) based on random distribution of triplets with observed mammalian base composition. $\triangle$ = fibrinogen; $\bigcirc$ = frequency in 53 other vertebrate proteins which have been completely sequenced and which have been depicted in this fashion by King and Jukes (1969). The fibrinogen amino acid frequencies were calculated from the compositions reported by Cartwright and Kekwick (1971). The ratios of aspartic acid/asparagine and glutamic acid/glutamine have been set arbitrarily to 1.5. For a discussion of the widely observed "arginine anomaly," see King (1971).

rat, however (Blombäck and Blombäck, 1968; Wooding and Doolittle, 1972). A phosphoserine residue occurs in the fibrinopeptide A of several higher primates, including man (Blombäck *et al.*, 1962; Doolittle *et al.*, 1971b), and also the dog (Osbahr *et al.*, 1964). Small amounts of phosphorus may also occur in parts of the fibrinogen molecule other than the fibrinopeptides (Blombäck *et al.*, 1963; Krajewski and Cierniewski, 1972), as well as may tyrosine-*O*-sulfate (Jevons, 1963).

Fibrinogen has no free sulfhydryl groups, all of its cysteine being involved in disulfide bridges. Henschen's data on bovine and human fibrinogen (Henschen, 1964b) indicate that there should be 28–29 disulfide bridges per 340,000 molecular weight, but the data of Cartwright and Kekwick (1971) suggest that the number might be as high as 32–34. On the other hand some investigators put the number as low as 21–22 (Latallo *et al.*, 1971).

Mammalian fibrinogens contain about 4% carbohydrate, mostly consisting of neutral hexoses, glucosamine, and sialic acid (Blombäck, 1958). In the case of the human molecule, the data of Mester and Szabadoz (1968) can be used to calculate that there are 19 galactose residues, 22 mannoses, 19 glucosamines, and 6 sialic acid groups for every 340,000 molecular weight (Spiro, 1973). Lamprey fibrinogen also contains a carbohydrate cluster on its fibrinopeptide B (Doolittle and Cottrell, 1974).

2. End Group Determinations

Amino terminal analysis has played an enormously important role in our understanding the conversion of fibrinogen to fibrin, proving without doubt that limited proteolysis is the triggering mechanism for fibrin formation (Bailey *et al.*, 1951). Beyond that, it was the quantitative determination of amino terminals of a variety of fibrinogens and fibrins which showed that the native fibrinogen molecule is a dimer, each particle of 340,000 molecular weight having three pairs of nonidentical polypeptide chains (Blombäck and Yamashina, 1958). Two of the three different chains were found to undergo a change in amino terminal as a result of thrombin-catalyzed fibrin formation, corresponding to the release of the fibrinopeptides A and B. By convention, the chains which lose the fibrinopeptides A are called the α chains and the ones which lose the fibrinopeptides B the β chains.[2] The chain whose amino terminal residue

---

[2] The International Committee on Nomenclature of Blood Clotting Factors has designated the fibrinogen chain with the fibrinopeptide A still attached Aα, and the chain with the fibrinopeptide B at its amino terminus Bβ. The corresponding chains from fibrin, after the removal of the fibrinopeptides, are called the α chain and β chain. In this article the Aα and Bβ chains are simply called the fibrinogen α chain and β chain.

remains unchanged is termed the γ chain. The formula $\alpha_2\beta_2\gamma_2$ apparently applies to all vertebrate fibrinogens (see also Section IX).

The amino terminals of fibrinogen α chains vary in the more than 50 species which have been examined, although there is a decided preference for alanine or threonine (Dayhoff, 1972). Similarly, although a wide variety of residues exists at the amino terminus of the β chains from various species, a disproportionate number of pyrrolidone carboxylic acid residues[3] ([Glu) has been found (Blombäck and Doolittle, 1963a,b; Mross and Doolittle, 1967; Wooding and Doolittle, 1972). Most mammalian γ chains have amino terminal tyrosine (Blombäck and Yamashina, 1958), although several exceptions have now been found, including leucine in the case of the tapir and arginine in the rhinoceros (O'Neil and Doolittle, 1975). The one lower vertebrate which has been studied has serine at the amino terminus of its γ chains (Doolittle *et al.,* 1963; Doolittle, 1965a).

The carboxy terminals of fibrinogens from six different mammals have been determined (Okude and Iwanaga, 1971). In four of these species, the α chain terminates with proline (ox, sheep, pig, and dog); in the other two it is valine (human and horse). All the β chains examined have carboxy terminal valine. In the case of the γ chains, pig and dog end with isoleucine, whereas the remaining four have carboxy terminal valine (Table III).

TABLE III

Amino and Carboxy Terminal Groups of Six Mammalian Fibrinogens[a]

	α Chain		β Chain		γ Chain	
	Amino	*Carboxy*	*Amino*	*Carboxy*	*Amino*	*Carboxy*
Ox	Glu	Pro	[Glu	Val	Tyr	Val
Sheep	Ala	Pro	Gly	Val	Tyr	Val
Pig	Ala	Pro	Ala	Val	Tyr	Ile
Human	Ala	Val	[Glu	Val	Tyr	Val
Dog	Thr	Pro	His	Val	Tyr	Ile
Horse	Thr	Val	Leu	Val	Tyr	Val

[a] Amino terminal data from Dayhoff (1972); carboxy terminal data from Okude and Iwanaga (1971).

[3] Nonstandard abbreviations used in this article include [Glu (pyrrolidone carboxylic acid), SDS (sodium dodecyl sulfate), and PAS (periodic acid-Schiff).

3. Structural Studies on Fibrinopeptides

The amino acid sequences of fibrinopeptides from a large number of species have been determined. Most of these have been accomplished in Blombäck's laboratory in Stockholm (see, e.g., Blombäck and Blombäck, 1968) or in the author's laboratory (Doolittle, 1970), and are tabulated in Dayhoff's "Atlas of Protein Sequence and Structure" (Dayhoff, 1972). These structures are exceptionally variable and have proved of great interest in the area of molecular phylogeny and evolution (Doolittle and Blombäck, 1964). On the other hand, some generalizations about structure–function relationship can be made on the basis of these data also. In spite of the great variability—which implies a nonspecific function which can be satisfied by a large number of amino acid combinations—certain features of these peptides have been conserved during the course of evolution. For example, the junctions split by thrombin are always arginyl-glycine bonds, in lower vertebrates as well as mammals (Doolittle, 1965a). Furthermore, all the fibrinopeptides examined bear a substantial negative charge (ranging from −2 to −6 in mammals), a property consistent with early notions that the fibrinopeptides prevent polymerization by the mutual electrostatic repulsion of individual fibrinogen molecules. This tendency toward electronegativity is also reflected in the occurrence of the sulfated tyrosines, the phosphorylated serines, and the pyrrolidone carboxylic acid terminal residues, and in the case of the lamprey fibrinopeptide B, sialic acid residues (Doolittle and Cottrell, 1974).

The lengths of the fibrinopeptides range from 13 to 21 residues in mammals, although they may be as long as 36–45 residues in lower vertebrates (Doolittle, 1965b; Gladner, 1968) or as short as six residues, as evidenced by the lamprey fibrinopeptide A (Doolittle and Cottrell, 1974). A number of substantial deletions, terminal and internal, have occurred during the evolution of these structures without apparent consequence to the parent fibrinogen molecule. In two closely related buffalo, for example, the only difference in the amino acid sequences of their fibrinopeptides A is an internal deletion of four residues (Mross and Doolittle, 1967). The fibrinopeptides B tend to be somewhat more changeable than the A peptides, including several large-scale deletions (Wooding and Doolittle, 1972), suggesting that their role is even less demanding than that of the A peptide.

In spite of this great tolerance for change, some amino acids have never been found in any of the fibrinopeptides examined. In this regard, cysteine, methionine, and tryptophan appear to have been selected against. In the case of cysteine, there could be an obvious disadvantage if a free sulfhydryl group existed in these presumably exposed locations, since bridge formation leading to premature polymerization would always be a threat. Similarly tryptophan and methionine might be thermodynamically undesirable in these polar charge clusters.

The liberated fibrinopeptides exhibit the characteristic spectrum of a random coil when examined by circular dichroism methods, although this may have no bearing on their natural configuration before release from the parent fibrinogen molecule (Doolittle, 1973).

4. Separation and Characterization of Subunits

In 1962 two laboratories independently reported the separation of the three nonidentical chains by chromatography after sulfitolysis of fibrinogen (Henschen, 1962; Clegg and Bailey, 1962). Henschen (1964a) was subsequently able to prepare the individual chains in sufficient quantity for a rigorous chemical characterization. Using similar procedures, McKee *et al.* (1966) determined the molecular weights of the individual chains from human fibrinogen and found them to add up to approximately 170,000, the accepted value for a half-molecule of fibrinogen. The individual values, which were determined by sedimentation equilibrium in the presence of 6 M guanidinium chloride, were α chain = 63,500, β chain = 56,000, and γ chain = 47,000. Subsequent studies employing SDS-gel electrophoresis have substantially borne out these values (McKee *et al.*, 1970).

The amino acid compositions of the three chains, while unremarkable, are significantly different from each other. Hence, the α chains from a variety of species all have considerably less tyrosine than the β and γ chains, but are richer in arginine and serine (Cartwright and Kekwick, 1971). γ Chains have significantly less proline than the other two chains, and β chains are richer with regard to methionine and cysteine. All three chains were reported to contain carbohydrate (Henschen, 1964c; Mills and Triantaphyllopoulos, 1969), although on SDS-gel electrophoresis only β chains and γ chains are PAS-positive (Pizzo *et al.*, 1972; Gaffney, 1972). In the case of the human γ chain, one carbohydrate attachment site has been located at asparagine-52 (Iwanaga *et al.*, 1968).

C. Enzymatic Dissection of the Fibrinogen Molecule

Fibrinogen can be proteolytically digested into a characteristic set of fragments by plasmin (fibrinolysin), and, for that matter, also by trypsin and chymotrypsin. Moreover, the action of all three enzymes follows a virtually identical course during the early stages of digestion, indicating

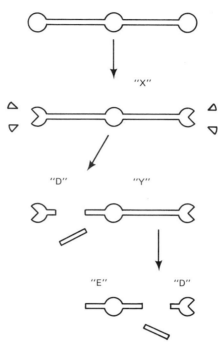

Fig. 4. Schematic depiction of the degradation of fibrinogen by plasmin showing how compatible the pattern of split products is with Hall and Slayter's model. Adapted from the description of Marder (1970).

that the pattern of breakdown is determined more by the vulnerability of the substrate than by the preferential affinities of the proteases (Mihalyi, 1970). Most studies have been performed using plasmin, however, primarily because it yields the most clearly defined set of terminal fragments.

The nomenclature used to define the plasmin-derived fragments goes back to an early study by Nuzzensweig *et al.* (1961), in which the major chromatographic peaks on a DEAE-cellulose column of exhaustively digested fibrinogen were labeled A, B, C, D, and E. As it turned out, D and E were large molecular weight fragments, but A, B, and C represented collections of smaller peptides. A consideration of the relative molecular weights and recoveries of D and E led to the conclusion that there were 2 moles of D per molecule of fibrinogen, but only 1 mole of E. The correspondence with the two terminal and one central globules of the Hall and Slayter model of fibrinogen was not immediately appreciated, however.

Later, Marder *et al.* (1969) examined the early stages of plasmin digestion and characterized a set of intermediate fragments which they termed X and Y. The existence of these high molecular weight materials was nicely interpreted in light of the Hall and Slayter model, as shown in Fig. 4. Briefly, the first intermediate to appear during the plasmin digestion is fragment X; it has a molecular weight of about 240,000 and is still fully clottable. Fragment X is then broken down into two major pieces, Y and D, the molecular weights of which are about 155,000 and 85,000, respectively. These two pieces are not clottable, but do inhibit fibrin formation when mixed into a system of polymerizing fibrin monomers (Marder and Shulman, 1969). Fragment Y is subsequently digested further into another molecule of D and a second product which is fragment E, the molecular weight of which is about 50,000. Fragment E does not inhibit fibrin formation when added to a polymerizing system. Several of the physicochemical properties of these major fragments are listed in Table IV.

The advent of SDS-gel electrophoresis has made the execution of studies dealing with the proteolytic fragmentation of large proteins a rather simple matter, and a very large number of investigators have joined in the assault on fibrinogen structure by way of its plasmin-derived fragments. The interpretation of the gel patterns is not always as simple as running the gels, however, and there is not universal agreement among all parties. What follows is a rather general distillation of some of these events without great pains being taken to cite individual

TABLE IV

Some Physicochemical Parameters of Fibrinogen Degradation Products[a]

	Fibrinogen	*Fragment X*	*Fragment Y*	*Fragment D*	*Fragment E*
Molecular weight (MW)	300,000	240,000	155,000	83,000	50,000
Translational diffusion coefficient $(D_{25,w})$	2.4	2.9	3.6	5.8	5.7
Sedimentation coefficient $(S_{25,w})$	8.3	7.9	6.5	5.5	3.3
Extinction coefficient $(E_{1\%})$	15.1	14.2	17.6	20.8	10.2

[a] Taken from Marder *et al.* (1969). The values have got to be regarded as approximate in the sense that these fragments may be slightly larger or smaller depending on the degree to which the plasmin degradation is allowed to proceed. Note also that the calculated molecular weight for fibrinogen is slightly lower than the usually accepted value (Table II).

contributions. The SDS-gel studies have also made it clear that X, Y, D, and E are very general fragment types, and the pattern of plasmin digestion is such that each of these is intrinsically heterogeneous. Thus, one can distinguish "early D," "middle D," "late D," etc., depending on the extent of the digestion and the exact conditions.

It is generally conceded that the conversion of fibrinogen to fragment X is the result of number of plasmin cleavages in the carboxy terminal half of the α chain. Simultaneously, a segment of about 40 residues is removed from the amino terminal end of the β chain (including the fibrinopeptide B) (Lahiri and Shainoff, 1973). The transition of X to Y and D, as well as the subsequent conversion of Y to D and E, is primarily the result of a cluster of plasmin hits not too far in from the amino terminals of all three chains. It is now clear that fragment E is a dimeric molecule comprised of segments of all three chains held together by disulfide bonds. Fragment D is a monomeric molecule and is also made up of segments of all three chains.

While most of the SDS-gel studies have confirmed and refined the sequence of events developed by the studies of Nuzzensweig *et al.* (1961) and Marder *et al.* (1969), there have been some other interpretations. In particular, Mosesson *et al.* (1973) contend that there is only one fragment D per molecule of fibrinogen and imply that the conformity with the Hall and Slayter model of fibrinogen is a figment of historical wishfulness. These authors believe that fragment D is *dimeric,* containing three *pairs* of nonidentical chain segments held together by disulfides. A schematic representation of their "Gatling gun" model is depicted in Fig. 5. So far they have not been able to convince the majority of other workers of the correctness of their scheme.

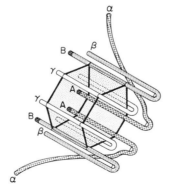

Fig. 5. Mosesson's "Gatling gun" model of fibrinogen. (Photograph courtesy of M. Mosesson.)

D. Chemical Fragmentation Studies

Cyanogen bromide digestion of human fibrinogen, which contains about 30 methionine residues per half-molecule, results in a very large number of fragments, but in a pioneering effort, B. Blombäck *et al.* (1968) were able to isolate a very interesting piece which contained both the fibrinopeptides A and B. The same fragment was also found to contain the amino terminal tyrosine of the γ chain and was therefore comprised of all three amino terminal segments bound together by disulfide links. The material contained about half of the cysteine (all in the form of disulfide) of fibrinogen, even though accounting for only 15% of the mass, and was accordingly referred to as the "disulfide knot" (DSK). As it turned out, the "knot" was actually dimeric and corresponds closely to the plasmin-derived fragment E (Marder, 1971).

The revelation that the disulfide knot was actually a dimer had a dramatic impact on the thinking of persons trying to integrate structure and function for the fibrinogen–fibrin conversion, for until that time it was generally believed that the fibrinopeptides A were at the extremities of an elongated molecule (see Section IV,A). Furthermore, the elucidation of its structure paved the way to a determination of the primary structure of fragment E.

A number of other major fragments have now been isolated from cyanogen bromide digests, including two which are rich in disulfide bonds (Timpl and Gollwitzer, 1973). The cyanogen bromide peptides of the separated chains are now being ordered in several laboratories. Cyanogen bromide fragmentation has also been used very effectively in the characterization of the plasmin-derived fragments D and E, and these two approaches in concert are being employed in an effort to determine the entire sequence of the fibrinogen molecule.

Summing to this point, fibrinogen is an atypical protein from the physicochemical point of view, and there is not universal agreement with regard to describing its general structure. The most widely accepted interpretation, however, is that the molecule has a nodular structure consisting of several independent domains. In particular, there is a central "knot" region which includes all six amino terminals (and therefore all four fibrinopeptides) (Figs. 6 and 7). Physicochemical data indicate that this region, which includes overlapping portions of fragment E and the disulfide knot, is open and extended (Table IV). In contrast, the domains which are the two fragments D are evidently compact, each being about the size and shape of a plasma albumin molecule. In keeping with this compactness, the fragments D have a number of intrachain disulfide

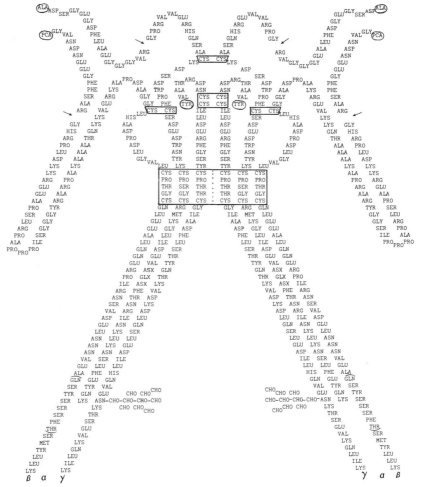

Fig. 6. The amino acid sequence of the central domain of human fibrinogen. The α chains begin with the amino terminal alanine residues of the fibrinopeptides A in the upper corners. The β chains originate at the PCA residues of the fibrinopeptides B, and the γ chains begin with the tyrosines near the upper middle. The structure as shown consists of 2 × 259 = 518 residues, and consists of overlapping portions of fragment E and the disulfide knot. Much of the sequence was determined by Blombäck's group in their studies on the latter (Blombäck and Blombäck, 1972), but the carboxy terminal 28 residues of the α chain and the carboxy terminal four residues of the β chain are from Takagi and Doolittle (1975b). CHO = carbohydrate residues.

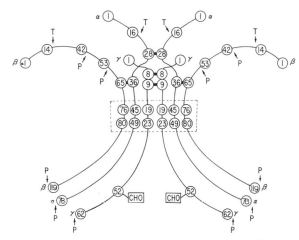

Fig. 7. A schematic rendering of the central domain of human fibrinogen showing some key locations (by residue number), including the six amino terminals (α, β, and γ), thrombin attack points (T), plasmin attack points (P), disulfide bridges, and carbohydrate (CHO) attachment points. Compare with Fig. 6.

bonds, as well as interchain connections. Each D fragment—which we prefer to call domain II—is evidently connected to the central domain (domain I) by a three-stranded rope. As was suggested long ago (Cohen, 1961), these polypeptide connectors may be the "coiled coils" responsible for the characteristic X-ray spacing observed in fibrinogen and fibrin preparations (Bailey *et al.*, 1943).

Finally, emanating from the terminal domains (domains II) at some point are the free-swimming carboxy terminal halves of the α chains. The amino acid composition of these appendages is typified by an excess of serine, glycine, and proline and a distinct deficit of nonpolar amino acids (Takagi and Doolittle, 1974b). The segments are very exposed and vulnerable to proteolysis by a host of proteases, and they apparently contribute significantly to the anomalous physical chemistry of the native molecule. In our laboratory we call them "the water wings." A schematic depiction of a molecule so comprised is rendered in Fig. 8.

IV. The Conversion of Fibrinogen into Fibrin

Aesthetics aside, the primary reason for studying the structure of fibrinogen is to understand its conversion into fibrin. In this regard, there is a large body of evidence which indicates that the individual units in fibrin differ chemically from fibrinogen only in that a few small peptides

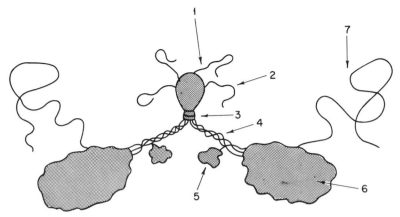

Fig. 8. Depiction of a fibrinogen molecule showing some key structural features. (1) Thrombin attack point for release of fibrinopeptide A; (2) thrombin attack point for release of fibrinopeptide B; (3) "disulfide girdle"; (4) three-stranded rope connecting domains I and II; (5) carbohydrate attached to γ chain; (6) domain II (fragment D); and 7, free-swimming α chain carboxy terminal halves. (Only one of the dimeric halves is numbered.)

(the fibrinopeptides) have been lost. There are also some physical data which suggest that the general shape of the molecule — whatever it may be — is not significantly changed during the transformation into fibrin. These inferences are based on certain X-ray studies which show that packed or precipitated fibrinogen demonstrates the same characteristic spacing as does fibrin (Bailey *et al.*, 1943; Stryer *et al.*, 1963). This viewpoint is also supported by comparisons of the proteolytic digestion of fibrinogen and fibrin which indicate that the vulnerability to plasmin, for example, follows the same pattern in both cases (Dudek *et al.*, 1970). Immunochemically, no unique antigenic differences have been reported for fibrin compared with fibrinogen, except for the absence of the fibrinopeptides, although it has been reported that the plasmin cleavage products of the two are distinguishable (Plow and Edgington, 1973).

On the other hand, there has to be a number of molecular adjustments made, no matter how subtle, in order for a soluble protein to be converted into a three-dimensional network kind of polymer. Moreover, the gelation process must involve a variety of different contacts during the growth of the network. Over the years a general dogma has emerged which states that the polymerization process can be divided into two parts (Ferry, 1952). First, there is a formation of intermediate polymers by an "end-to-end" association of the individual units (although the "end-to-end" process may actually involve staggered overlaps of a "side-by-side" nature), and, then, a second stage involving the lateral aggregation of the intermediate polymers. The latter stage is known to be very sensitive to environmental conditions, including pH, ionic strength, the presence of certain small molecules, etc. For example, "coarse clots," which are white and opaque, are thought to involve more lateral aggregation than "fine clots," which are transparent. In general, the latter tend to develop at high pH and high ionic strength (Ferry and Morrison, 1947), although all gradations between fine and coarse can occur. Physiologically the situation is also influenced by clot stabilization (Section V).

A. Release of the Fibrinopeptides

The thrombin-catalyzed conversion of fibrinogen to fibrin is accompanied by the release of two pairs of polar peptides, referred to as the fibrinopeptides A and B (Lorand, 1952; Bettelheim and Bailey, 1952). In those mammalian species which have been studied, the release of the fibrinopeptide A occurs very much faster than the release of the B peptide. In fact, only the fibrinopeptide A need be released from mammalian fibrinogen for gelation to ensue, as evidenced by the fact that fibrin gels can be formed by the catalytic action of certain snake venom enzymes which apparently release only the fibrinopeptide A (Blombäck et al., 1957; Esnouf and Tunnah, 1967). A similar result can be obtained in certain instances where distantly related heterologous thrombins are used to clot the fibrinogen (Doolittle et al., 1962).

On the other hand, the release of the fibrinopeptide B alone may not be sufficient to induce the gelation of mammalian fibrinogen, as implied by the finding that the amino terminal segment of the β chain, including the fibrinopeptide B, is lost during the conversion of fibrinogen to fragment X (Lahiri and Shainoff, 1973). It is possible, of course, that the plasmin-catalyzed removal of the β chain amino terminal segment also removes a potential polymerization site at the same time, although it should be recalled that fragment X can be clotted by thrombin treatment removing the fibrinopeptides A. An enzyme in copperhead snake venom reportedly cleaves the fibrinopeptide B preferentially; clotting was not observed until a significant amount of fibrinopeptide A was also removed (Herzig et al., 1970). In some lower creatures, fibrin can be formed by the release of the fibrinopeptide B only, however. For example, in the case of lamprey fibrinogen, mammalian thrombins induce clot formation after the release of only the fibrinopeptides B (Doolittle, 1965a), even though the parental β chain is distinctly homologous to mammalian β chains (Section IX).

The role of the fibrinopeptides is generally thought to be one of electrostatic fending, although the distinction between this simple repulsive function and the unmasking of definite contact sites is a subtle one. It must be remembered that the fibrinopeptides are highly variable from species to species, indicating a very nonspecific function which can be accomodated by a wide assortment of amino acid combinations. In this regard, fibrinogen can be "gelled" by stoichiometric amounts of protamine sulfate, presumably by the neutralization of the fibrinopeptides or other negative charge clusters. Electron microscopy of polymers formed by this method has revealed a characteristic fibrin spacing of approximately 230 Å (Stewart and Niewarowski, 1969).

When it became apparent that the triggering event for the transformation of fibrinogen into fibrin was the mere removal of a few polar peptides, a number of simple electrostatic models were offered in explanation of the subsequent associative events. In particular, Ferry and his colleagues showed how the release of negative charge clusters from either the center or the end of an elongated fibrinogen molecule could lead to the formation of a staggered molecular overlap of the sort postulated for the formation of intermediate polymers (Fig. 9). These models were in keeping with Ferry's general supposition (Ferry, 1952) that the association of fibrin monomers is the result of overcoming long-range repulsive forces by accommodating short-range attractive forces in a manner similar to that predicated by Debye (1949) for micelle formation.

The subsequent discovery that fibrinogen is a dimeric molecule led to some elegant electric birefringence studies on the fibrinogen–fibrin conversion which unfortunately gave rise to the mistaken notion that the fibrinopeptides A were at the opposite ends of an elongated fibrinogen molecule (Haschemeyer, 1963). These experiments depended on lowering the pH of the system to halt thrombin action at early stages in the transformation process, and the results were apparently due to an artifact stemming from a structural deformation of fibrinogen at low pH (Doolittle *et al.,* 1974b).

Kinetic Aspects

Apart from the relative rates of release of the fibrinopeptides A and B, the kinetic aspects of the thrombin–fibrinogen reaction remain unclear. It is still not known whether "one-hit" or "two-hit" kinetics better describe the situation. This is to ask, must every fibrinogen molecule have both fibrinopeptides A removed before it becomes a part of a growing chain, or can the release of a single peptide A lead to incorporation, with the second fibrinopeptide A actually being released from the growing chain?

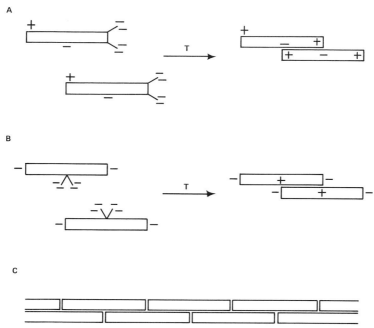

Fig. 9. Schematic depiction of events leading to formation of intermediate polymers formed from staggered overlaps of individual monomeric units. In sequence A the fibrino-peptides would be disposed at one end of the fibrinogen molecule, whereas in sequence B they would be clustered in the middle of the molecule. In either case, a staggered overlap could occur leading to the intermediate polymer depicted in C. (Redrawn from Ferry *et al.,* 1954.)

B. Polymerization

Fibrin polymerization can be studied independently of the thrombin-catalyzed release of the fibrinopeptides by dispersing unstabilized fibrin in suitable unfolding solvents and then restoring the system to more or less physiological conditions. Some of the solvents which have been used—for example, concentrated urea or guanidine solutions—may actu-ally denature the individual molecular units (Gollwitzer *et al.,* 1970; Belitser *et al.,* 1971), and some caution must be exhibited in evaluating many such studies. On the other hand, a few systems appear mild enough that the reaggregated fibrin can be regarded as authentic. The most popular of these systems involves dispersal of fibrin in 1 *M* sodium bromide at pH 5.3; reaggregation is attained by diluting the system with a suitable neutral buffer.

The polymerization of fibrin under these conditions is a highly ex-

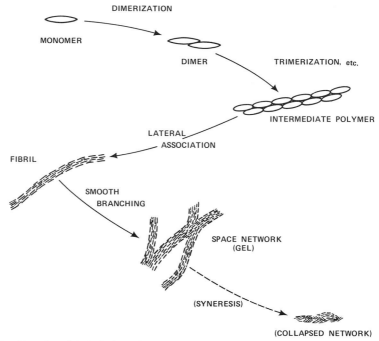

DIMERIZATION

MONOMER

DIMER

TRIMERIZATION, etc.

INTERMEDIATE POLYMER

LATERAL
ASSOCIATION

FIBRIL

SMOOTH
BRANCHING

SPACE NETWORK
(GEL)

(SYNERESIS)

(COLLAPSED NETWORK)

Fig. 10. Pictorial depiction of associative steps occurring during fibrin formation.

othermic reaction (Sturtevant *et al.,* 1955). It likely involves a variety of
weak forces, including extensive hydrogen bonding, dipole–dipole interactions, and hydrophobic interactions. It must be appreciated that not
all of these interactions are necessarily between neighboring molecules
in the polymer; some of the heat release is likely due to *intramolecular*
rearrangements and interactions with solvent.

The detailed nature of the kinds of intermolecular association remains
obscure. Although chemical derivatization of a number of different
amino acid side chains can interfere with polymerization, usually it is not
possible to distinguish specific blocking effects from general structural
distortions. Furthermore, although the arrangement of the individual
units within the polymer must be very specific—as evidenced not only
by the characteristically observed fibrin repeat unit, but also by other
restrictions apparent from clot stabilization studies (Section V)—there
may still be a variety of contact sites involved at different stages of clot
development (Fig. 10).

With regard to the location of the contact sites, it will be recalled that
the fragments Y and D are nonclottable but inhibit fibrin polymerization
(Section III,C). Presumably these derivatives of fibrinogen (or fibrin)

can become involved in the growing polymer, but, lacking two binding sites themselves, effect chain termination. As we shall see, the initial cross-linking site for fibrin stabilization is located on fragment D (domain II), and there is reason to think that these sites are also primary contact points in nonstabilized fibrin (Section V). On the other hand, fragment E derived from fibrinogen does not interfere with fibrin polymerization. It must be emphasized that the triggering event for the fibrinogen to fibrin transformation is the release of fibrinopeptides from the central domain, even though major contact sites have so far only been identified on the terminal domains (fragment D) (Kudryk *et al.*, 1974).

V. Fibrin Stabilization

A. Cross-linking by Factor XIII

Under normal conditions, the blood plasma of vertebrates contains the inactive precursor of an enzyme which can "stabilize," or strengthen, fibrin gels by the introduction of covalent bonds between neighboring molecules in the polymer. The responsible protein, which is activated by the thrombin-catalyzed removal of a specific peptide, is officially called Factor XIII, although a variety of other names has been used in the past, including fibrin-stabilizing factor, Laki-Lorand factor, fibrinase, fibrinoligase, and cross-linking enzyme. The active enzyme is a calcium-dependent, sulfhydryl-type transglutaminase (Folk and Chung, 1973). The proenzyme is a contaminant of almost all fibrinogen preparations unless special care is taken to remove or destroy it, although it remains inactive in the absence of calcium ions. Its presence is often turned to advantage, however, since nonstabilized and stabilized fibrin can be prepared from the same fibrinogen batches simply by clotting one with thrombin dissolved in a buffer containing EDTA and the other with thrombin dissolved in a buffer containing calcium ions and a little cysteine.

Activated Factor XIII (= XIIIa) stitches neighboring molecules together by covalently joining the side chains of specific lysine residues with the side chains of certain glutamine acceptors. The result is an ϵ-(γ-glutamyl)lysine cross-link (Fig. 11). Under optimum conditions as many as six of these bonds may be introduced per mole of fibrin monomer (which is, of course, a dimeric molecule) (Pisano *et al.*, 1971), although clot stabilization—as determined by its resistance to dispersal in various solvents capable of dissolving noncross-linked fibrin—may occur after the formation of as few as 2–3 of the bonds per mole.

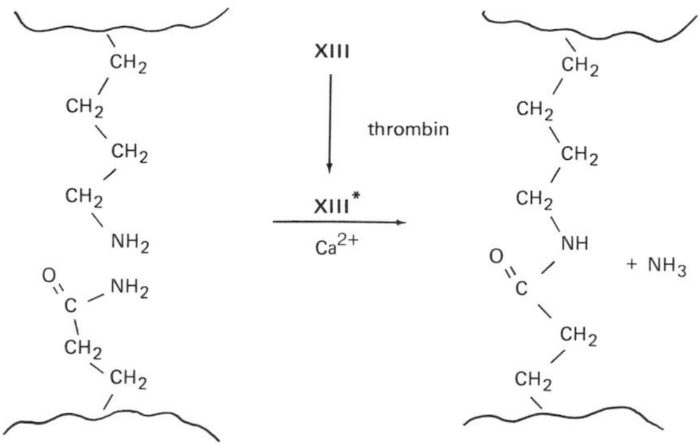

Fig. 11. Formation of ε-(γ-glutamyl)lysine cross-links by condensation of glutamine and lysine side chains.

As a result of this cross-linking, fibrin formed under physiological conditions has somewhat different properties than that formed from the action of purified thrombin on fibrinogen (Robbins, 1944; Laki and Lorand, 1948). Not only is it more resistant to fibrinolysis, but it is also mechanically stronger and ought to be better able to bear the brunt of less specific collisional events *in vivo*. On the other hand, stabilized fibrin does not appear to be morphologically different from the noncross-linked type when viewed in the electron microscope (Kay and Cuddigan, 1967), and it is unlikely that any major structural rearrangement occurs in the polymer during the incorporation of the cross-links.

B. Structural Significance of Fibrin Cross-links

Interest in fibrin cross-linking extends beyond the stabilization process itself, inasmuch as information about the geometry and structure of cross-linked regions should offer insights into how fibrin units are packed together during the polymerization process. In this regard, the first cross-links to be introduced into fibrin during the stabilization process are between γ chains of neighboring molecules (Chen and Doolittle, 1969; Takagi and Iwanaga, 1970). Subsequently, there is a more sluggish introduction of multiple cross-links between α chains (McKee *et al.,* 1970), only a small number of these chains being involved by the time all the γ chains have been cross-linked. These events are nicely visualized by the use of SDS-gels which clearly show that the end product of γ chain cross-linking is a γ–γ dimer (after reduction of interchain disulfide bonds) but that α chains can be progressively tied into covalently bound multimers (Fig. 12).

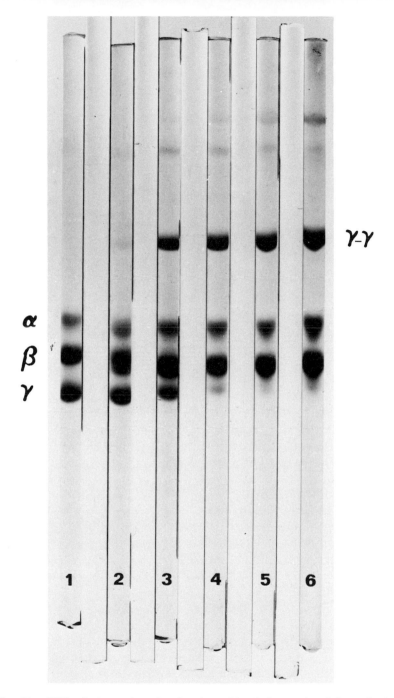

Fig. 12. SDS-gel electrophoresis of polypeptide chains produced by reduction of bovine fibrin forming under cross-linking conditions and poisoned at various time intervals by the addition of a urea-SDS-mercaptoethanol mixture. (1) zero time; (2) 1.5 min; (3) 5 min; (4) 10 min; (5) 25 min; and (6) 40 min. Note disappearance of γ chains concomitant with appearance of γ–γ dimers. α Chain dimers are strongest in (3); α chain trimers are strong in (6). Patterned on the experiments of McKee *et al.* (1970).

HUMAN

```
                    5                    10                   15                   20
... Leu – Thr – Ile – Gly – Glu – Gly – Gln – Gln – His – His – Leu – Gly – Gly – Ala – Lys – Gln – Ala – Gly – Asp – Val – COOH
                                          ↑                                          ↓
      HOOC – Val – Asp – Gly – Ala – Gln – Lys – Ala – Gly – Gly – Leu – His – His – Gln – Gln – Gly – Glu – Gly – Ile – Thr – Leu ...
             20                    15                   10                   5
```

BOVINE

```
                    5                    10                   15                   20
... Leu – Ala – Ile – Gly – Glu – Gly – Gln – Gln – His – Gln – Leu – Gly – Gly – Ala – Lys – Gln – Ala – Gly – Asp – Val – COOH
                                          ↑                                          ↓
      HOOC – Val – Asp – Gly – Ala – Gln – Lys – Ala – Gly – Gly – Leu – Gln – His – Gln – Gln – Gly – Glu – Gly – Ile – Ala – Leu ...
             20                    15                   10                   5
```

Fig. 13. Amino acid sequences of carboxy terminal segments of γ chains showing locations of reciprocal cross-links (arrows) between antiparallel neighboring chains (Chen and Doolittle, 1971).

The complete structure and surrounding amino acid sequences of the γ–γ cross-linking unit have been determined (Chen and Doolittle, 1970, 1971). As it happens, the γ chain cross-linking sites are located in the extreme carboxy terminal segments of those chains, the joined molecules being oriented in an antiparallel fashion and bonded by two reciprocal cross-links (Fig. 13). The cross bridges are only eight residues apart, and space-filling models indicate that opposing α-helical segments would fit together very well. It is important to note that virtually *all* γ chains become paired in this highly restrictive manner, indicating that each of the units in the fibrin polymer has an equivalent orientation.

The argument has been made (Doolittle *et al.,* 1972) that the γ chain cross-linking sites are also primary contact sites in nonstabilized fibrin, the inference being that Factor XIII simply stitches together segments which are already in position. It seems significant that this is a very conservative region of the molecule, there being only three amino acid differences between human and bovine in a 27-residue string available for comparison (Sharp *et al.,* 1972). By contrast, the fibrinopeptides of these two species differ in 17 of 30 comparable residues.

Because the fibrinogen molecule and its fibrin counterpart are dimeric in themselves, the finding of γ–γ dimers might conceivably have been *intramolecular* and not *intermolecular*. Accordingly, advantage was taken of the observed differences between the human and bovine sequences and an experiment performed in which hybrid fibrin was made from a mixture of human and bovine fibrinogen. The demonstration of hybrid cross-linking units clearly established the intermolecular nature of γ–γ dimers in cross-linked fibrin (Doolittle *et al.,* 1971a).

Finally, studies on the plasmin digestion of cross-linked fibrin have demonstrated that the γ–γ cross-linking sites reside in fragment D (Pizzo

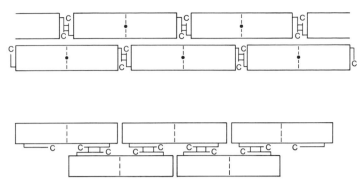

Fig. 14. Schematic representation showing two different ways reciprocal γ–γ dimers could be involved in the formation of intermediate polymers involving staggered overlaps.

et al., 1973; Kopec *et al.,* 1973), thereby positioning the γ chain carboxy terminals in that domain. The linkages themselves might be at the very ends of those domains or back nearer the central region, either case allowing reciprocal linkage (Fig. 14).

Significance of α Chain Cross-linking

The fact that α chains can become involved in multimeric crosslinked systems (McKee *et al.,* 1970) implies that either the donor and acceptor sites are spatially distant — so that different parts of a given chain can be attached to at least two other α chains — or that there are two or more donor–acceptor systems per chain. In fact, there is now good evidence for the latter, two acceptor sites having been reported by a number of laboratories (Chen, 1970; Pisano *et al.,* 1971). Both of these acceptor sites are located in the carboxy terminal half of the α chain (Finlayson and Mosesson, 1973; Ferguson *et al.,* 1974; Takagi and Doolittle, 1974b). Since this is also a portion of the molecule which is exceptionally vulnerable to degradation by various proteolytic enzymes, including plasmin, α chain cross-linking may be compromised in many situations (Mattock and Esnouf, 1971). Its contribution to fibrin stabilization is still not entirely clear, but if, as has been suggested (Doolittle *et al.,* 1972), the α chain cross-links are primarily involved in the stage of polymerization whereby intermediate polymers are laterally bound together — whereas γ chain cross-linking binds the individual units within the intermediate polymer — then only a relatively small number of α chain cross-links ought to increase the overall stabilization very much.

VI. Fibrinolysis

Although an individual's ability to form durable blood clots may be of vital importance, there also has to be some mechanism for clearing away those clots when they are no longer needed or for dissolving any loose fibrin which might break away into the general circulation. In this regard, the complicated system responsible for the generation of thrombin has its counterpart in a system geared to the generation of the enzyme plasmin (fibrinolysin), and, indeed, the two systems may be coupled in some subtle way. Like thrombin, plasmin is converted from an inactive precursor which circulates in the plasma (Robbins and Summaria, 1973). Also, both enzymes belong to the "active serine" class of protease and are clearly descended from the trypsinogen–chymotrypsinogen family (Hartley, 1970). In this regard, it is interesting to note that thrombin always strikes preferentially at arginyl targets—and even then, only in special situations—whereas plasmin has a decided preference for lysine sites (Weinstein and Doolittle, 1972). Trypsin, as is well known, is much less discriminating, cleaving virtually all arginyl and lysyl peptide bonds.

We have already commented on the large number of *in vitro* studies on the plasmin digestion of fibrinogen—primarily aimed at elucidating the structure of the latter molecule—and although a significant amount of fibrinogenolysis does indeed occur *in vivo*, the physiologically more important event must be the plasmin digestion of fibrin (as opposed to fibrinogen). As noted previously, the products produced by the plasmin digestion of fibrin are remarkably similar to those obtained from fibrinogen (Dudek *et al.*, 1970). The fragments obtained from the digestion of cross-linked fibrin are also similar, with the notable exception of those fragments which are actually involved in the cross-linking (Section V). On the other hand, the rate of digestion of cross-linked fibrin is significantly slower, and the possibility exists that access routes for the enzyme are more congested or less readily cleared (Gormsen *et al.*, 1967).

Although emphasis is usually put on those features of the fibrinogen molecule which might lend themselves to a ready transition to a polymeric system (its being dimeric, for example), it bears mentioning that the molecular design seems also drafted to afford easy reversal of the process by proteolytic digestion. In effect, the fibrinogen molecule seems to have evolved in a manner consistent with the dynamic balance which typifies the maintenance of intravascular fluidity while simultaneously retaining a potential for clot formation. Thus, not only can fibrinogen be gelled by the cleavage of only two peptide bonds (out of approximately 3000!) per molecule, but the ensuing gel can be rendered soluble by the splitting of a very small number of bonds also (Weinstein and Doolittle, 1972). Presumably, the cleavages that count most are those that occur between the fragments D and E. It can be expected that not every unit in the polymer has to be attacked and that lysis (i.e., dissolution of the clot as a separate phase) may occur at a point when a significant number of intermediate polymers remain, corresponding in essence to the occurrence of intermediate polymers during fibrin polymerization. Under most conditions these soluble remnants would be digested further, of course, until the terminal D and E core fragments are all that remain.

Possible Aftereffects of Lysis Products

The breakdown products of fibrin, as well as fibrinogen, might conceivably have further physiological significance, dealing directly or indirectly with hemostasis or wound repair. The terminal core fragments are large enough that they should not readily pass the kidney, and the general frugality of nature as expressed through evolution makes it attractive to search for secondary roles "after-the-fact." Indeed, a variety of effects have been claimed for one or another of these split products, including antipolymerant and antithrombin activity (Latallo *et al.*, 1964), inhibition of thrombin generation (Takaki *et al.*, 1972), interference with platelet aggregation (Stachurska *et al.*, 1971), stimulation of fibrinogen biosynthesis (Barnhart *et al.*, 1970), and even leukocyte chemotactic effects (Stecher and Sorkin, 1972).

Of all these, there is universal agreement that split products (whether derived from fibrinogen or fibrin) can inhibit fibrin polymerization *in vitro* by terminating chain growth. How influential this inhibition might be in maintaining intravascular fluidity under physiological circumstances remains a matter of conjecture. As for the other effects reported, it remains to be seen how many of them will bear the test of time and further scrutiny.

VII. Biosynthesis of Fibrinogen

As far as has been determined, the bulk of mammalian fibrinogen — if not all — is synthesized in the liver. More precisely, immunofluorescent studies have demonstrated that it is synthesized and stored in hepatocytes (Barnhart and Forman, 1963). So far very little is known of the molecular dynamics of fibrinogen biosynthesis, and it is still unclear as to whether the three nonidentical chains are synthesized independently and then combined, or whether one long chain is translated, folded, and

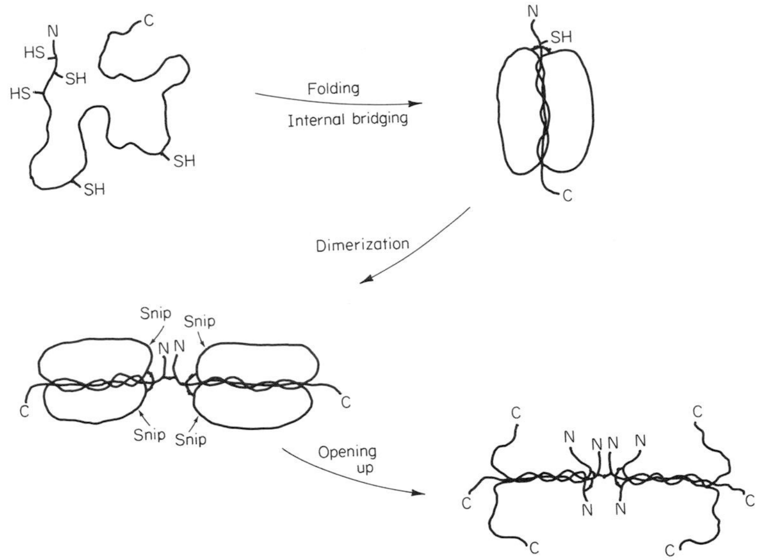

Fig. 15. Hypothetical scheme for assembly of fibrinogen molecule starting with large molecular weight precursor chain that is snipped into constituent nonidentical chains after folding. Snipping could occur either before or after joining of half-molecules (Doolittle, 1973).

then snipped appropriately to yield the final equivalent of a half-molecule (Fig. 15). The reason for speculating that the latter might be the case lies not only with the inherent complications of synchronizing the assembly of a six-chained structure — and, indeed, no one has been able to reassemble a fibrinogen molecule after breaking the interchain disulfide bonds — but also because of the ease with which fibrinogen is denatured. The molecule seems to lack the innate stability that many proteins have which are folded *de novo;* instead, it seems to be poised in some metastable state ready to collapse upon the least provocation, as though some of its struts had been kicked away after its original assembly. It must be noted, nonetheless, that so far there is no experimental basis for a precursor fibrinogen molecule (profibrinogen), and that this is not for a lack of looking.

Regulation of Fibrinogen Biosynthesis

The amounts of fibrinogen in the plasma can vary widely. Like a number of other plasma proteins, fibrinogen is an "acute phase" protein, its concentration being markedly elevated in the wake of various inflammatory or traumatic experiences suffered by the individual. The basis of this phenomenon remains mysterious, but it is known that fibrinogen synthesis can be stimulated by the administration of a variety of hormones, and especially corticotropin (Atencio *et al.,* 1969). Other experiments have indicated that fibrinogen and fibrin degradation products may be agents for signaling the release of stored fibrinogen and inducing the synthesis of additional material (Barnhart *et al.,* 1970), although contrary evidence has been reported (Otis and Rapaport, 1973).

VIII. Genetics of Fibrinogen

In a sense, any discussion of the genetics of a system ought to start with a few words about the genes involved. In the case of fibrinogen, however, it is not yet known how many genes are involved. At first glance, it might be assumed *a priori* that there is simply one gene for each of the three nonidentical chains in the molecule. But, as noted in the previous section, it is not impossible that a single gene might be translated into a very long polypeptide chain and then processed into the functional half-molecule. On the other hand, regardless of the primary gene to polypeptide chain correspondence, there are other possibilities for multiplicity. For example, is there a separate gene system for a fetal fibrinogen molecule? Similarly, is platelet fibrinogen coded for by the same gene system as plasma fibrinogen? Or, on another tack, does any of the well-known heterogeneity of plasma fibrinogen have a genetic basis, as might arise either from "minor" genes or polymorphic alleles?

A. Human Afibrinogenemia and Dysfibrinogenemias

Congenital fibrinogen abnormalities among humans are relatively rare, although this is at least partly attributable to their not having been looked for very much in the past. Two quite different situations exist and are distinguished as follows. Afibrinogenemia is a "total" absence of fibrinogen as determined by immunological means as well as by the absence of a clottable molecule (Girolami *et al.,* 1971). It can be classified clinically — and perhaps often confused with — hypofibrinogenemia, in which cases there is a very small amount of fibrinogen, usually detectable only by immunological means (Barbui *et al.,* 1972). Dysfibrinogenemia, on the other hand, is a situation in which a defective fibrinogen molecule is present. It may be clottable to varying degrees depending on the nature of the molecular change, but it is almost fully cross-reactive in an immunological sense, since fibrinogen has a variety of antigenic determinants, not all of which would likely be disturbed by a mutant geometry. In the most severe circumstances the affected molecule may never form a clot; in mild situations it may clot slowly upon the addition of thrombin *in vitro,* but behave within normal limits under physiological circumstances when calcium ion and Factor XIII are present to help the situation to completion.

The majority of abnormal fibrinogens studied to date exhibit defective polymerization in a reaggregation system (von Felten *et al.,* 1966), but a few are defective only in that the fibrinopeptides A are slow to be released (Gralnick *et al.,* 1971). The former type usually inhibits the polymerization of normal fibrinogen or reaggregating fibrin systems, presumably by becoming involved in growing fibers themselves. As a consequence, an individual heterozygous for a dysfibrinogenemia may actually be worse off than a person heterozygous for afibrinogenemia, since the latter is characterized only by a somewhat lowered fibrinogen level, all the molecules being perfectly functional. The dysfibrinogenemic carrier, however, has a mixed population of molecules, which not only makes chemical characterization of the abnormal molecule difficult, since it must be purified away from the normal (von Felten *et al.,* 1969), but also because the interference in polymerization by the abnormal molecules can lead to slower clotting. In the antiquated language of classic genetics, the dysfibrinogenemics are *dominant* in severe cases or *codominant* in mildly affected molecules. Afibrinogenemia, on the other hand, is hardly ever detected in a heterozygote except during a study of the family tree of a homozygote, and in classic parlance would be called a *recessive.* In both cases, there is agreement that no evidence exists for any sex-linkage of the genes involved, females being afflicted about as often as males.

In only one case so far has an amino acid replacement been identified in a variant human fibrinogen (M. Blombäck *et al.,* 1968), one of the residues in the disulfide knot of human fibrinogen Detroit having undergone an arginine to serine substitution. The location of the replacement is just two residues away from the amino terminal glycine of the fibrin α chain, a site predicted as a polymerization site by Bailey and Bettelheim (1955). Although the possibility of other structural changes in this molecule cannot be ruled out (Mammen *et al.,* 1969), it appears likely that this single amino acid replacement is responsible for the virtual abolition of fibrin polymerization in the homozygous individual studied. This might be because the peptide segment actually represents a contact site, or it might be that the loss of the positively charged arginine side chain has changed the distribution of charge sufficiently that electrostatic alignment of the polymerizing molecules is hampered. The change might

TABLE V

A Listing of Some "Variant" Human Fibrinogens with References to the Original Literature[a]

Variant	References	Variant	References
Amsterdam	Jansen and Vreeken, 1971	Metz	Soria *et al.*, 1972
Baltimore	Beck *et al.*, 1965	Montreal	Lacombe *et al.*, 1973
Bethesda I	Gralnick *et al.*, 1971	Parma	Imperato and Dettori, 1958
Bethesda II	Gralnick *et al.*, 1973	Paris I	Ménaché, 1964
Cleveland I	Forman *et al.*, 1968	Paris II	Samama *et al.*, 1969
Cleveland II	Crum *et al.*, 1974	Philadelphia	Martinez *et al.*, 1974
Detroit	Mammen *et al.*, 1969	St. Louis	Sherman *et al.*, 1972
Giessen	Krause *et al.*, 1973	Troyes	Soria *et al.*, 1972
Iowa City	Jacobsen and Hoak, 1973	Zurich	von Felten *et al.*, 1969

[a] As it is used here, the term "variant" human fibrinogen applies to fibrinogens which are slow to clot or do not clot upon the addition of exogenous thrombin. With the exception of fibrinogen Detroit (see text), the amino acid replacements responsible for the defective clotting have not been determined.

also have effected a large-scale conformational shift affecting contact sites elsewhere in the molecule. Recently it has been reported that the defect in fibrinogen Paris I is associated with its γ chain (Budzynski *et al.*, 1974). The affected molecules polymerize poorly and cannot be cross-linked into γ–γ dimers, in accord with earlier suggestions that the γ chain cross-linking site in fibrinogen ought also to be a primary polymerization site (Doolittle *et al.*, 1972).

A complete listing of abnormal fibrinogens has been assembled by Ménaché (1973); a more limited tabulation is presented in Table V. Although the field is still a long way from the remarkable correlation of structural changes and dysfunctions achieved in the case of human hemoglobin (Perutz and Lehmann, 1968), further structural studies on those variant fibrinogens already identified as well as on others as yet undiscovered ought to provide critical information about those features of the molecule which are associated with specific events in the conversion to fibrin.

B. Platelet Fibrinogen

Mammalian blood platelets contain a thrombin-clottable protein — platelet fibrinogen — independent of any plasma fibrinogen adsorbed to the external surface of the platelet (Nachman, 1965; Solum and Lopaciuk, 1969). Platelet fibrinogen cross-reacts with antibodies produced against plasma fibrinogen, but a variety of reports have indicated that it differs significantly from plasma fibrinogen with regard to hydrodynamic properties, mobility on SDS-gels, clottability by thrombin and susceptibility to attack by plasmin (Ganguly, 1972). Its very existence has served as a convenient possibility for rationalizing some of the widely observed heterogeneity in plasma fibrinogen preparations (Henschen and Edman, 1972). Some investigators have attributed the bulk of the observed differences between platelet and plasma fibrinogen to degradation by the highly active proteolytic systems in platelets, but others have expressed the belief that the two fibrinogen molecules are fundamentally different in origin as well as structure (James and Ganguly, 1973). It has been reported that fibrinogen can be synthesized in platelets, although the data remain sketchy and debatable (Rosiek *et al.,* 1969). It has also been claimed that no exchange occurs between plasma fibrinogen synthesized in the liver and the platelet variety (Castaldi and Caen, 1965). Finally, immunological evidence has also been presented which purports to show structural differences between the two types of molecule (Plow and Edgington, 1974).

In spite of this array of data seeming to demonstrate the individuality of platelet fibrinogen, there is really little doubt that the two fibrinogens are products of the same gene system. First and foremost, the amount of fibrinogen in platelets from persons with afibrinogenemia is greatly reduced (Nachman and Marcus, 1968). Second, if great care is taken to reduce proteolysis during storage and isolation of the platelet fibrinogen, many of the observed differences disappear or are greatly reduced (Fig. 16). Finally, the amino acid compositions of human fibrinopeptides A and B isolated from platelet fibrinogen are identical with those from human plasma fibrinogen (Doolittle *et al.,* 1974a). Inasmuch as the fibrinopeptides are among the most changeable peptide structures known, it would be anticipated that amino acid differences should have been found in these regions if they existed at all. The fact that they are identical argues strongly for a single genetic system.

Whether or not the platelet fibrinogen is synthesized in the platelet, however, is something which ought to be pursued more thoroughly. It is entirely possible that fibrinogen, as well as a number of other plasma proteins found in platelets, becomes a part of the platelet system at an early step in the development of the platelet, before or during its budding off from the parental megakaryocyte. There is also some basis for believing that its accumulation there may have something to do with binding to thrombasthenin, the contractile protein of platelets, since platelet fibrinogen levels are reported to be very low in persons afflicted with thrombasthenia (Nachman and Marcus, 1968).

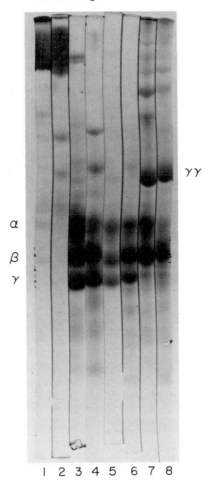

Fig. 16. SDS-gel electrophoresis (6% polyacrylamide) of human plasma and platelet fibrinogens and fibrins: (1) plasma fibrinogen, unreduced; (2) platelet fibrinogen, unreduced; (3) plasma fibrinogen, reduced; (4) platelet fibrinogen, reduced; (5) fibrin (reduced) prepared from plasma fibrinogen; (6) fibrin (reduced) prepared from platelet fibrinogen; (7) cross-linked fibrin (reduced) prepared from plasma fibrinogen; and (8) cross-linked fibrin (reduced) prepared from platelet fibrinogen (Doolittle *et al.,* 1974a).

C. Fetal Fibrinogen

The possible existence of a fetal fibrinogen, analogous to fetal hemoglobin, was first reported by Burstein *et al.* (1954). Those workers observed that the fibrin clot of the newborn is more transparent and less compressible than the adult type, the implication being that the starting fibrinogen molecules were different. The difference in gelation was sensitive to pH, however, being most severe at pH 8.6 but hardly detectable at pH 6.9. The issue was pursued subsequently by Künzer (1961) and his colleagues who noted that, whereas newborn children frequently have low amounts of other clotting factors, their fibrinogen levels are usually the same as occur in the adult (Künzer, 1964).

Witt and her co-workers (1969) isolated fibrinogen from human cord blood, and although its overall amino acid composition was indistinguishable from the adult type, it eluted somewhat later upon DEAE-cellulose chromatography. Fingerprints of tryptic digests — a formidable task for a molecule containing approximately 190 arginines and lysines per half molecule — revealed at least three different peptides among the 40–50 that stained most strongly. Further studies (Witt and Müller, 1970) resulted in the finding that the fetal fibrinogen has almost twice as much inorganic phosphorus per mole as the adult type, and it is possible that the different peptides observed on fingerprints were due to phosphorylation of peptides which are not phosphorylated in the adult type. Fetal fibrinogen was found to have the same hexose content as adult fibrinogen (Witt and Müller, 1970). Consistent with earlier findings, these workers found a pH dependence for the thrombin-catalyzed conversion of fetal fibrinogen to fibrin which was different from the adult type, clotting being significantly retarded at moderately high pH (Witt *et al.*, 1969).

Mills and Karpatkin (1972), investigating the notion that human fetal plasma (cord blood) is slow to clot upon the addition of thrombin, concluded that the delay is due to a greater content of preformed fibrin in cord blood fibrinogen preparations. Their finding that fibrinogen from cord blood — when care is taken to exclude preformed fibrin — is indistinguishable from adult fibrinogen upon SDS-gel electrophoresis, and isoelectric focusing challenges the existence of a distinctive fetal fibrinogen in humans. Loly *et al.* (1971) had previously come to the same conclusion after an exhaustive comparison of sheep fetal and adult fibrinogens, no significant differences being found.

IX. Evolution of the Fibrinogen–Fibrin System

Blood coagulation in all vertebrates follows the same fundamental plan, culminating in a fibrinogen to fibrin conversion which is effected by fibrinopeptide removal. Thrombin from any vertebrate species will clot the fibrinogen of virtually any other, although the clotting times involved vary more or less inversely with the evolutionary relationship of the species involved. In extreme cases, thrombins from distantly related creatures may effect clotting by releasing only one of the two sets of fibrinopeptides (Doolittle *et al.,* 1962; Doolittle, 1965a). These heterologous interactions of thrombin and fibrinogen are classic manifestations of the general phenomenon loosely referred to as "species specificity" in which interacting macromolecules from a given organism seem to be co-adapted for maximum effectiveness.

In spite of the general cross-reactivity of thrombins and fibrinogens from different vertebrate classes, immunological cross-reactivity is usually limited to a single vertebrate class (Kenton, 1933; Hektoen and Welker, 1927). For example, antibodies raised against mammalian fibrinogen do not precipitate avian fibrinogens and vice-versa, indicating that the superficial aspects of their structures have been prone to substantial variation during evolution. An illustration of this propensity for change has already been encountered in our discussion of the fibrinopeptides, which are among the most variable peptide structures studied.

For the most part, the physicochemical properties of those vertebrate fibrinogens which have been examined all seem to be very similar, and the same purification schemes which have been developed for mammalian fibrinogens have been applied to plasmas of all vertebrate classes (Finlayson and Mosesson, 1964). Surveys of many vertebrate fibrins using SDS-gel electrophoresis have revealed that the molecular weights of γ and β chains have remained fairly constant during mammalian evolution, but α chains vary substantially (Schwartz *et al.,* 1973; Doolittle, 1973). Among mammals the largest α chains are found to exist among the equines (horses, donkeys, and mules), increasing the apparent molecular weight of an $\alpha_2\beta_2\gamma_2$ fibrinogen unit to approximately 380,000 for these creatures (Fig. 17).

A. Lamprey Fibrinogen

The characteristic six-chained fibrinogen structure comprised of two pairs of three nonidentical polypeptides exists even in the most primitive vertebrate extant, the lamprey (Doolittle, 1965a). This molecule can be clotted by mammalian thrombins, although in so doing the mammalian thrombins only release a set of fibrinopeptides corresponding to mammalian fibrinopeptide B. This is a large peptide ($n = 36$ residues) with a covalently attached carbohydrate cluster (Doolittle and Cottrell, 1974). The B designation was originally made because the peptide contains the rare amino acid tyrosine-*O*-sulfate, a residue which also occurs in many

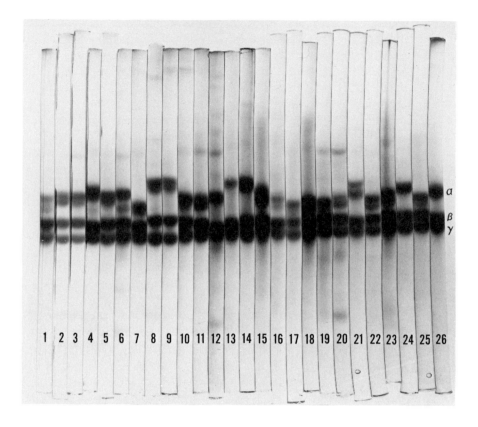

Fig. 17. SDS electrophoresis gels of individual α, β, and γ chains produced upon reduction of fibrins from 26 selected mammalian species representing five orders (Primates, Perissodactyls, Carnivores, Artiodactyls, and Proboscids). (1) Human, (2) chimpanzee, (3) gorilla, (4) orangutan, (5) siamang, (6) cebus monkey, (7) slow loris, (8) horse, (9) donkey, (10) rhinoceros, (11) tapir, (12) golden jackal, (13) black bear, (14) collared peccary, (15) vicuna, (16) muntjak, (17) elk, (18) pronghorn, (19) sheep, (20) ibex, (21) impala, (22) Grant's gazelle. (23) Persian gazelle, (24) yak, (25) water buffalo, and (26) Indian elephant. In many cases the α chain appears as a doublet; this may be due to ancillary degradation during fibrin formation, or it may reflect inherent polymorphism. Most of the gels represent individual animal specimens (Doolittle, 1973).

mammalian fibrinopeptides B; further sequence studies on the parent molecule side of the junction split have borne out this assignment (Fig. 18). Lamprey thrombin clots lamprey fibrinogen by releasing both fibrinopeptides A and fibrinopeptides B; the A peptide only has six residues. As in all fibrinopeptides examined to date, the carboxy terminus is arginine. It is remarkable that the lamprey fibrinopeptides are so very

Human α	...Gly-Val-Arg	Gly-Pro-Arg-Val-Val-Glu-Arg...
Bovine α	...Gly-Val-Arg	Gly-Pro-Arg-Leu-Val-Glx-Arg...
Lamprey α	...Ser-Leu-Arg	Gly-Pro-Arg-Leu- ? -Glx-Glx...

Human β	...Ser-Ala-Arg	Gly-His-Arg-Pro-Leu-Asp-Lys...
Bovine β	...Gly-Ala-Arg	Gly-His-Arg-Pro-Tyr-Asx-Lys...
Lamprey β	...Asp-Val-Arg	Gly-Val-Arg-Pro-Leu-Pro- ? ...

Fig. 18. Comparison of amino acid sequences cleaved by thrombins in α and β chains of human, bovine, and lamprey fibrinogens. Mammalian thrombins cleave the lamprey β chain but not the lamprey α chain during *in vitro* clotting (Doolittle and Cottrell, 1975).

different from those found in mammals, while the amino terminal portions of fibrin exposed upon their release are almost identical to mammalian types (Fig. 18).

On SDS-gels the α chains of lamprey fibrinogen appear to be oversized relative to mammalian types (Doolittle, 1973; Murtaugh *et al.,* 1974), even though other data suggest that lamprey fibrinogen has about the same molecular weight as mammalian fibrinogen (Doolittle *et al.,* 1962; Murtaugh *et al.,* 1974). In spite of their homologous amino terminals, lamprey α chains have a very distinctive amino acid composition, 45% of the residues being threonine, serine, or glycine. It may be that this unusual amino acid composition is responsible for the anomalous migration on SDS-gels (Doolittle and Cottrell, 1975).

Cross-linking of lamprey fibrin occurs along the same lines as occurs in mammalian systems, γ–γ dimers forming very quickly, followed by the slow incorporation of α chains into multimer units (Doolittle and Wooding, 1974). The fibrinogen of this ancient beast continues to be an object of much study, and it may well be that significant insights into the mechanism of fibrin formation will be gained by discovering which molecular features have been most rigorously conserved over the past 400 million years.

B. Where Did Vertebrate Fibrinogen Come From?

Given that all vertebrates extant today have a *bona fide* fibrinogen molecule, the question arises as to where the molecule evolved from in the first place. Ascidians and other protochordates seem not to have an extracellular protein comparable to vertebrate fibrinogen, and although some invertebrates have a circulating protein which can be gelled under

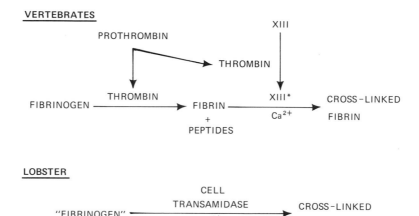

Fig. 19. Comparison of vertebrate and lobster blood coagulation systems. The complex sequence of events leading to the transformation of prothrombin to thrombin in vertebrates has been omitted. Similarly, the events provoking the disruption of the coagulocytes containing the transamidase (transglutaminase) which clots lobster fibrinogen have not been included.

appropriate circumstances, the systems seem to have evolved independently. For example, some crustaceans, including the lobster, have a protein in their blood which is referred to as "fibrinogen" and which can be "clotted" by a calcium-dependent enzyme found in certain blood cells (coagulocytes) (Fig. 19). The fibrinogen has a completely different structure from vertebrate fibrinogen, however (Table VI). Moreover, the gelation is effected by the direct introduction of covalent bonds, no pep-

TABLE VI

A Comparison of Some Properties of Lobster and Vertebrate Fibrinogens

	Lobster[a]	Vertebrate[b]
Molecular weight (MW)	420,000	340,000
Sedimentation coefficient ($s_{20,w}$)	14.5	7.9
Diffusion coefficient ($D_{20,w}$)	2.9	2.0
Partial specific volume ($\bar{v}$)	0.71	0.71–0.72
Extinction coefficient ($E^{1\%}_{1\,cm,280}$)	12.5	15.8
Polypeptide chains	2	2×3
Amino terminal end groups	Leucine	Variable

[a] Fuller and Doolittle (1971a); Doolittle and Fuller (1972).
[b] See also Table I.

tide material being released in the process. It is interesting, nonetheless, that the covalent bonds are ε-(γ-glutamyl)lysine bonds, the same as are introduced into vertebrate fibrin during stabilization (Fuller and Doolittle, 1971b). That this is not such an unexpected coincidence is now better appreciated as the virtual ubiquity of tissue enzymes capable of introducing such links is becoming known (Folk and Chung, 1973). The blood cells of the horseshoe crab, *Limulus polyphemus,* contain a coagulable protein ("coagulogen") which has a molecular weight of the order of 25,000 (Solum, 1973). Its gelation is apparently provoked by an endotoxin-initiated catalysis of another intracellular protein.

If the vertebrate fibrinogen molecule is not directly related to invertebrate analogs, this still leaves unanswered the question as to where its ancestry does lie. The amino acid sequence studies performed on mammalian fibrinogen so far have not yet revealed any segments which are obviously related to the known sequences of other fibrous proteins such as keratin, myosin, or collagen, although some intriguing physical similarities to prekeratin have been pointed out recently (Skerrow, 1974). The possibility exists that fibrinogen may be related to one or more of the other thrombin-sensitive proteins involved in blood clotting, including Factors V, VIII, and/or XIII. In the last named case, however, a detailed comparison of the amino acid sequences in the thrombin-attacked segments failed to show any significant sign of common ancestry other than the arginyl-glycine cleavage site itself (Takagi and Doolittle, 1974a). Moreover, should any indication of common ancestry surface for any of these proteins, it would seem more likely that these descended from fibrinogen rather than the other way around.

There is reasonable cause for thinking that the three nonidentical chains (α, β, and γ) are themselves homologous, some regions of these chains having very similar sequences. In particular, all three chains have one pentapeptide skein in the disulfide knot where the sequences are all . . . . CYS-PRO-Thr/Ser-Thr/Gly-CYS . . . . (Blombäck and Blombäck, 1972). It is not impossible that this unusual arrangement evolved independently in all three chains, but it seems highly unlikely. Also, it has been reported that α and β chains are immunologically cross-reactive (Gollwitzer *et al.,* 1972). Moreover, the very fact that thrombin releases fibrinopeptides from the amino termini of the α and β chains served as a basis for conjecture that these two chains were descended from a common ancestor (Doolittle, 1970). On the other hand, the very different amino acid compositions of the α and β chains, the cross-linking of α chains but not β chains, and the unusual vulnerability of α chains to proteolysis, all argue for very different structures and functions and against common ancestry.

X. Some Clinical Aspects

The fibrinogen–fibrin transformation has widespread importance in very many medical situations involving potential or actual hemorrhagic or thrombotic occurrences. Although this section could not possibly describe any of those clinical problems in a proper manner, it does seem appropriate to comment on a few areas in which a better understanding of the molecular events could not fail to prove beneficial.

As a starting place, we can note that in normal healthy persons the clotting of the blood plasma *in vitro* — either by endogenously generated or exogenous thrombin — leads to a total consumption of fibrinogen or any fibrinogen derivatives which might be present. On the other hand, in many traumatic situations, including those typified by a consumptive coagulopathy where many of the clotting factors are greatly reduced, the *serum* may contain significant amounts of fibrinogen and/or fibrinogen-related substances. These latter have been reported to be soluble fibrin monomers, fibrinogen–fibrin monomer complexes, and/or intermediate polymers, as well as the degradation products called fragments X, Y, D, and E.

The tests used for establishing the presence of these substances fall into two classes, immunological and nonimmunological. The former depend on the interaction of these substances with antibodies raised in animals to fibrinogen, fibrin or the various degradation products. They range all the way from relatively insensitive simple immunodiffusion tests to very sensitive fixation tests with latex beads coated with antifibrinogen antibodies (Garvey and Black, 1972) and a scheme in which fibrinogen is adsorbed to tanned red cells (Merskey *et al.*, 1966) (TRCHII = tanned red cell hemagglutination inhibition immunoassay).

Among the nonimmunological assays are the ethanol-gelation test (Godal and Abildgaard, 1966), which purportedly causes soluble fibrinogen–fibrin complexes to gel, the protamine sulfate precipitation method (Sanfellippo *et al.*, 1971), which also aims at soluble large molecular weight fibrinogen derivatives (compare Section IV,A), and the staphylococcal clumping test (Allington, 1967). The latter is based on the casual observation that fibrinogen alone among the plasma proteins can cause certain strains of *Staphylococcus aureus* to agglutinate.[4] Quite apart from the usefulness of the staphylococcal clumping test for the clinical determination of fibrinogen and its derivatives (including fragments X and Y, but probably not D and E) (Marder *et al.*, 1971), the phenom-

---

[4] The clumping factor should not be confused with the quite different situation in which certain staphylococcal strains excrete a coagulase which can initiate a clotting reaction under appropriate circumstances.

enon itself merits intensive study since it focuses on some very unique structural feature of the fibrinogen molecule. Whatever it is that causes the clumping, it is quite stable in a physical sense (Sternberger and Hörmann, 1974). Interestingly enough, not all (but most) species have fibrinogens capable of this action (Duthie, 1954; Lewis and Wilson, 1973).

In all of the above cases, the presence of the fibrinogen-related materials in serum is regarded as presumptive evidence of recent intravascular clotting, especially when combined with a knowledge of low levels of other clotting factors. Disseminated intravascular clotting can be initiated by a wide variety of agents, among the most common of which can be mentioned bacterial infections, endotoxins released from dying bacteria, general tissue damage, pregnancy complications, and many others. Other indices of *in vivo* thrombin activity include radioimmunoassays designed specifically to measure free fibrinopeptide A (Nossel *et al.,* 1971).

The clinical sector of fibrinogen–fibrin research extends well beyond more efficient tests for the detection of disseminated intravascular coagulation, of course. The entire natural histories of pulmonary embolisms, cerebral strokes, and coronary thromboses are interwoven with the dynamics of fibrin deposition and propagation. The introduction of ^{125}I-labeled fibrinogen for monitoring fibrinogen metabolism and scanning for potential emboli has become very popular, although a degree of caution about conclusions is still warranted (Krohn *et al.,* 1972). On the surgical front, tissue damage, clotting, and wound healing are naturally related, and an obvious objective is to insure good fibrin deposition at wound sites while minimizing fibrin formation elsewhere. In the area of prosthetic devices, the search continues for materials which will not serve as such attractive sites for fibrin deposition. Again, thromboembolic complications are very common in malignant disease, in many cases as a direct result of a hyperfibrinogenemia (Brugarolas *et al.,* 1972). Finally, the importance of fibrin formation in many natural events — birth and repair of the cord stump, menstrual cessation, the simple bumps and bruises of everyday life — must be appreciated. For although some afibrinogenemics do indeed reach adulthood without major catastrophe (Section VIII), it is a chancy business fraught with risk.

XI. Concluding Remarks

In the preceding pages I have attempted to interweave some chemical and biological — and even some medical — aspects of the fibrinogen–fibrin transformation. This event, common to all vertebrates, plays a significant role in preventing blood loss among the sick and healthy alike. The principal molecule in this drama is fibrinogen, an entity artfully designed by natural selection for one special happening, whereby an individual molecule is activated once in its lifetime in order to become a part of a fibrin polymer. Beyond that, the molecule is adapted in such a way that an efficient fibrinolysis may subsequently ensue. Although much has been learned about these events in recent years, much remains undetermined. And although the entire amino acid sequence of the human fibrinogen molecule will soon be established,[5] the real interest is in the three-dimensional structure. For therein lie the answers to the questions about the nature and location of the contact sites and the conditions which actually allow polymerization upon release of the fibrinopeptides. Several other matters, such as those having to do with the molecule's biosynthesis and evolution, ought soon to be clarified. And with all these answers and insights, perhaps it will be possible to more intelligently modulate the transformation of fibrinogen into fibrin in those medical situations where it is a primary or complicating factor.

REFERENCES

Allington, M. J. (1967). *Brit. J. Haematol.* **13,** 550.

Atencio, A. C., Chao, P.-Y., Chen, A. Y., and Reeve, E. B. (1969). *Amer. J. Physiol.* **216,** 773.

Bailey, K., and Bettelheim, F. R. (1955). *Brit. Med. Bull.* **11,** 50.

Bailey, K., Astbury, W. T., and Rudall, K. M. (1943). *Nature (London)* **151,** 716.

Bailey, K., Bettelheim, F. R., Lorand, L., and Middlebrook, W. R. (1951). *Nature (London)* **167,** 233.

Barbui, T., Porciello, P. I., and Dini, E. (1972). *Thromb. Diath. Haemorrh.* **28,** 129.

Barnhart, M. I., and Forman, W. B. (1963). *Vox Sang.* **8,** 461.

Barnhart, M. I., Cress, D. C., Noonan, S. M., and Walsh, R. T. (1970). *Thromb. Diath. Haemorrh., Suppl.* **39,** 143.

Beck, E. A., Charache, P., and Jackson, D. P. (1965). *Nature (London)* **208,** 143.

Belitser, V. A., Manjakov, V. P., and Varetskaja, T. V. (1971). *Biochim. Biophys. Acta* **236,** 546.

Belitser, V. A., Varetska, T. V., and Manjakov, V. P. (1973). *Thromb. Res.* **2,** 567.

Bettelheim, F. R. (1954). *J. Amer. Chem. Soc.* **76,** 2838.

Bettelheim, F. R., and Bailey, K. (1952). *Biochim. Biophys. Acta* **9,** 578.

Birnboim, M. H., and Lederer, K. (1972). *Polym. Prep., Amer. Chem. Soc., Div. Polym. Chem.* **13,** 203.

Blombäck, B. (1958). *Ark. Kemi* **12,** 99.

Blombäck, B., and Blombäck, M. (1956). *Ark. Kemi* **10,** 415.

Blombäck, B., and Blombäck, M. (1968). *In* "Chemotaxonomy and Serotaxonomy" (J. G. Hawkes, ed.), p. 3. Academic Press, New York.

---

[5] At least five laboratories around the world are currently conducting major sequencing studies on fibrinogen. At the time of this writing, approximately one-third of the 1500 residues in a half-molecule of human fibrinogen have been positioned.

Blombäck, B., and Blombäck, M. (1972). *Ann. N.Y. Acad. Sci.* **202**, 77.

Blombäck, B., and Doolittle, R. F. (1963a). *Acta Chem. Scand.* **17**, 1816.

Blombäck, B., and Doolittle, R. F. (1963b). *Acta Chem. Scand.* **17**, 1819.

Blombäck, B., and Yamashina, I. (1958). *Ark. Kemi* **12**, 299.

Blombäck, B., Blombäck, M., and Nilsson, J. M. (1957). *Thromb. Diath. Haemorrh.* **1**, 76.

Blombäck, B., Blombäck, M., Edman, P., and Hessel, B. (1962). *Nature (London)* **193**, 883.

Blombäck, B., Blombäck, M., and Searle, J. (1963). *Biochim. Biophys. Acta* **74**, 148.

Blombäck, B., Blombäck, M., Henschen, A., Hessel, B., Iwanaga, S., and Woods, K. R. (1968). *Nature (London)* **218**, 130.

Blombäck, M., Blombäck, B., Mammen, E. F., and Prasad, A. S. (1968). *Nature (London)* **218**, 134.

Brown, M. E., and Rothstein, F. (1967). *Science* **155**, 1017.

Brugarolas, A., Mink, I. B., Elias, E. G., and Mittelman, A. (1972). *Surg. Gynecol. Obstet.* **135**, 75.

Budzynski, A. Z., Marder, V. J., Ménaché, D., and Guillin, M.-C. (1974). *Nature (London)* **252**, 66.

Burstein, M., Lewi, S., and Walter, P. (1954). *Sang* **25**, 102.

Cartwright, T., and Kekwick, R. G. O. (1971). *Biochim. Biophys. Acta* **236**, 550.

Castaldi, P. A., and Caen, J. (1965). *J. Clin. Pathol.* **18**, 579.

Chen, R. (1970). Ph.D. Dissertation, University of California, San Diego.

Chen, R., and Doolittle, R. F. (1969). *Proc. Nat. Acad. Sci. U.S.* **63**, 420.

Chen, R., and Doolittle, R. F. (1970). *Proc. Nat. Acad. Sci. U.S.* **66**, 472.

Chen, R., and Doolittle, R. F. (1971). *Biochemistry* **10**, 4486.

Clegg, J. B., and Bailey, K. (1962). *Biochim. Biophys. Acta* **63**, 525.

Cohen, C. (1961). *J. Polym. Sci.* **49**, 144.

Cohn, E. J., Strong, L. E., Hughes, W. L., Jr., Mulford, D. J., Ashworth, J. N., Melin, M., and Taylor, H. L. (1946). *J. Amer. Chem. Soc.* **68**, 459.

Crum, E. D., Shainoff, J. R., Graham, R. C., and Ratnoff, O. D. (1974). *J. Clin. Invest.* **53**, 1308.

Davie, E. W., and Hanahan, D. J. (1976). *In* "The Plasma Proteins" (F. W. Putnam, ed.), 2nd ed., Vol. III. Academic Press, New York.

Dayhoff, M. O., ed. (1972). "Atlas of Protein Sequence and Structure," Vol. 5. Nat. Biomed. Res. Found., Washington, D.C.

Debye, P. (1949). *J. Phys. Colloid Chem.* **53**, 1.

Doolittle, R. F. (1965a). *Biochem. J.* **94**, 735.

Doolittle, R. F. (1965b). *Biochem. J.* **94**, 742.

Doolittle, R. F. (1970). *Thromb. Diath. Haemorrh., Suppl.* **39**, 25.

Doolittle, R. F. (1973). *Advan. Protein Chem.* **27**, 1.

Doolittle, R. F., and Blombäck, B. (1964). *Nature (London)* **202**, 147.

Doolittle, R. F., and Cottrell, B. A. (1974). *Biochem. Biophys. Res. Commun.* **60**, 1090.

Doolittle, R. F., and Cottrell, B. A. (1975). *Fed. Proc., Fed. Amer. Soc. Exp. Biol.* **34**, 289 (abstract).

Doolittle, R. F., and Fuller, G. M. (1972). *Biochim. Biophys. Acta* **263**, 805.

Doolittle, R. F., and Wooding, G. L. (1974). *Biochim. Biophys. Acta* **271**, 277.

Doolittle, R. F., Oncley, J. L., and Surgenor, D. M. (1962). *J. Biol. Chem.* **237**, 3123.

Doolittle, R. F., Lorand, L., and Jacobsen, A. (1963). *Biochim. Biophys. Acta* **69**, 161.

Doolittle, R. F., Schubert, D., and Schwartz, S. A. (1967). *Arch. Biochem. Biophys.* **18**, 456.

Doolittle, R. F., Chen, R., and Lau, F. (1971a). *Biochim. Biophys. Res. Commun.* **44**, 94.

Doolittle, R. F., Wooding, G. L., Lin, Y., and Riley, M. (1971b). *J. Mol. Evol.* **1**, 74.

Doolittle, R. F., Cassman, K. G., Chen, R., Sharp, J. J., and Wooding, G. L. (1972). *Ann. N.Y. Acad. Sci.* **202**, 114.

Doolittle, R. F., Takagi, T., and Cottrell, B. A. (1974a). *Science* **185**, 368.

Doolittle, R. F., Troll, M., and Cottrell, B. A. (1974b). *Circulation* **50**, III-283 (abstr.).

Dudek, G. A., Kloczewiak, M., Budzyński, A. Z., Latallo, Z. S., and Kopeć, M. (1970). *Biochim. Biophys. Acta* **214**, 44.

Duthie, E. S. (1954). *J. Gen. Microbiol.* **10**, 427.

Edsall, J. T., and Lever, W. F. (1951). *J. Biol. Chem.* **191**, 735.

Esnouf, M. P., and Tunnah, F. W. (1967). *Brit. J. Haematol.* **13**, 581.

Ferguson, E. W., Ball, A. P., and McKee, P. A. (1974). *Fed. Proc., Fed. Amer. Soc. Exp. Biol.* **33**, 217 (abstr.).

Ferry, J. D. (1952). *Proc. Nat. Acad. Sci. U.S.* **38**, 566.

Ferry, J. D., and Morrison, P. R. (1947). *J. Amer. Chem. Soc.* **69**, 388.

Ferry, J. D., Katz, S., and Tinoco, I., Jr. (1954). *J. Polym. Sci.* **12**, 509.

Finlayson, J. S., and Mosesson, M. W. (1963). *Biochemistry* **2**, 42.

Finlayson, J. S., and Mosesson, M. W. (1964). *Biochim. Biophys. Acta* **82**, 415.

Finlayson, J. S., and Mosesson, M. W. (1973). *Thromb. Res.* **2**, 467.

Folk, J. E., and Chung, S. J. (1973). *Advan. Enzymol.* **38**, 109.

Forman, W. B., Boyer, M. H., and Ratnoff, O. D. (1968). *J. Lab. Clin. Med.* **72**, 455.

Fuller, G. M., and Doolittle, R. F. (1971a). *Biochemistry* **10**, 1305.

Fuller, G. M., and Doolittle, R. F. (1971b). *Biochemistry* **10**, 1311.

Gaffney, P. J. (1972). *Biochim. Biophys. Acta* **263**, 453.

Ganguly, P. (1972). *J. Biol. Chem.* **247**, 1809.

Garvey, M. B., and Black, J. M. (1972). *J. Clin. Pathol.* **25**, 680.

Girolami, A., Zacchello, G., and D'Elia, R. (1971). *Thromb. Diath. Haemorrh.* **25**, 460.

Gladner, J. A. (1968). *In* "Fibrinogen" (K. Laki, ed.), p. 87. Dekker, New York.

Godal, H. C., and Abildgaard, U. (1966). *Scand. J. Haematol.* **3**, 342.

Gollwitzer, R., Karges, H. E., Hörmann, H., and Kuhn, K. (1970). *Biochim. Biophys. Acta* **207**, 445.

Gollwitzer, R., Timpl, R., Becker, U., and Furthmayr, H. (1972). *Eur. J. Biochem.* **28**, 497.

Gormsen, J., Fletcher, A. P., Alkjaersig, N., and Sherry, S. (1967). *Arch. Biochem. Biophys.* **120**, 654.

Gralnick, H. R., Givelber, H. M., Shainoff, J. R., and Finlayson, J. S. (1971). *J. Clin. Invest.* **50**, 1819.

Gralnick, H. R., Givelber, H. M., and Finlayson, J. S. (1973). *Thromb. Diath. Haemorrh.* **29**, 562.

Hall, C. E., and Slayter, H. S. (1959). *J. Biophys. Biochem. Cytol.* **5**, 11.

Hammarsten, O. (1879). *Arch. Gesamte Physiol. Menschen Tiere* **19**, 563.

Hartley, B. S. (1970). *Phils. Trans. Roy. Soc. London, Ser. B* **257**, 77.

Haschemeyer, A. E. V. (1963). *Biochemistry* **2**, 851.

Hektoen, L., and Welker, W. H. (1927). *J. Infec. Dis.* **40**, 706.

Henschen, A. (1962). *Acta Chem. Scand.* **16**, 1037.

Henschen, A. (1964a). *Ark. Kemi* **22**, 1.

Henschen, A. (1964b). *Ark. Kemi* **22**, 355.

Henschen, A. (1964c). *Ark. Kemi* **22**, 375.

Henschen, A., and Edman, P. (1972). *Biochim. Biophys. Acta* **263**, 351.

Herzig, R. H., Ratnoff, O. D., and Shainoff, J. R. (1970). *J. Lab. Clin. Med.* **76**, 451.

Imperato, C., and Dettori, A. G. (1958). *Helv. Paediat. Acta* **13**, 380.

Iwanaga, S., Blombäck, B., Gröndahl, N. J., Hessel, B., and Wallen, P. (1968). *Biochim. Biophys. Acta* **160**, 280.

Jacobsen, C. D., and Hoak, J. C. (1973). *Thromb. Res.* **2**, 261.
Jakobsen, E., and Kierulf, P. (1973). *Thromb. Res.* **3**, 145.
James, H. L., and Ganguly, P. (1973). *Biochim. Biophys. Acta* **328**, 448.
Janssen, C. L., and Vreeken, J. (1971). *Brit. J. Haematol.* **20**, 287.
Jevons, F. R. (1963). *Biochem. J.* **89**, 621.
Johnson, P., and Mihalyi, E. (1965). *Biochim. Biophys. Acta* **102**, 476.
Kay, D., and Cuddigan, B. J. (1967). *Brit. J. Haematol.* **13**, 341.
Kazal, L. A., Amsel, S., Miller, O. P., and Tocantins, L. M. (1963). *Proc. Soc. Exp. Biol. Med.* **113**, 989.
Kenton, H. B. (1933). *J. Immunol.* **25**, 461.
King, J. L. (1971). *In* "Molecular Evolution" (E. Schoffeniels, ed.), Vol. 2, p. 3. North-Holland Publ., Amsterdam.
King, J. L., and Jukes, T. H. (1969). *Science* **164**, 788.
Kopeć, M., Teisseyre, E., Dudek-Wojciechowska, G., Kloczewiak, M., Pankiewicz, A., and Latallo, Z. S. (1973). *Thromb. Res.* **2**, 283.
Köppel, G. (1966). *Nature (London)* **212**, 1608.
Köppel, G. (1967). *Z. Zellforsch. Mikrosk. Anat.* **77**, 443.
Krajewski, T., and Cierniewski, Cz. (1972). *Biochim. Biophys. Acta* **271**, 174.
Krause, W. H., Heene, D. L., and Lasch, H. G. (1973). *Thromb. Diath. Haemorrh.* **29**, 547.
Krohn, K., Sherman, L., and Welch, M. (1972). *Biochim. Biophys. Acta* **285**, 404.
Kudryk, B. J., Collen, D., Woods, K. R., and Blombäck, B. (1974). *J. Biol. Chem.* **249**, 3322.
Künzer, W. (1961). *Klin. Wochenschr.* **39**, 536.
Künzer, W. (1964). *Deut. Med. Wochenschr.* **89**, 1005.
Lacombe, M., Soria, J., Soria, C., D'Angelo, G., Lavallee, R., and Bonny, R. (1973). *Thromb. Diath. Haemorrh.* **29**, 536.
Lahiri, B., and Shainoff, J. R. (1973). *Biochim. Biophys. Acta* **303**, 161.
Laki, K. (1951). *Arch. Biochem. Biophys.* **32**, 317.
Laki, K., and Lorand, L. (1948). *Science* **108**, 280.
Latallo, Z. S., Budzynski, A. Z., and Kowalski, E. (1964). *Nature (London)* **203**, 1184.
Latallo, Z. S., Ducek, G. A., and Kloczewiak, M. (1971). *Scand. J. Haematol., Suppl.* **13**, 37.
Lederer, K. (1972). *J. Mol. Biol.* **63**, 315.
Lederer, K., and Finkelstein, A. (1970). *Biopolymers* **9**, 1553.
Lewis, J. H., and Wilson, J. H. (1973). *Thromb. Res.* **3**, 419.
Loly, W., Israels, L. G., Bishop, A. J., and Israels, E. D. (1971). *Thromb. Diath. Haemorrh.* **26**, 526.
Lorand, L. (1952). *Biochem. J.* **52**, 200.
McKee, P. A., Rogers, L. A., Marler, E., and Hill, R. L. (1966). *Arch. Biochem. Biophys.* **116**, 271.
McKee, P. A., Mattock, P., and Hill, R. L. (1970). *Proc. Nat. Acad. Sci. U.S.* **66**, 738.
Mammen, E. F., Prasad, A. J., Barnhart, M. I., and Au, C. C. (1969). *J. Clin. Invest.* **48**, 235.
Marder, V. J. (1970). *Thromb. Diath. Haemorrh., Suppl.* **39**, 187.
Marder, V. J. (1971). *Scand. J. Haematol., Suppl.* **13**, 21.
Marder, V. J., and Shulman, N. R. (1969). *J. Biol. Chem.* **244**, 2120.
Marder, V. J., Shulman, N. R., and Carroll, W. R. (1969). *J. Biol. Chem.* **244**, 2111.
Marder, V. J., Matchett, M. O., and Sherry, S. (1971). *Amer. J. Med.* **51**, 71.
Martinez, J., Holburn, R. R., Shapiro, S. S., and Erslev, A. J. (1974). *J. Clin. Invest.* **53**, 600.

Mattock, P., and Esnouf, M. P. (1971). *Nature (London) New Biol.* **233,** 277.

Ménaché, D. (1964). *Thromb. Diath. Haemorrh., Suppl.* **13,** 173.

Ménaché, D. (1973). *Thromb. Diath. Haemorrh.* **29,** 525.

Merskey, C., Kleiner, G. J., and Johnson, A. J. (1966). *Blood* **28,** 1.

Mester, L., and Szabadoz, L. (1968). *C. R. Acad. Sci., Ser. D* **226,** 34.

Mihalyi, E. (1965). *Biochim. Biophys. Acta* **102,** 487.

Mihalyi, E. (1970). *Thromb. Diath. Haemorrh., Suppl.* **39,** 43.

Mills, D. A., and Karpatkin, S. (1972). *Fed. Proc., Fed. Amer. Soc. Exp. Biol.* **31,** 261 (abstr.).

Mills, D. A., and Triantaphyllopoulos, D. C. (1969). *Arch. Biochem. Biophys.* **135,** 28.

Mosesson, M. W., and Sherry, S. (1966). *Biochemistry* **5,** 2829.

Mosesson, M. W., Finlayson, J. S., and Galanakis, D. K. (1973). *J. Biol. Chem.* **248,** 7913.

Mosher, D. F., and Blout, E. R. (1973). *J. Biol. Chem.* **248,** 6896.

Mross, G. A., and Doolittle, R. F. (1967). *Arch. Biochem. Biophys.* **122,** 674.

Murtaugh, P. A., Halver, J. E., and Gladner, J. A. (1974). *Biochim. Biophys. Acta* **359,** 415.

Nachman, R. L. (1965). *Blood* **25,** 703.

Nachman, R. L., and Marcus, A. J. (1968). *Brit. J. Haematol.* **15,** 181.

Nossel, H. L., Younger, L. R., Wilner, G. D., Procupez, T., Canfield, R. E., and Butler, V. P., Jr. (1971). *Proc. Nat. Acad. Sci. U.S.* **68,** 2350.

Nuzzensweig, V., Seligman, M., Pelmont, J., and Grabar, P. (1961). *Ann. Inst. Pasteur, Paris* **100,** 377.

Okude, M., and Iwanaga, S. (1971). *Biochim. Biophys. Acta* **251,** 185.

O'Neil, P. B., and Doolittle, R. F. (1975). In preparation.

Osbahr, A. J., Jr., Colman, R. W., Laki, K., and Gladner, J. A. (1964). *Biochem. Biophys. Res. Commun.* **14,** 555.

Otis, P. T., and Rapaport, S. I. (1973). *Proc. Soc. Exp. Biol. Med.* **144,** 124.

Pennell, R. B. (1960). *In* "The Plasma Proteins" (F. W. Putnam, ed.), 1st ed., Vol. 1, Chapter 2, pp. 9–50. Academic Press, New York.

Perutz, M. F., and Lehmann, H. (1968). *Nature (London)* **219,** 902.

Pisano, J. J., Finlayson, J. S., Peyton, M. P., and Nagai, Y. (1971). *Proc. Nat. Acad. Sci. U.S.* **68,** 770.

Pizzo, S. V., Schwartz, M. L., Hill, R. L., and McKee, P. A. (1972). *J. Biol. Chem.* **247,** 636.

Pizzo, S. V., Schwartz, M. L., Hill, R. L., and McKee, P. A. (1973). *J. Biol. Chem.* **248,** 4574.

Plow, E., and Edgington, T. S. (1973). *J. Clin. Invest.* **52,** 273.

Plow, E., and Edgington, T. S. (1974). *Fed. Proc., Fed. Amer. Soc. Exp. Biol.* **33,** 218 (abstr.).

Pouit, L., Marcille, G., Suscillon, M., and Hollard, D. (1972). *Thromb. Diath. Haemorrh.* **27,** 559.

Robbins, K. C. (1944). *Amer. J. Physiol.* **142,** 581.

Robbins, K. C., and Summaria, L. (1973). *Thromb. Diath. Haemorrh., Suppl.* **54,** 167.

Rosiek, O., Wegrzynowicz, A., Sawicki, Z., and Kopeć, M. (1969). *Folia Haematol. (Leipzig)* **92,** 553.

Samama, M., Soria, J., Soria, C., and Bousser, J. (1969). *Nouv. Rev. Fr. Hematol.* **9,** 817.

Sanfellippo, M. J., Stevens, D. J., and Koenig, R. R. (1971). *Amer. J. Clin. Pathol.* **56,** 166.

Scheraga, H. A., and Laskowski, M., Jr. (1957). *Advan. Protein Chem.* **12,** 1.

Schwartz, M. L., Pizzo, S. V., Sullivan, J. B., Hill, R. L., and McKee, P. A. (1973). *Thromb. Diath. Haemorrh.* **29,** 313.

Seegers, W. H., Nieft, M. L., and Vandenbelt, J. M. (1945). *Arch. Biochem.* **7**, 15.
Sharp, J. J., Cassman, K. G., and Doolittle, R. F. (1972). *FEBS (Fed. Eur. Biochem. Soc.) Lett.* **25**, 334.
Sherman, L. A., Gaston, L. W., Kaplan, M. E., and Spivack, A. R. (1972). *J. Clin. Invest.* **51**, 590.
Shulman, S. (1953). *J. Amer. Chem. Soc.* **75**, 5846.
Siegel, B. M., Mernan, J. P., and Scheraga, H. A. (1953). *Biochim. Biophys. Acta* **11**, 329.
Skerrow, D. (1974). *Biochem. Biophys. Res. Commun.* **59**, 1311.
Solum, N. O. (1973). *Thromb. Res.* **2**, 55.
Solum, N. O., and Lopaciuk, S. (1969). *Thromb. Diath. Haemorrh.* **21**, 428.
Soria, J., Soria, C., Samama, M., Poirot, E., and Kling, C. (1972). *Thromb. Diath. Haemorrh.* **27**, 619.
Spiro, R. G. (1973). *Advan. Protein Chem.* **27**, 349.
Stachurska, J., Latallo, Z., and Kopeć, M. (1971). *Thromb. Diath. Haemorrh.* **23**, 91.
Stecher, V. K., and Sorkin, E. (1972). *Int. Arch. Allergy Appl. Immunol.* **43**, 879.
Sternberger, A., and Hörmann, H. (1974). *Thromb. Res.* **4**, 753.
Stewart, G. J., and Niewiarowski, S. (1969). *Biochim. Biophys. Acta* **194**, 462.
Stryer, L., Cohen, C., and Langridge, R. (1963). *Nature (London)* **197**, 793.
Sturtevant, J. M., Laskowski, M., Jr., Donnelly, T. H., and Scheraga, H. A. (1955). *J. Amer. Chem. Soc.* **77**, 6168.
Takagi, T., and Doolittle, R. F. (1974a). *Biochemistry* **13**, 750.
Takagi, T., and Doolittle, R. F. (1974b). *Circulation* **50**, III-284 (abstr.).
Takagi, T., and Doolittle, R. F. (1975a). *Biochemistry* **14**, 940.
Takagi, T., and Doolittle, R. F. (1975b). In preparation.
Takagi, T., and Iwanaga, S. (1970). *Biochem. Biophys. Res. Commun.* **38**, 129.
Takaki, A., Ishiguro, M., and Funatsu, M. (1972). *Proc. Jap. Acad.* **48**, 528.
Timpl, R., and Gollwitzer, R. (1973). *FEBS (Fed. Eur. Biochem. Soc.) Lett.* **29**, 92.
Tooney, N. M., and Cohen, C. (1972). *Nature (London)* **237**, 23.
von Felten, A., Duckert, F., and Frick, P. G. (1966). *Brit. J. Haematol.* **12**, 667.
von Felten, A., Frick, P. G., and Straub, P. W. (1969). *Brit. J. Haematol.* **16**, 353.
Walker, L., and Catlin, A. (1971). *Thromb. Diath. Haemorrh.* **26**, 99.
Ware, A. G., Guest, M. M., and Seegers, W. H. (1947). *Arch. Biochem.* **13**, 231.
Weinstein, M. J., and Doolittle, R. F. (1972). *Biochim. Biophys. Acta* **258**, 577.
Witt, I., and Müller, H. (1970). *Biochim. Biophys. Acta* **221**, 402.
Witt, I., Müller, H., and Kunzer, W. (1969). *Thromb. Diath. Haemorrh.* **22**, 101.
Wooding, G. L., and Doolittle, R. F. (1972). *J. Hum. Evol.* **1**, 553.

4 / Structure and Function of Glycoproteins

John R. Clamp

I. Introduction

Glycoproteins are a class of proteins containing covalently linked carbohydrate. They are extremely widely distributed in nature, occurring in all the living kingdoms that have been examined from viruses (Hughes, 1973; Krantz *et al.,* 1974) to animals. In animals, glycoproteins occur as an integral part of cell membranes and structural tissues and are also free in the various body fluids and secretions. Thus virtually all the plasma proteins are glycoproteins. The most important exception in man is albumin, the plasma protein in the highest concentration, and this is a further interesting characteristic of this protein. Other plasma proteins that appear to be devoid of carbohydrate are minor constituents such as retinol-binding protein (Haupt and Heide, 1972) and prealbumin (Peterson, 1971).

The term "glycoprotein" is relatively old, being coined toward the end of the last century when it was realized that in some materials carbohydrate and protein were in inseparable association. Although this was originally discovered with mucin (mucus glycoprotein) it was not long before this was found to be true of many proteins.

The earliest studies on glycoproteins in plasma were of course limited to broad and heterogeneous fractions. Thus carbohydrate was found to be associated with the proteins precipitated by various denaturation procedures and could only be released from the precipitate by vigorous hydrolysis (Mörner, 1893; Pavy, 1893; Krakow, 1897). In addition, the protein fraction that was not precipitated under these conditions was also shown to be glycoprotein in nature. This fraction was called "seromucoid" (Zanetti, 1897, 1903) and consists principally of α_1-acid glycoprotein or orosomucoid. Presumably the reason that this fraction resists denaturation is because of its high carbohydrate content which is in the region of 40%.

One of the first relatively pure plasma proteins to be isolated and shown to be a glycoprotein was probably IgG (Hewitt, 1934; Pappenheimer et al., 1940; Smith et al., 1946). The field has developed rapidly over the last few years and now the list of plasma proteins that have been isolated and found to contain carbohydrate numbers close to 60.

By the late 1930's, it began to be appreciated just how widespread and important glycoprotein and related material were, with the result that the first classifications of these substances began to appear (Meyer, 1938; Blix, 1940; Stacey, 1943). Classification reached its most elaborate form (Meyer, 1945) with the division of glycoproteins quite arbitrarily into "mucoids" and "glycoids" corresponding to proteins with N-acetylhexosamine contents greater than or less than 4%, respectively. Finally the term "mucoprotein" which up to that time had been used synonymously with "glycoprotein" (Stacey, 1946) was given the restricted meaning of the easily split association between acid mucopolysaccharide and protein (Winzler, 1958). However, nature is no respecter of human classification systems and it is not surprising that this diverse group of functionally evolved proteins should defy rigid classification when the only property most of them have in common is the presence of carbohydrate. Recent classifications therefore have tended to divide carbohydrate-containing materials into broad, general groups. Table I shows a simplified

TABLE I

Some Types of Glycoconjugate[a]

Type of glycoconjugate	Characteristics of glycoconjugate
I. Glycolipid	Carbohydrate linked to lipid such as phosphatidic acid or sphingosine derivatives
II. Proteoglycan	Glycosaminoglycan (mucopolysaccharide) linked to protein. The carbohydrate component (glycosaminoglycan) has the following characteristics (Lindahl and Rodén, 1972): a. Carbohydrate units tend to be large, containing more than 50 monosaccharide residues b. Most of the carbohydrate is present as a repeating disaccharide unit c. Hexosamine is always present, as is hexuronic acid (with one exception)
III. Glycoprotein[b]	The carbohydrate component has the following characteristics: a. Carbohydrate units tend to be small, containing less than 25 monosaccharide residues b. The carbohydrate units have little or no repeating structure c. The types of monosaccharide present include fucose, mannose, galactose, glucose (in collagen), N-acetylglucosamine, N-acetylgalactosamine, and sialic acid. Hexuronic acid is rarely, if ever a component
A. Structural-type glycoproteins	Examples: Collagen, membrane glycoproteins and so on
B. Mucus-type glycoproteins	Examples: Mucus, blood group substances a. Carbohydrate content is usually more than 50% b. The carbohydrate units are usually O-glycosidically linked to protein c. Of the monosaccharides listed above, the mannose content is usually low or absent d. The protein component has a high content of threonine, serine, and proline
C. Plasma-type glycoproteins	Examples: immunoglobulins, transferrin, and so on a. Carbohydrate content is usually less than 50% b. The carbohydrate units are usually N-glycosidically linked to protein c. Of the monosaccharides listed above, the N-acetylgalactosamine content is usually low or absent

[a] This table is principally concerned with human material. Glycoconjugates may be defined as carbohydrate covalently linked to lipid, protein, or related materials, but excluding nucleic acids.

[b] The terms "structural-type," "mucus-type," and "plasma-type" are merely used as general headings as the major source representative of that type of glycoprotein.

classification from Gottschalk (1972). The definitions are of necessity vague and are merely intended to give some idea of the general properties of the groups. In these names the final part of the word usually represents the important part of the glycoconjugate. Thus in a proteoglycan, the carbohydrate is most important whereas in a glycoprotein the protein component tends to dominate the overall properties. The plasma glycoproteins are typical in this respect. They have precise molecular weights, most of them can be denatured by the usual techniques and they tend to have specific biological roles.

Despite the fact that plasma contains a large number of glycoproteins, only a few of them have been studied in any detail with regard to the carbohydrate moiety. Inevitably, those that have been studied have tended to be the ones that are present in plasma in the greatest amount; can be isolated with relative ease; advantage is taken of some disease in which there is an increased amount of some glycoprotein in plasma (immunoglobulins in multiple myeloma or macroglobulinemia); or in which a plasma glycoprotein appears in some other body fluid (α_1-acid glycoprotein in urine in nephrosis).

The list of such glycoproteins includes α_1-acid glycoprotein, transferrin, haptoglobin, ceruloplasmin, immunoglobulins, and α_2-macroglobulin. As a result, the remainder of this chapter is, to a large extent, a comparative study of the glycoprotein nature of these few plasma proteins.

II. Aspects of Component Carbohydrate

A. Monosaccharide Chemistry

Glycoproteins contain a range of monosaccharides which in the case of plasma glycoproteins includes fucose, mannose, galactose, N-acetylglucosamine, N-acetylgalactosamine, and sialic acid. Before these are discussed in detail, it would be helpful to consider some general aspects of carbohydrate chemistry that are relevant. For example, those who are not familiar with the field often find the degree of isomerism confusing. Thus mannose and galactose are isomeric structures, both being aldohexoses, which also includes sugars such as glucose. In fact there are 16 stereoisomers in the aldohexose series arising from the 4 asymmetric centers as can be deduced from the general formula: $CHO(CHOH)_4CH_2OH$. The problem then is to explain the relationship between these isomers in a way that gives some idea of the three-dimensional structures. These structures must, however, be represented two-

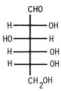

Fig. 1.   The Fischer acyclic representation of D-glucose.

dimensionally on paper and this need has given rise to a number of conventions often misunderstood by those inexperienced in carbohydrate chemistry.

For example, there are valid stereochemical reasons why glucose is the commonest sugar in nature and it is therefore convenient to use it for illustrative purposes, although this monosaccharide does not appear to be present in most plasma glycoproteins. Glucose is often drawn as shown in Fig. 1. This is known as the acyclic Fischer formula or convention and there is no resemblance whatever between the drawing and any conformation that the molecule could adopt in solution. The convention is that the monsaccharide is drawn with the most oxidized group at the top and the most reduced group at the bottom, then each carbon atom in turn is viewed as if the horizontal bonds are coming toward the viewer, out of the paper; whereas the vertical bonds to the neighboring carbon atoms are going away from the viewer, into the paper. It will perhaps be easier to understand this by considering the simplest "sugar" with an asymmetric center, namely, glyceraldehyde. This is shown in various representations in Fig. 2. The Fischer formula is shown in Fig. 2a and corresponding to this are two attempts to make the molecule appear stereoscopic. In the Fischer convention if the hydroxyl group is on the right then the asymmetric center is said to have the D configuration. Figure 2 therefore is D-glyceraldehyde and this is the reference sugar for all monosaccharides in two respects. First, any asymmetric carbon atom which when viewed according to the above convention has a similar orientation of hydrogen and hydroxyl groups is said to have the D configu-

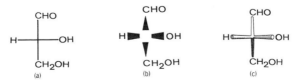

Fig. 2.   Three different ways of representing the molecule of D-glyceraldehyde. On the left is the Fischer acyclic formula (2a). The other two drawings are attempts to represent the molecule in a more stereoscopic fashion either by wedge-shaped bonds (center) or with a wire model (right).

ration. The second point is a consequence of the fact that one could, in theory, derive every aldose sugar from glyceraldehyde by a series of addition reactions, thereby building up the molecules from the aldehyde group. The penultimate carbon atom would in every case have the same configuration, namely, D, because it was derived from C-2 of D-glyceraldehyde. All these aldoses are therefore said to belong to the D family or series. L-Glyceraldehyde would give rise to a corresponding family of aldoses, all belonging to the L series. The prefix D or L placed before a monosaccharide defines the configuration of the penultimate carbon atom and therefore the family or series that the monosaccharide belongs to.

It should now be clear that the acyclic Fischer formula for D-glucose shown in Fig. 1 is concerned only to show the relationship of one asymmetric center to another. The penultimate carbon atom C-5 has the D-configuration and this fixes the molecule as a D sugar. C-2 and C-4 are similarly D, whereas C-3 has the L configuration.

A more realistic representation of the open-chain form of D-glucose is shown in Fig. 3. This is known as the zigzag representation. The carbon chain is placed in the plane of the paper and the H and OH groups then either come out of (wedge-shaped bonds) or enter (dotted bonds) the plane of the paper.

Very little of D-glucose exists in solution in the acyclic or open-chain form. The aldehyde group at C-1 is very reactive and when it comes into contact with an OH group, a hemiacetal bond is formed according to the following reaction:

$$-CHO + HO \longrightarrow -CHOH-O-$$

Thus the molecule cyclizes with the creation of another asymmetric center on C-1, and for historical reasons the two stereoisomers, called anomers, are designated as α and β. The α anomer has the same configuration as the penultimate reference carbon atom (C-5 in hexoses), so that in the D series "α" means that C-1 has the D configuration. Conversely, in the L sugars "α" means that C-1 has the L configuration.

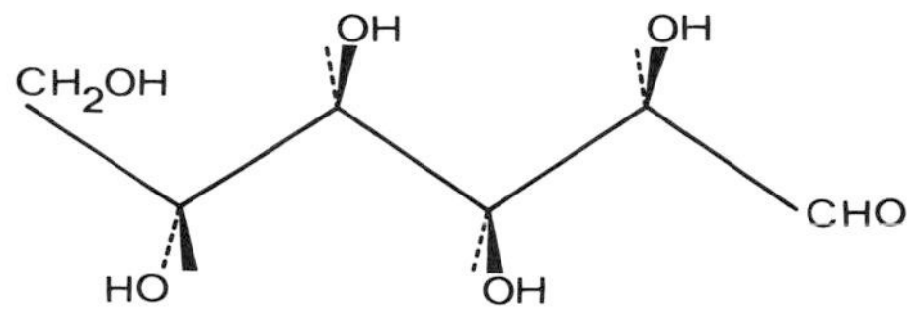

Fig. 3. A zigzag representation of the open-chain form of D-glucose. The wedge-shaped bonds are assumed to be coming out of the plane of the paper toward the viewer, whereas the dotted bonds are going away from the viewer. Hydrogen atoms have been omitted.

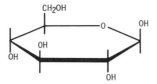

Fig. 4. The Haworth cyclic formula for β-D-glucopyranose. Hydrogen atoms have been omitted.

If the aldehyde group reacts with the C-4 hydroxyl, a five-membered oxygen-containing ring is formed and this is the furanose form of the sugar. There is a great deal of bond strain in the furanose ring and so this is energetically unfavorable. However, the six-membered or pyranose ring which is formed when the aldehyde group reacts with the C-5 hydroxyl has little bond strain and is the favored form. For this reason probably all the monosaccharides that occur in glycoproteins are pyranosides. These are often represented by the Haworth formula as shown in Fig. 4 for α-D-glucopyranose. The Haworth formula is unsatisfactory because it neither shows clearly the relationships between asymmetric centers as does the Fischer formula, nor does it give a reasonable idea of the three-dimensional structure of the ring. The pyranose ring can exist in six boat conformations and two chair conformations, but only the chair conformations are important in the context of this chapter. Figure 5 shows the *C1* chair for β-D-glucopyranose and it can be seen that the bulky hydroxyl groups are all in the plane of the ring, that is they are "equatorial." This means that these groups are as widely spaced as possible and consequently any interference between them is at a minimum. On the other hand, in the *IC* chair form (Fig. 6) the hydroxyl groups are all perpendicular to the plane of the ring ("axial") and are therefore rela-

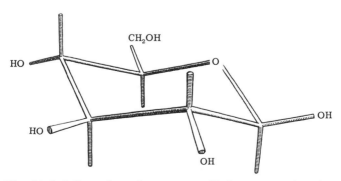

Fig. 5. The *C1* chair form of β-D-glucopyranose. Hydrogen atoms have been omitted.

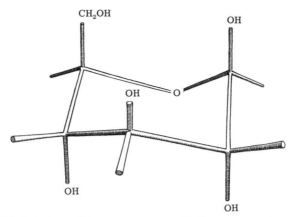

Fig. 6. The *1C* chair form of β-D-glucopyranose. Hydrogen atoms have been omitted.

tively crowded. It is not surprising that β-D-glucopyranose exists to a large extent in the *C1* chair conformation. It is probable that in glycoproteins the D-mannose, D-galactose, *N*-acetyl-D-glucosamine (2-acetamido-2-deoxy-D-glucose), and *N*-acetyl-D-galactosamine (2-acetamido-2-deoxy-D-galactose) residues all exist in the *C1* chair conformation whereas the L-fucosyl (6-deoxy-L-galactose) and sialyl (*N*-acetyl-neuraminic acid) residues are present in the *1C* conformation (Yu and Leeden, 1969).

B. The Monosaccharides Present in Glycoproteins

The monosaccharides that are commonly present in plasma glycoproteins have been listed in the previous paragraph. The structures of these various monosaccharides are given according to the Fischer acyclic convention in Fig. 7. These are discussed below very briefly under a general heading for each type of monosaccharide. In this discussion the configurational sign will be omitted for the sugars.

1. Hexoses

In the strict sense all the monosaccharides listed, apart from sialic acid, are hexoses. However, this term is usually applied to sugars with no functional groups other than hydroxyl groups and the potential aldehyde group and is thus often qualified as "neutral" or "simple" hexoses.

Two hexoses have been identified in most plasma glycoproteins and these are mannose and galactose.

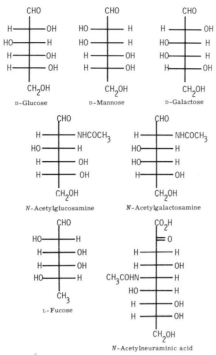

Fig. 7.   The Fischer acyclic formulas of the monosaccharides commonly present in plasma glycoproteins. D-Glucose is included for comparison.

Mannose was first identified in plasma glycoproteins by Dische (1928) and at almost the same time by Rimington (1929). Soon afterward, galactose was first shown to be present in plasma proteins (Bierry, 1934). These early workers had a formidable task in identifying particular monosaccharides. Apart from the problem of isolating the monosaccharide from such a complex mixture after hydrolysis, a suitable chemical derivative, usually a phenylosazone, had then to be prepared from whose melting point the sugar was identified. Nowadays, with a battery of chromatographic procedures at his disposal, the biochemist has a much simpler problem. Although the identification of hexoses may be easier, the estimation (quantitation) of each hexose still presents problems. Thus the ratio of mannose to galactose in transferrin varies from 2:1 to 1:2 depending on the laboratory making the estimation. It is hoped that these problems will largely disappear with the adoption of recent methods of carbohydrate analysis based upon automated ion-exchange chromatography or upon gas-liquid chromatography.

Glucose has often been reported in plasma glycoproteins. It is certainly present in structural glycoproteins (Beisswenger and Spiro, 1970) and not surprisingly in the collagen-like stretch (Reid, 1974) of the C1q component of complement (Calcott and Müller-Eberhard, 1972). Apart from C1q, it is probably true to say that so far glucose has never been shown unequivocally to be present in any well-characterized plasma glycoprotein.

2. Deoxyhexoses

Only one deoxyhexose has been identified in plasma glycoproteins and that is L-fucose. The full name for this monosaccharide is 6-deoxy-L-galactose. The "6-deoxy-" prefix indicates that C-6 carries no hydroxyl group and is in fact a methyl group, hence the earlier name for this type of monosaccharide—"methylpentose." The methyl group may be of fundamental importance in the overall properties of this sugar, for example, in conferring a small area with hydrophobicity, perhaps for interaction with some part of the adjacent protein and thereby act as a mechanism for orientation of the oligosaccharide unit on the glycoprotein surface. Alternatively the group may interact with cell membranes either before or after secretion from the cell.

3. N-Acetylhexosamines

This type of monosaccharide has been called "*N*-acetylhexosamine" rather than "hexosamine" to emphasize the fact that it almost certainly occurs exclusively as the acetylated derivative in glycoproteins. Alternative names that are sometimes used for these sugars are "aminohexoses" with "acetamidohexoses" for the corresponding acetylated derivative. There are two monosaccharides of this type in plasma glycoproteins and these are *N*-acetylglucosamine and *N*-acetylgalactosamine. The full names for these are 2-acetamido-2-deoxy-D-glucose and 2-acetamido-2-deoxy-D-galactose, respectively. Every plasma glycoprotein contains *N*-acetylglucosamine and in addition some of them contain *N*-acetylgalactosamine. The result is that there is about 10 times as much of the former sugar than of the latter in pooled plasma glycoproteins.

4. Sialic acids

Sialic acid was first obtained from two quite different sources. Blix (1936) heated bovine submaxillary gland mucin in aqueous solution and succeeded in isolating a crystalline acid, later called "sialic acid." Two years later he showed (Blix, 1938) that similar material was present in certain lipid fractions of ox brain. Independently Klenk (1941) investigating a glycolipid (ganglioside) from human brain isolated a substance which he called "neuraminic acid."

The relationship among sialic acid, neuraminic acid, and similar compounds named after their sources was soon established and the confused nomenclature revised by general agreement (Blix *et al.*, 1957). The parent, unsubstituted compound was called neuraminic acid, the full name for which is 5-amino-3,5-dideoxy-D-*glycero*-D-*galacto*nonulosonic acid. The N- or O-substituted derivatives are known collectively as "sialic acids."

Human glycoproteins appear to contain only *N*-acetylneuraminic acid (Odin, 1955), but animal glycoproteins contain a range of other derivatives (Schauer *et al.*, 1974) including *N*-glycollyl and *O*-acetyl or *O*-glycollyl derivatives which may be present at positions 4, 7, or 8.

The function of sialic acid is presumably to provide the major source of negative charge in glycoproteins.

C. Oligosaccharide Chemistry

The investigation of oligosaccharide structure presents formidable problems when compared to that of proteins. For example, one can calculate the number of possible isomers in simple peptides and saccharides. Thus two alanine residues give rise to a single dipeptide but two glucose residues can be linked together to give 11 different disaccharides. Even this number is a lower limit because it assumes that both the glucose molecules are in the preferred chair conformation. If one increases the number of residues to three the differences become even more striking. Three alanines give only a single tripeptide but three glucoses give rise to nearly 200 trisaccharides. When one considers the usual type of oligosaccharide unit in a glycoprotein the number of possible isomers becomes astronomical. Thus a unit containing 1 fucose, 3 mannose, 2 galactose, 4 *N*-acetylglucosamine, and 2 sialic acid residues can exist in over 10^{24} different isomeric forms. The reason for this state of affairs is that a hexopyranose molecule can be substituted at so many positions, namely, at C-2, C-3, C-4, and C-6, and in addition can be mono-, di-, tri-, or tetrasubstituted. Apart from these possibilities of substitution, the monosaccharide itself is of course always linked through C-1 to the next residue in the chain. The monosaccharide involved in the linkage to protein is the potential "reducing end group." Terminal sugars that are not themselves substituted are "nonreducing end groups." A linear oligosaccharide has one nonreducing end group whereas a branched oligosaccharide has one for each branch.

In order to characterize an oligosaccharide unit completely the following information must be obtained:

i. Complete carbohydrate analysis
ii. Molecular weight of unit
iii. Sequence of residues
iv. Positions of linkages
v. Anomeric configurations

There are no really satisfactory methods available for obtaining all this information.

Methods of carbohydrate analysis have improved somewhat in the last few years. Procedures are now available using automated ion-exchange chromatography (Kennedy, 1974) or gas-liquid chromatography (g.l.c.) (Clamp, 1974; Clamp *et al.,* 1972). Using g.l.c. it is possible to separate and estimate, in a single procedure, all the monosaccharides that commonly occur in glycoproteins. Thus the chromatogram for IgM is given in Fig. 8 showing the presence of fucose, mannose, galactose, *N*-acetylglucosamine, and sialic acid.

The techniques used for the structural investigation of oligosaccharides include periodate oxidation, methylation, partial degradation (partial hydrolysis), and the use of specific glycosidases.

Periodic acid or its salts will cleave the carbon–carbon bond between vicinal hydroxyl groups, creating the corresponding aldehyde groups. Thus periodate oxidation studies can provide a variety of information. The consumption (uptake) of periodate is a direct measure of the number of bonds cleaved and therefore of the number of vicinal hydroxyl groups in the original material. Monosaccharides that survive ox-

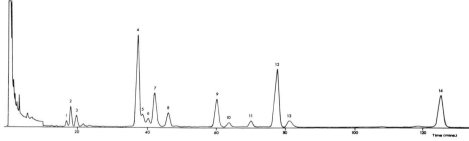

Fig. 8. Gas chromatogram of the monosaccharides present in IgM. Peaks are identified as follows: 1,2,3 fucose; 4,6 mannose; 5,7,8 galactose; 9 mannitol (internal standard); 10,11,12,13 *N*-acetylglucosamine; 14 sialic acid. Monosaccharides are run as *O*-trimethylsilyl derivatives of the methyl glycosides. Most sugars therefore give rise to a characteristic multiple peak pattern corresponding to the isomeric forms.

idation must be substituted, the minimum requirement for a hexose being substitution at C-3. If the periodate-oxidized material is then reduced, the aldehyde groups are converted to the corresponding alcohols and this renders the adjacent glycosidic linkage labile to mild acid hydrolysis. After hydrolysis additional hydroxyl groups are uncovered and become susceptible to further periodate oxidation. These cycles of oxidation, reduction, and mild acid hydrolysis are known as Smith degradation (Smith and Unrau, 1959).

In methylation techniques, the oligosaccharide is reacted under conditions that will convert all the free hydroxyl groups to the methyl derivative. Any monosaccharide that is substituted therefore will, upon cleavage of the oligosaccharide, have a free hydroxyl group in that position. The various partially and fully methylated derivatives of each monosaccharide are now identified and estimated. The problems in this technique are first to completely methylate the oligosaccharide, second to cleave the oligosaccharide without splitting off any methyl groups, and third to identify and estimate all the possible methyl derivatives of every monosaccharide.

Partial hydrolysis or partial degradation studies depend upon splitting the oligosaccharide into smaller fragments such as di-, tri-, and tetrasaccharides which can be more easily investigated. Knowledge of these fragments allows conclusions to be drawn about the overall structure. The problems here are the inadequacy of chemical methods for the specific cleavage of oligosaccharides, and the identification and estimation of the fragments when they are produced.

Glycosidases are being increasingly used for the investigation of oligosaccharide structure. Specific exoglycosidases release the appropriate monosaccharide if it is in a nonreducing end group position. With well-characterized glycosidases both positive and negative results provide important structural information. The sequential use of such exoglycosidases with adequate controls can determine the sequence of monosaccharides in an oligosaccharide.

An exciting possibility is the discovery of endoglycosidases, usually endo-*N*-acetylhexosaminidases, which are capable of splitting the oligosaccharide internally at specific linkages (Nishigaki *et al.,* 1974; Tarentino and Maley, 1974). Such enzymes, when their substrate specificities are fully worked out, will be invaluable in the structural investigation of oligosaccharide units from glycoproteins.

All these techniques are usually carried out, not on the intact glycoprotein, but upon glycopeptides isolated therefrom. The glycopeptides are produced in most cases by exhaustive proteolysis of the glycoprotein, either with an enzyme of wide specificity such as pronase or by a combination of proteinases. The glycopeptides are then isolated by ion-exchange chromatography or by exclusion chromatography.

III. Carbohydrate Content of Plasma Glycoproteins

There are a number of problems when one attempts to tabulate data about plasma glycoproteins. Thus it is very difficult to establish the relationship between minor constituents of plasma which have been isolated by different workers and only partially characterized. It is also a problem to reconcile divergent values obtained by different laboratories for the same glycoprotein. Such values include not only carbohydrate analysis, but also plasma concentration, molecular weight, and so on.

Where results vary, a mean has been taken of a selection of the more recent values. The results are given in Table II.

IV. Oligosaccharide Units of Plasma Glycoproteins

A. Introduction

Any discussion of the oligosaccharide units of human plasma glycoproteins cannot help referring to a glycoprotein that is not derived from plasma and is not even a human or mammalian glycoprotein. The protein of course is hen ovalbumin which has been a model system for glycoprotein biochemists for the past 40 years. There are a number of reasons for this. Thus it can be easily prepared in a pure form from a readily available source. Even more important is the fact that the glycoprotein contains only a single oligosaccharide unit and this unit is small, containing an average of eight monosaccharide residues, and simple, consisting of just mannose and *N*-acetylglucosamine. It is not surprising, therefore, that many of the important milestones in glycoprotein biochemistry have been reached through studies on ovalbumin and thus this protein, together with the related ovomucoid, are often mentioned in the succeeding sections.

B. Linkage between Carbohydrate and Protein

In mammals, oligosaccharide units are probably always linked through their reducing end groups to protein. The linkages involved may be divided into two broad groups, namely, "N-glycosidic" and "O-glycosidic." In the former, the anomeric carbon atom of the monosac-

TABLE II

Carbohydrate Content of Some Human Plasma Glycoproteins

Glycoprotein[a]	Concn. (gm/liter)	Molecular weight	Carbohydrate content (%)[b]									References
			Fuc	Man	Total Hex	Gal	GlcNAc	Total HexNAc	GalNAc	Sialic acid	Total carbohydrate	
Ceruloplasmin	0.4	160,000	0.2	1.4		1.4	2.5		0.0	1.7	7	Holtzmann et al. (1967)
Complement system												
Clq	0.02	410,000 400,000	0.1	3.2c	7.0	3.2	0.8		0.0	0.3	8 10	Reid et al. (1972) Calcott and Müller-Eberhard (1972)
C3 (β_1C-globulin)	3.5	185,000	0.2		1.8			0.6		0.5	3	Müller-Eberhard et al. (1960)
C4 (β_1E-globulin)	0.3	230,000	0.1		1.9			1.4		1.0	4	Haupt et al. (1970) Heide and Schwick (1973)
Corticosteroid-binding globulin[d]	0.028	51,700	1.5		11.5			11.0		4.1	28	Muldoon and Westphal (1967)
Fibrinogen	4.0	330,000	0.0	1.0		1.1		1.0		0.5	7	Mester and Szabados (1968)
Gc-globulin	n.g.	50,800	0.2		2.0			2.0		0.0	4	Schultze and Heremans (1966)
Haptoglobin	1.5	99,000	0.2	2.8		2.8	5.4		0.0	4.6	16	Gerbeck et al. (1967)
Hemopexin	1.0	70,000	n.g.	3.8		3.1	9.4		0.0	6.9	23	Hrkal and Müller-Eberhard (1971)
Immunoglobulins												
IgG	13.0	150,000	0.2	1.0		0.5	1.0		0.0	0.2	3	Clamp and Johnson (1972)
IgA	2.5	160,000	0.2	1.7		1.3	1.6		0.7	1.3	7	
IgM	1.3	900,000	0.3	3.6		1.2	3.3		0.0	1.9	10	
IgD	0.2	180,000	0.1	2.0		1.3	1.8		1.2	3.1	9	
IgE	0.001	190,000	0.8	3.7		1.8	4.3		0.0	2.5	13	
Lipoproteins												
Very low density lipoproteins apoproteins	1.0	15,000,000 7 to 10,000								3.0		Brown et al. (1970)

(continued)

TABLE II (*Continued*)

Carbohydrate Content of Some Human Plasma Glycoproteins

Glycoprotein[a]	Concn. (gm/liter)	Molecular weight	Carbohydrate content (%)[b]									References
			Fuc	Man	Total Hex	Gal	GlcNAc	Total HexNAc	GalNAc	Sialic acid	Total carbo-hydrate	
Low density lipoproteins apoproteins	3.5	2,500,000										Margolis and Langdon (1966)
		500,000	n.g.		3.2		1.2		0.0	0.4		Marshall and Kummerow (1962)
											5	Margolis (1969)
			0.3		2.7		1.2		0.0	1.3	3	Gotto et al. (1972)
High density lipoproteins (HDL)												
HDL2	1.0	400,000										
HDL3	2.5	170,000										Scanu (1969)
Apoproteins		21,000	0.6	0.4		0.4	1.8		0.0	0.5	4	Scanu (1966)
Plasminogen	2.9	89,000	n.g.		1.5			n.g.		n.g.	n.g.	Robbins et al. (1965)
Prothrombin	0.15	70,000	n.g.		3.4		3.1		0.0	2.8	9	Kisiel and Hanahan (1973); Lanchantin et al. (1968)
Thyroxine-binding α-globulin	0.01	36,500	0.0	2.3		2.5	6.0		0.0	3.7	14	Sterling et al. (1971)
Transcortin	0.04	55,700	0.3	2.9		2.9	5.1		0.0	3.3	14	Schneider and Slaunwhite (1971)
Transferrin	3.0	76,000	0.0	1.5		1.0	2.2		0.0	1.4	6	Jamieson (1965b); Spik and Montreuil (1969)
α1-Acid glycoprotein	0.3	40,000	0.7	5.2		8.7	13.5		0.0	11.5	40	Hughes and Jeanloz (1966); Schultze et al. (1962)
α1-Antichymotrypsin	0.2	68,000	0.8		11.0			8.0		7.0	27	Heimburger and Haupt (1965)
α1-Antitrypsin	3.0	54,000	0.2		5.0		3.6			3.4	12	Heide and Schwick (1973)

Glycoprotein										Reference
α_1-Glycoprotein (9.5 S)	0.055	308,000	0.1	5.5		3.7		3.5	12	Haupt et al. (1972)
Tryptophan-poor α_1 T-glycoprotein	n.g.	58,000	0.3	5.5		4.5		3.4	14	Haupt and Heide (1964)
α_2-HS-glycoprotein	1.0	49,000	0.3	3.4	2.6	4.0	0.0	5.0	15	Poortmans et al. (1967); Schmid and Bürgi (1961)
Zn-α_2-glycoprotein	n.g.	41,000	0.2	4.2	2.8	4.0	0.0	7.0	18	Bürgi and Schmid (1961)
Histidine-rich 3.8 S α_2-glycoprotein	0.09	58,500	0.0	3.2	3.2	4.4		3.5	14	Heimburger et al. (1972)
α_2-Macroglobulin	2.5	900,000	0.4	2.3	1.5	3.7	0.0	2.0	10	Bourrillon et al. (1968); Dunn and Spiro (1967a)
4 S α_2-β_1-Glycoprotein	0.0002	60,000	0.5	4.1	4.1	9.9	0.0	7.1	26	Iwasaki and Schmid (1970)
8 S α_3-Glycoprotein	0.04	220,000	0.4	11.0		10.8		9.2	31	Haupt et al. (1971)
Sialic acid-free β_1-Glycoprotein	0.002	31,000	1.1	8.7	7.5	15.5	0.0	0.0	30	Labat et al. (1969)
β_2-Glycoprotein I	n.g.	40,000	0.3	7.8		6.2		4.5	19	Haupt and Heide (1965)
β_2-Glycoprotein II	n.g.	60,000	0.2	2.2		1.8		1.5	6	Haupt and Heide (1965)
β_2-Glycoprotein III	0.07	35,000	0.1	2.5		2.0		5.5	10	Heide and Schwick (1973); Schwick et al. (1968)

[a] The glycoproteins are arranged alphabetically in the case of named proteins and according to electrophoretic mobility in other cases. Total carbohydrate is given to the nearest whole number. Results in the literature quoted as "hexosamine" and so on, are calculated as the N-acetyl derivative. Abbreviations are as follows: Fuc, fucose; Man, mannose; Hex, hexose; Gal, galactose; GlcNAc, N-acetylglucosamine; HexNAc, N-acetylhexosamine; GalNAc, N-acetylgalactosamine; n.g., not given in literature.

[c] Glucose.

[d] See transcortin.

charide is linked through nitrogen to a carboxyl group of the amino acid side chain (—C1—NH—CO—). In this type of linkage, the sugar involved is always N-acetylglucosamine and the amino acid is always asparagine. Of course after acid hydrolysis the asparagine is identified as aspartic acid and is therefore referred to as aspartic acid in the literature and here. This linkage was first postulated by Johansen *et al.* (1961).

In the O-glycosidic type of linkage the anomeric carbon atom is attached through oxygen to a hydroxyamino acid in an ether (acetal) linkage (—C1—O—CH$_2$—). In this type of linkage both the monosaccharide and the amino acid may vary. A summary of these linkages is shown in Table III.

In order to establish the type of linkage present in a glycoprotein, three aspects of the problem must be investigated. These are to determine first the amino acid involved, second the monosaccharide involved, and third the details of the linkage itself.

It is comparatively easy to determine the amino acid involved in the linkage since exhaustive proteolysis of the glycoprotein produces glycopeptides, some of which contain only the linkage amino acid. Ovalbumin was the first glycoprotein in which aspartic acid was shown to be involved in the carbohydrate linkage (Cunningham *et al.*, 1957); Jevons, 1958; Johansen *et al.*, 1958). This observation was soon extended to the plasma proteins and aspartic acid was implicated in glycopeptides from IgG (Rosevear and Smith, 1958; Clamp and Putnam, 1964), α_1-acid glycoprotein (Kamiyama and Schmid, 1962a,b; Eylar, 1962), and transferrin (Jamieson, 1964, 1965b; Spik *et al.*, 1965a,b).

Few attempts have been made to use corresponding procedures to identify the linkage monosaccharide although Hughes and Jeanloz (1966) in a study of α_1-acid glycoprotein used glycosidase incubation and periodate oxidation techniques to isolate material with only N-acetylglucosamine remaining attached to peptide. The usual procedure to establish the linkage, however, is to take advantage of the fact that the carbohydrate–amino acid bond is marginally more stable to acid hydrolysis than other glycosidic linkages. Glycopeptides are therefore prepared containing just aspartic acid and these are subjected to controlled acid hydrolysis. In this manner the N-acetylglucosamine-aspartic acid compound was isolated from ovalbumin (Marks *et al.*, 1962, 1963; Bogdanov *et al.*, 1962, 1964; Yamashina *et al.*, 1963, 1965). Similar studies were carried out on human plasma proteins such as α_1-acid glycoprotein (Yamashina *et al.*, 1965; Wagh *et al.*, 1969). Other techniques have been used to isolate this compound such as a series of Smith degradations (Makino and Yamashina, 1966).

N-Acetylglucosamine could in theory be linked to any one of three reactive groups in aspartic acid, namely, the 1- or the 4-carboxyl groups

TABLE III

Types of Linkage between Carbohydrate and Protein in Some Human Glycoconjugates

Type of linkage	Monosaccharide involved	Amino acid involved	Occurrence
N-Glycosidic	*N*-Acetylglucosamine	Aspartic acid	Probably all plasma glycoproteins
O-Glycosidic	Xylose	Serine	Certain proteoglycans
	Galactose	5-Hydroxy-lysine	C1q; collagen
	N-Acetylgalactosamine	Serine and/or threonine	Mucus glycoproteins; IgA; IgD; membrane glycoproteins (rabbit IgG; fetuin)

or the 2-amino group. The 1-carboxyl and the 2-amino groups are unlikely because carbohydrate-linked aspartic acid is always found internally in a peptide chain. However, more conclusive evidence was obtained from studies on glycopeptides. In these, involvement of the 1-carboxyl group could be excluded because a phenylthiohydantoin could be made without release of carbohydrate (Fletcher *et al.,* 1963). Similarly, the 2-amino group must be unsubstituted because a 2,4-dinitrophenyl derivative could be prepared (Johansen *et al.,* 1961; Yamashina and Makino, 1962). By exclusion therefore of the other linkage possibilities the 4-carboxyl group is involved (Fig. 9) which was the original suggestion (Johansen *et al.,* 1961; Bogdanov *et al.,* 1962).

No exception has been found to the rule that in mammalian glycoproteins when aspartic acid is attached to carbohydrate the link is N-glycosidic in type and the monosaccharide involved is *N*-acetylglucosamine. As a result, when glycopeptides are isolated containing just aspartic acid most workers assume the nature of the linkage and do

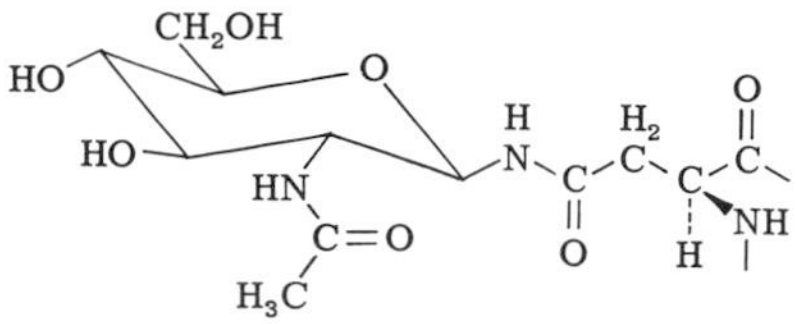

Fig. 9. Structure of the N-glycosidic bond between *N*-acetylglucosamine and aspartic acid. The hydrogen atoms on the monosaccharide have been omitted.

not attempt to characterize it further. This could be a dangerous assumption and the easiest method to obtain more information about the linkage is to incubate the aspartic acid-containing glycopeptide with a specific enzyme. This enzyme, called 4'-L-aspartylglycosylamine amidohydrolase abbreviated to amidohydrolase in this discussion, has been isolated from a variety of sources including sheep epididymis (Murakami and Eylar, 1965; Clamp et al., 1966), ram testis (Roston et al., 1965), pig serum (Makino et al., 1968) or kidney (Kohno and Yamashina, 1969), hen oviduct (Plummer et al., 1968; Tarentino and Maley, 1969), and snails (Kaverzneva, 1966). Roston et al. (1965) appeared to suggest in their paper that the enzyme was active against intact ovomucoid. Most studies with the enzyme, however, agree that the linkage is only hydrolyzed when both the 1-carboxyl and 2-amino groups of aspartic acid are unsubstituted.

Amidohydrolase has been used to investigate the linkage in glycopeptides from ovalbumin (Clamp et al., 1966) and from plasma proteins such as α_1-acid glycoprotein (Yamauchi et al., 1968).

All the plasma glycoproteins that have been investigated in detail contain N-glycosidic type of linkages. The O-glycosidic linkage on the other hand is unusual in plasma glycoproteins. Table III lists the linkages of this type and of these, only the N-acetylgalactosamine-serine/threonine and the galactose-hydroxylysine have been demonstrated in plasma glycoproteins. The former was first shown to be present in an IgAl globulin (Dawson and Clamp, 1967a,b, 1968), and the latter in C1q (Calcott and Müller-Eberhard, 1972).

The techniques used to establish an O-glycosidic linkage differ to some extent from those described above for N-glycosides. The isolation of an N-acetylgalactosamine-containing glycopeptide which also contains serine and/or threonine but little or no aspartic acid is of course suggestive of this type of linkage but it is not conclusive. However the O-glycosidic linkage is susceptible to chemical cleavage by alkali in the β-elimination reaction. β-Hydroxy-α-amino acids with substituted carboxyl and amino groups possess a labile acidic hydrogen atom on C-2. In the presence of base this is removed as a proton and the bonding electrons move into and create a double bond between C-2 and C-3 of the amino acid. This process is facilitated by the carbohydrate as a satisfactory departing group. The reaction is illustrated in Fig. 10. The overall result is that the oligosaccharide unit is released and the hydroxyamino acid is converted to an $\alpha\beta$ unsaturated amino acid. This base-catalyzed elimination reaction is usually carried out in the presence of an excess of reducing agent such as sodium borohydride. The liberated reducing end group is thus converted to the corresponding glycitol and the unsaturated amino acid is converted to the corresponding saturated one, name-

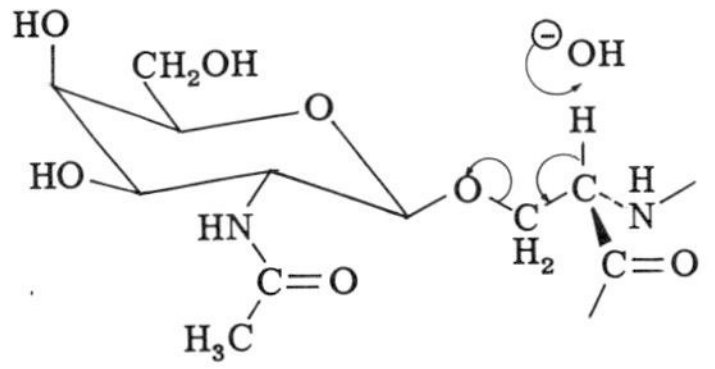

Fig. 10. Structure of the O-glycosidic bond between *N*-acetylgalactosamine and serine. The hydrogen atoms on the monosaccharide have been omitted. The arrows show the mechanism of the alkali-catalyzed β-elimination reaction.

ly, alanine from serine and α-aminobutyric acid from threonine. This technique therefore would confirm a suspected O-glycosidic linkage by the liberation of the oligosaccharide unit and should identify the linkage amino acid. In practice, interpretation of the results is a little more difficult because there is some elimination and conversion of hydroxyamino acids not carrying oligosaccharide units.

C. Types of Oligosaccharide Units

Three types of oligosaccharide units have been found in plasma glycoproteins. Two of these are N-glycosidically linked and can be further subdivided into "simple" and "complex" (Clamp and Johnson, 1972). The third type is O-glycosidically linked. Each type has certain characteristics, although these are by no means rigidly exclusive.

The simple unit contains just mannose and *N*-acetylglucosamine. The *N*-acetylglucosamine content is low, being less than 3 and usually only 2 residues. The mannose content is greater than this and may be as high as 11 residues. This unit is probably not as highly branched as the complex unit.

The complex unit usually contains fucose, mannose, galactose, *N*-acetylglucosamine, and sialic acid. The *N*-acetylglucosamine content is generally 3 or more residues which is equal to, or more than, the mannose content. The unit tends to be highly branched.

O-Glycosidically linked units have so far only been identified in the immunoglobulins and in C1q. Units of the *N*-acetylgalactosamine-serine/threonine type have been found in IgA1 (Dawson and Clamp, 1968; Baenziger and Kornfeld, 1974b), the heavy chain disease proteins Cra (Clamp *et al.,* 1968) and Zuc (Frangione and Milstein, 1969), and rabbit IgG (Smyth and Utsumi, 1967). The unit contains, apart from *N*-acetylgalactosamine, galactose and often sialic acid and some of them also contain mannose. The C1q component of complement appears to contain a disaccharide unit consisting of glucosyl-galactose in which the galactose residue is O-glycosidically linked to hydroxylysine (Calcott and Müller-Eberhard, 1972). Thus the collagen-like amino acid sequence in C1q (Reid, 1974) contains oligosaccharide units similar to those of collagen (Spiro, 1967).

D. Structure of Oligosaccharide Units

In order to present carbohydrate structures, which are by nature complex, some form of abbreviation must be employed. The usual method, as with amino acids, is to represent a monosaccharide by its first three letters. An exception to this rule is glucose, represented by "Glc" because "Glu" could be confused with the abbreviation for glutamic acid. N-Acetylglucosamine is written GlcNAc and similarly for N-acetylgalactosamine (GalNAc) and N-acetylneuraminic acid (NeuNAc). The anomeric configuration is placed immediately after the monosaccharide together with details of the linkage. Thus "Galβ1-4GlcNAc" means that the galactose is β-linked from C-1 to C-4 of N-acetylglucosamine. Where a position of linkage is uncertain, it will be written for example as 3/4/6, meaning that the linkage could be at C-3, C-4, or C-6. In the following discussion it is assumed that all monosaccharides are in the pyranose form and have the D-configuration apart from fucose which is assumed to have the L-configuration.

There have been very few investigations carried out upon the structure of O-glycosidically linked oligosaccharide units. A glycopolypeptide was isolated from IgA1 myeloma globulin (Dawson and Clamp, 1968) which contained 3 residues of galactose and 3 of N-acetylgalactosamine together with 5 residues of proline, 4 of serine, and 3 to 4 of threonine (Dawson and Clamp, 1967a). This glycopolypeptide could not be broken down to smaller units presumably because of the high content of proline and so it was not possible to decide whether there were 3 units consisting of Galβ1-3/4GalNAc or one unit containing all the carbohydrate. This problem has been resolved by Baenziger and Kornfeld (1974b), who found 5 units attached to serine in the hinge region of their IgA1 myeloma globulin. One of these consisted of just GalNAc whereas the other 4 had the structure Galβ1-3GalNAc. A similar unit occurs in the hinge region of rabbit IgG (Fanger and Smyth, 1972). The human heavy chain disease proteins Zuc (Frangione and Milstein, 1969) and Cra (Clamp *et al.,* 1968) also contain O-glycosidically linked units even though they are derived from IgG. However, they are a product of abnormal cells synthesizing an aberrant protein, which presumably contains the recognition peptide for N-acetylgalactosaminyl transferase. The composition of these various units is given in Table IV.

TABLE IV

Composition of O-Glycosidically Linked Oligosaccharide Units in Plasma Glycoproteins

| Glycoprotein | Carbohydrate content[a] (moles/mole) | | | | | References |
	Mannose	Galactose	Glucose	Sialic acid	N-Acetylgalactosamine	
IgA1	0	1 or 3	0	0 or 1	1 or 3	Dawson and Clamp (1968)
	0	0 to 1	0	0	1	Baenziger and Kornfeld (1974b)
Clq	0	1	1	0	0	Calcott and Müller-Eberhard (1972)
Rabbit IgG	0	1	0	0 to 2	1	Fanger and Smyth (1972)
"Cra"[b]	1	2	0	0 to 3	1	Clamp et al. (1968)

[a] Results are given to the nearest whole number.
[b] Heavy chain disease protein.

TABLE V

Composition of Some Simple Oligosaccharide Units in Plasma Glycoproteins

| | Carbohydrate content[a] (moles/mole) | | |
Glycoprotein	Mannose	N-Acetylglucosamine	References
IgA	4	3	Dawson and Clamp (1968a)
IgM	6	1	Spragg and Clamp (1969)
	5	2	Spragg and Clamp (1969)
	6	2	Spragg and Clamp (1969)
	2	2	Jouanneau et al. (1970)
	6	3	Jouanneau et al. (1970)
	6	2	Johnson and Clamp (1971)
	7	2	Johnson and Clamp (1971)
	8	2	Johnson and Clamp (1971)
	5	2	Shimizu et al. (1971)
	8	2	Shimizu et al. (1971)
	11	3	Shimizu et al. (1971)
	5	2	Hickman et al. (1972)
	6	2	Hickman et al. (1972)
	7	2	Hickman et al. (1972)
	3	1–2	Hurst et al. (1973)
	3–4	2	Hurst et al. (1973)
IgE	6	2	Baenziger et al. (1974a)

[a] Results are given to the nearest whole number.

As mentioned in a previous section, the N-glycosidically linked units can be divided into simple and complex. Simple units have been found in IgG (J. R. Clamp, unpublished findings), IgA (Dawson and Clamp, 1968), and IgM (Clamp et al., 1967; Spragg and Clamp, 1969; Jouanneau et al., 1970; Johnson and Clamp, 1971; Hickman et al., 1972; Hurst et al., 1973). The analyses of these various groups is given in Table V. From these results certain conclusions can be drawn about these simple units. The N-acetylglucosamine content is always low, never being more than three residues and usually only two. The mannose content, on the other hand, can be very high. It is always greater than the N-acetylglucosamine content and may be as high as 11 residues. There are differences between the structures proposed for this type of unit. Largely on the basis of results from periodate oxidation studies, Dawson and Clamp (1968) and Johnson and Clamp (1971) suggested that the simple unit was unbranched. Dawson and Clamp (1968) proposed that the sequence of mannose residues was attached to an inner region consisting of GlcNAcβ1-3/4GlcNAcβ1-3/4GlcNACβ1-

Asp, whereas Johnson and Clamp (1971) proposed that the sequence of mannose residues was attached to GlcNAcβ1-3Manα1-3Manα1-3/4GlcNAcβ1-Asp. On the other hand Hickman *et al.* (1972), largely on the basis of methylation studies, suggested that the simple unit was branched although their structure agreed with that of Dawson and Clamp (1968) in having *N*-acetylchitobiose linked to aspartic acid.

The overall structure was as follows:

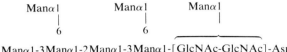

Baenziger *et al.* (1974a) have studied the simple unit from IgE using glycosidase incubations, periodate oxidation and methylation techniques. Their structure was similar to that proposed for IgM units by Hickman *et al.* (1972) in being branched, but differed from those given above in not having an *N*-acetylchitobiose entity linked to aspartic acid. In this respect it was closer to the structure given by Johnson and Clamp (1971) for an IgM unit. The overall structure is as follows:

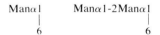

This structure differs from the others in that the anomeric configuration assigned to two of the mannose residues is β, and is α for one of the *N*-acetylglucosamine residues. This point is discussed later.

The simple unit appears in some ways to be an extension or a development of the core region of the complex unit. Possibly, therefore, similar initial structures are biosynthesized in both cases, but these are further developed in separate ways depending presumably upon the position of the unit in the overall molecule. Thus two IgM glycoproteins, which contain both simple and complex units, have the simple units in corresponding positions (Shimizu *et al.*, 1971).

The complex type of oligosaccharide unit has been found in a number of plasma glycoproteins, a selection of which are shown in Table VI. The *N*-acetylglucosamine content of complex units tends to be equal to or greater than the mannose content which in turn is greater than the galactose content. The reason for the relative amounts of each monosaccharide follows from the structure of the complex unit.

The discussion of the structure of the complex oligosaccharide unit is easier if the "core" and "periphery" of the unit are dealt with separately.

TABLE VI

Composition of Some Complex Oligosaccharide Units in Plasma Glycoproteins

| Glycoprotein | Carbohydrate content[a] (moles/mole) | | | | | References |
	Fuc	Man	Gal	GlcNAc	NeuNAc	
Ceruloplasmin	0–1	2–4	1–3	2–3	1–2	Jamieson (1965a)
Haptoglobin	–	2	4	4	2	Cheftel *et al.* (1965)
IgG	0–1	2–3	1–2	4	0–1	Clamp and Putnam (1964)
IgA1	0–1	3	2	3–4	0–2	Dawson and Clamp (1968)
	0–1	3	2	4	2	Baenziger and Kornfeld (1974a)
	0	3	2	4	0	Moore and Putnam (1973)
	0	3	2	5	1	Baenziger and Kornfeld (1974a)
IgM	0–1	3–4	2	4–5	1	Hickman *et al.* (1972)
	0–1	2–6	1–2	2–3	p	Hurst *et al.* (1973)
	1	3–4	1–2	3–5	0–2	Johnson and Clamp (1971)
	0–1	1–3	1–2	2–4	0–2	Jouanneau *et al.* (1970)
	0–1	1–3	1–2	2–5	0–2	Shimizu *et al.* (1971)
	0–1	3	1–2	3–4	0–2	Spragg and Clamp (1969)
IgE	1	3	2	4	1–2	Baenziger *et al.* (1974a,b)
Transferrin	–	4	2	4	2	Jamieson *et al.* (1971)
α_1-Acid glycoprotein	0–1	3	4	6	–	Wagh *et al.* (1969)
	0–1	2	2–5	3–6	2–4	Yamauchi *et al.* (1968)
α_2-Macroglobulin	0–1	3	2–3	3	0–2	Bourrillon *et al.* (1968)
	0–1	3	2	5	1–2	Dunn and Spiro (1967b)

[a] Abbreviations are as in Table II and in the text; "p" means the monosaccharide is present but not estimated.

There is general agreement about the structure of the periphery of complex units. The sequence of residues is as follows:

$$\text{NeuNAc}\alpha 2\text{-}2/3/4/6\text{Gal}\beta 1\text{-}4\text{GlcNAc-}$$

The only variability appears to be in the attachment of sialic acid to galactose which can be to any one of the free hydroxyl groups. Thus the linkage can be to C-2 in α_1-acid glycoprotein (Isemura and Schmid, 1971) and IgG (Rothfus and Smith, 1963), to C-3 in fetuin (Spiro, 1964) and IgA (Dawson and Clamp, 1968), to C-3, C-4, or C-6 in α_1-acid glycoprotein (Eylar and Jeanloz, 1962a; Jeanloz and Closse, 1963; Isemura and Schmid, 1971), and to C-6 in IgA1 (Baenziger and Kornfeld, 1974a), IgE (Baenziger *et al.*, 1974b), and transferrin (Jamieson *et al.*, 1971). Sialic acid has up to now always been found in a terminal position except when two residues are linked together (Kühn and Gauhe, 1965). There is a possibility that in some glycoproteins two sialic acid residues may be linked to different positions of the same galactose (Dawson and Clamp, 1968). The sialic acid is readily removed either by mild acid hydrolysis (Yamashina, 1956) or by the use of neuraminidase from a variety of microorganisms such as *Clostridium perfringens* (Labat and Schmid, 1969) and *Vibrio cholerae* (Montreuil and Biserte, 1959; Marshall and Porath, 1965) which have both been used on α_1-acid glycoprotein with the interesting observation that the sialic acid was released at different rates, presumably because of differences in position or linkage. Thus Isemura and Schmid (1971) have suggested that some sialic acid residues may be linked to N-acetylglucosamine. Similarly, neuraminidase from *Corynebacterium diphtheriae* has been used to release all the sialic acid from ceruloplasmin and transferrin (Jamieson, 1965a, 1966).

Fucose is also in a terminal position as a nonreducing end group, although there is much less certainty about its position in the overall oligosaccharide structure. This monosaccharide is also released under relatively mild conditions of acid hydrolysis (Yamashina, 1956). Fucose is usually attached to an internally located N-acetylglucosamine residue, such as the one involved in linkage to aspartic acid. This has been shown in IgA (Dawson and Clamp, 1968; Baenziger and Kornfeld, 1974a), IgM (Spragg and Clamp, 1969; Hickman *et al.*, 1972), and IgE (Baenziger *et al.*, 1974b). Alternatively it may be similar to sialic acid in attachment to galactose. After the removal of sialic acid, galactose becomes susceptible to enzymatic release. Interestingly, β-galactosidase does not release all of the galactose from sialic acid-free α_1-acid glycoprotein whether the enzyme is derived from *Diplococcus pneumoniae* (Hughes and Jeanloz, 1964a) or from *C. perfringens* (Chipowsky and McGuire, 1969). Similarly the exposed N-acetylglucosamine cannot all be released enzymatically (Hughes and Jeanloz, 1964b), although this may be due to enzyme limitations because Chipowsky and McGuire (1969), using a different N-acetylglucosaminidase, found that the theoretical amount of monosaccharide was released. These sequential enzyme studies have been confirmed by partial acid hydrolysis in which N-acetyllactosamine (Galβ1-4GlcNAc) has been isolated (Eylar and Jeanloz, 1962a). Similarly, the results from periodate oxidation are consistent with the above data, since all the sialic acid and fucose is oxidized together with most of the galactose whereas the N-acetylglucosamine survives (Popenoe, 1958, 1959; Eylar and Jeanloz, 1962b; Willard, 1962). The galactose results would be compatible with a small number of residues substituted at C-3 or disubstituted, and N-acetylglucosamine would be resistant if substituted at C-4.

There is much less agreement about the structure of the central or core region of the complex units. All the core structures agree in containing 2 N-acetylglucosamine residues although the mannose content varies from 3 for α_2-macroglobulin (Dunn and Spiro, 1967b), α_1-acid glycoprotein (Wagh *et al.,* 1969), IgA (Dawson and Clamp, 1968; Baenziger and Kornfeld, 1974a) and IgM (Spragg and Clamp, 1969) to 4 for IgM (Hickman *et al.,* 1972), transferrin (Jamieson *et al.,* 1971), and IgE (Baenziger *et al.,* 1974b). This difference probably reflects some intrinsic structural variation which is discussed later.

There are two further points of difference between the structures proposed for the core region. A number of structures include an N-acetylchitobiose unit linked to aspartic acid (GlcNAcβ1-4GlcNAc-Asp), for example, in IgG (Kornfeld *et al.,* 1971) IgA1 (Baenziger and Kornfeld, 1974a), and IgE (Baenziger *et al.,* 1974b), whereas others have one or more mannose residues attached to the linkage N-acetylglucosamine, for example, in IgA (Dawson and Clamp, 1968), IgM (Spragg and Clamp, 1969), α_1-acid glycoprotein (Wagh *et al.,* 1969), and transferrin (Jamieson *et al.,* 1971). It is unlikely that the core region invariably contains an internally linked N-acetylglucosamine residue in addition to the linkage residue as for example in an N-acetylchitobiose sequence. If this were so, the complex unit would always have an N-acetylglucosamine content that is two residues greater than the galactose content (assuming that the majority of peripheral regions have the sequence: Galβ1-4GlcNAc). The isolation from IgA of units containing 2 galactose residues which varied in their N-acetylglucosamine content from 3 to 4, together with other evidence, led Dawson and Clamp (1968) to place the second hexosamine in the core as a branch off the main sequence. This kind of evidence together with that for the sequence of mannose residues emphasizes the other point of difference in the postulated structures, namely, in the degree and positions of branching. A few of the proposed core structures are given in Table VII, and these are probably representative of most of the postulated structures for this type of unit. It is not possible to be certain whether the differences shown in Table VII are real or imagined. Unfortunately the limitations inherent in present methods of structural investigation mean that no one structure can be advanced with certainty. On the other hand, it is possible that

TABLE VII

Structure of the Core Region of Complex Oligosaccharide Units from Some Human Plasma Glycoproteins

Glycoprotein	References	Structure
IgA IgM	Dawson and Clamp (1968) Spragg and Clamp (1969)	Manα1-2/4Manα1-2/4Manα1-3/4GlcNAcβ1-Asp $\qquad\qquad\qquad\qquad\qquad$ |$_{3/4}$ $\qquad\qquad\qquad\qquad$ GlcNAcβ1
Transferrin	Jamieson et al. (1971)	Manα1-2/4Manα1-2/4/6Manα1-2/4/6Manα1-3/4GlcNAcβ1-Asp $\qquad\qquad\qquad\qquad\qquad\qquad\qquad\qquad$ | $\qquad\qquad\qquad\qquad\qquad\qquad\qquad$ GlcNAcβ1
α₁-Acid glycoprotein	Wagh et al. (1969)	Manα1-3/4GlcNAcβ1-2/4Manα1-3/4/6GlcNAcβ1-Asp $\qquad\qquad\qquad\qquad\qquad\qquad\qquad$ |$_{6/4/3}$ $\qquad\qquad\qquad\qquad\qquad\qquad$ Manα1
IgM	Hickman et al. (1972)	Manα1-3Man-⎤ $\qquad\qquad\qquad$ ⎬ [GlcNAc-GlcNAc]-Asp $\qquad\qquad$ Man-⎦ $\quad$ Manα1 $\qquad$ | $\qquad$ 6
IgA1 IgE	Baenziger and Kornfeld (1974a) Baenziger et al. (1974b)	Manα1-3Manβ1-4GlcNAcβ1-4GlcNAcβ1-Asp $\quad$ Manα1 $\qquad$ | $\qquad$ 6

considerable variations exist in core structures and are important in the creation of unique oligosaccharide units perhaps for clearance recognition and other purposes.

The use of specific glycosidases enables the anomeric configurations of individual monosaccharides to be assigned. In most cases fucose, mannose, and sialic acid are α-linked whereas galactose and N-acetylglucosamine are β-linked. However, recently it has become recognized that some monosaccharides may have the alternative anomeric configuration and this would of course have a profound effect on the overall structure of the oligosaccharide unit. Thus an α-linked N-acetylglucosamine residue has been demonstrated in a simple unit from IgE (Baenziger et al., 1974a). In addition, it now appears that in many glycoproteins the mannose residue attached to the asparagine-linked N-acetylchitobiose moiety has the β configuration as for example in IgE (Baenziger et al., 1974b).

The peripheral trisaccharide units are usually attached to the mannose residues of the core region, either to those in a "terminal" or external position or to internally located residues. Thus Hickman et al. (1972) postulate that in IgM there are peripheral moieties attached to two of the core terminal mannose residues, and similar findings were reported by Wagh et al. (1969) for α_1-acid glycoprotein except that in this case both external mannose residues carried two peripheral moieties. Transferrin (Jamieson et al., 1971), IgA (Dawson and Clamp, 1968), and IgM (Spragg and Clamp, 1969) contain, in addition to an externally attached moiety as outlined above, one that is linked to an internally located mannose residue. This trisaccharide moiety in transferrin is linked through a second N-acetylglucosamine to the mannose residue (Jamieson et al., 1971). The sequential use of neuraminidase, galactosidase and N-acetylglucosaminidase removes most of the peripheral moieties, in for example, α_1-acid glycoprotein thereby exposing core mannose residues which are themselves susceptible to mannosidase (Li, 1966). The substitution of these mannose units may be the reason why more than half the mannose content of the complex unit is resistant to periodate oxidation (Sato et al., 1967).

E. Heterogeneity of Oligosaccharide Units

The term "heterogeneity" has been used in a number of senses to describe differences in the carbohydrate of glycoproteins. Thus it has been used to describe differences between glycoproteins from different individuals or for glycoproteins that contain more than one type of oligosaccharide unit. The term is best reserved for those differences that exist in the oligosaccharide units within a glycoprotein family from a single individual.

Heterogeneity may be subdivided into the following types:

(a) *Site heterogeneity.* This may occur within a single symmetrical molecule or exist between different molecules
   (i) Unmatched units
   (ii) Mismatched units
(b) *Compositional heterogeneity.* Variations in the carbohydrate content of oligosaccharide units
   (i) Peripheral or microheterogeneity
   (ii) Central or core heterogeneity
(c) *Structural heterogeneity* (*isomerism*). Affecting sequence of residues, positions of linkage, anomeric configuration, and so on.

Examples of site heterogeneity in which there are unmatched oligosaccharide units have been found in a number of glycoproteins. For example, ribonuclease occurs as two species, one of which is glycosylated whereas the other is not (Plummer and Hirs, 1964). The immunoglobulins are symmetrical molecules consisting of two heavy chains and two light chains, and an unmatched unit has been found within a single molecule. Thus rabbit IgG has been shown (Smyth and Utsumi, 1967; Fanger and Smyth, 1972) to contain an O-glycosidically linked unit attached to a threonine residue on one heavy chain but not in the corresponding position on the other heavy chain. Other plasma glycoproteins show site heterogeneity with unmatched units, for example, this occurs among the different forms of ceruloplasmin (Rydén, 1971).

Another type of site heterogeneity that could theoretically occur is that of mismatched units. Thus a simple unit might be attached to an aspartic acid residue in one polypeptide chain whereas a complex unit is present at the corresponding site on another chain. This would be difficult to detect except during protein sequence studies, but might be suspected in a glycopeptide preparation whose analysis is an average of the two types. In two IgM proteins that have been examined in detail (Shimizu *et al.*, 1971) the two simple units and three complex units occur in corresponding positions. This would indicate that the development of a unit into simple or complex is precisely determined.

The biosynthesis of oligosaccharides is fundamentally different to that of polypeptides. Oligosaccharides are built up by the stepwise addition of monosaccharide residues catalyzed by specific glycosyl transferases. The control of the synthesis therefore resides in the presence of specific enzymes and the availability of activated monosaccharide intermediates, that is, the nucleotide derivatives. There is no template mechanism although the transferases may be organized into one or more polyenzyme systems around a recognition site for the efficient completion of particular oligosaccharide units (Roseman, 1970). The explanation of compositional heterogeneity has been that it is a built-in consequence of the biosynthetic method although this idea is now being challenged (see Section V). An alternative explanation, though much less likely, is that the oligosaccharide units may be modified after completion by various glycosidases. These enzymes are known to occur intracellularly and in various extracellular fluids and may release peripheral residues.

Compositional heterogeneity may affect either the core region of the units or the peripheral residues. Peripheral or microheterogeneity affecting the sialic acid residues is easy to detect because of the effect it has upon the charge of the glycoprotein molecule and this has been shown by electrophoresis (Schmid *et al.*, 1962) and by isoelectric focusing (Beeley, 1971). Some of the variation in sialic acid content may be due to the lability of the glycosidic linkage of this monosaccharide. Residues are therefore lost under relatively mild conditions during the various preparative procedures or perhaps even upon standing in solution under the influence of the monosaccharide's inherent acidity. The fucose content of a unit may also vary and carbohydrate analyses of oligosaccharide units rarely show the presence of an integral number of fucose residues. Thus complex units have been isolated from IgA1 entirely devoid of this monosaccharide (Moore and Putnam, 1973; Baenziger and Kornfeld, 1974a). Similarly, the galactose and *N*-acetylglucosamine content of units may vary, usually within limits, but sometimes the whole peripheral sequence appears to be missing, as for example, in α_2-macroglobulin (Dunn and Spiro, 1967b).

There appears to be much less compositional variation in the core region of complex units, although the mannose content which is usually 3 in IgM glycopeptides may vary between 2 (Shimizu *et al.*, 1971) and 4 (Spragg and Clamp, 1969), and the content of *N*-acetylglucosamine may vary between 3 and 5.

The distinction between "peripheral" and "core" residues is harder to draw in simple units although these also show compositional heterogeneity. Thus the content of mannose may vary from 5 to 11 and that of *N*-acetylglucosamine from 2 to 3.

The same type of heterogeneity affects O-glycosidically linked units, particularly in the attachment of sialic acid. In IgA1 the content of this monosaccharide may be 0 or 1 (Dawson and Clamp, 1968) and in rabbit IgG may be 1 or 2 (Fanger and Smyth, 1972). Galactose may also be missing so that the unit consists of just *N*-acetylgalactosamine (Baenziger and Kornfeld, 1974b).

Compositional heterogeneity is relatively easy to detect. The isolation of glycopeptides with sufficient peptide still attached will establish the position or site identity of that oligosaccharide unit. Variation in the carbohydrate content must therefore be due to heterogeneity within the unit. Similar results can be obtained during protein sequence studies. Structural heterogeneity within a unit, which is really a form of isomerism, is much more difficult to detect because of the inherent difficulties of structural investigations. Thus incomplete release of monosaccharides during glycosidase incubations may have many explanations other than variations in sequence of residues. Similarly nonintegral results of periodate oxidation or methylation studies are usually attributed to methodological difficulties rather than interpreted as evidence of structural heterogeneity. Nevertheless, variation in the linkage of sialic acid to galactose in α_1-acid glycoprotein as discussed above may be regarded as an example of structural heterogeneity affecting linkage positions. Where some other technique can be used to detect differences between oligosaccharide structures, then such differences can be found. For example, serological techniques will detect differences in nonreducing end groups of the oligosaccharide units of mucus-type glycoproteins (blood group substances). These differences are genetically controlled through the presence or absence of specific glycosyltransferases. In addition the blood group substances contain a core structure that also shows structural heterogeneity. Thus in type 1 units galactose is β-linked to the 3 position of N-acetylglucosamine whereas in type 2 units the attachment is to the 4 position (Watkins, 1966). The fact that "heterogeneity" in blood group substances is not haphazard but genetically controlled suggests that this may be true of glycoproteins in general.

F. Number and Sites of Oligosaccharide Units in Plasma Glycoproteins

The number of oligosaccharide units varies considerably between different plasma glycoproteins. For example, in the human immunoglobulin family the number of units in each protein molecule is 2 for IgG and 50 for IgM. However, the molecular weights of these two glycoproteins are quite different and a more satisfactory way of representing the "density" of oligosaccharide units is to relate the molecular weight to the number of units as shown in Table VIII. On this basis, α_1-acid glycoprotein has one unit for every 8000 or so of molecular weight and at the other extreme, IgG has a unit for every 75,000. One could say, therefore, that the density of units is 10 times greater in the former glycoprotein than in the latter, and that both are widely removed from the average density which is 1 unit/31,000. The average density is equivalent to an oligosac-

TABLE VIII

Types, Number, and Sites of Oligosaccharide Units in Some Human Plasma Glycoproteins

Glycoprotein	Polypeptide chains		Site of carbohydrate	Number and types of oligosaccharide units[a]			MW^b / No. of units	References
	No.	Types		N linked		O linked		
				S type	C type			
Ceruloplasmin	1 or 4	α; β			9–10		16,000	Jamieson (1965a)
Fibrinogen	6	Aα; Bβ; γ	Bβ; γ		8		41,000	Gaffney (1972)
Haptoglobin 1–1	4	α; β	β		7–8		13,000	Cheftel et al. (1965)
					6–7		15,000	Gerbeck et al. (1967)
IgG	4	Heavy; light	Heavy		2		75,000	Clamp and Putnam (1964)
IgA (monomer)	4	Heavy; light	Heavy	1	3	2 or 6	27,000	Dawson and Clamp (1968)
				0	4	10	12,000	Baenziger and Kornfeld (1974a,b)
IgM (monomer)	4	Heavy; light	Heavy	4	6		18,000	Shimizu et al. (1971)
IgE	4	Heavy; light	Heavy	2	6		24,000	Baenziger et al. (1974a)
Transferrin	1				2		38,000	Jamieson et al. (1971)
α₁-Acid glycoprotein	1				4		10,000	Wagh et al. (1969)
					5		8,000	Schmid et al. (1971)
					6		7,000	Yamauchi et al. (1968)
α₁-Macroglobulin	20–25				35		26,000	Bourrillon et al. (1968); Razafimahaleo et al. (1969)
α₁-Antitrypsin	1				31		29,000	Dunn and Spiro (1967b)
					4		13,500	S. K. Chan (personal communication, 1974)

[a] Types of oligosaccharide units are abbreviated as follows: N linked, N-glycosidically linked; O linked, O-glycosidically linked; S type, simple type; C type, complex type.

[b] Molecular weight divided by number of oligosaccharide units.

charide unit for about every 200 amino acids. However, this gives only an approximate idea of the density of units in any glycoprotein. For example, α_1-acid glycoprotein has a stretch of 65 amino acids carrying 4 oligosaccharide units (Schmid *et al.,* 1971). Even this density of 1 unit for every 16 amino acids does not match that of the mucus glycoproteins which have on average 3 to 4 times as many oligosaccharide units.

The attachment of N-glycosidically linked units is always to a sequence of amino acids containing the tripeptide Asn-X-Ser/Thr where X represents some other amino acid and Ser/Thr means either serine or threonine (Marshall, 1972). Almost any amino acid can occur in position X (Table IX), although some are rather rare, for example, aromatic amino acids and proline. This has been pointed out by Marshall (1972) who suggests that hydrogen bonding is necessary between the OH group of the hydroxyamino acid and the carbonyl group of asparagine. Possibly, therefore, the aromatic amino acids sterically hinder

TABLE IX

Tripeptide Sequences in Glycopeptides from Some Human Plasma Glycoproteins

X	Asn-X-Ser	Asn-X-Thr
Ala	IgM (Putnam *et al.,* 1973)	α_1-Acid glycoprotein (Schmid *et al.,* 1971)
		IgM (Putnam *et al.,* 1973)
Asx	IgM (Hurst *et al.,* 1973)	Ceruloplasmin (Rydén and Eaker, 1974)
Gly		α_1-Acid glycoprotein (Schmid *et al.,* 1971)
Ile	IgM (Putnam *et al.,* 1973)	
Leu		Ceruloplasmin (Rydén and Eaker, 1974)
Lys	α_1-Acid glycoprotein (Schmid *et al.,* 1971)	α_1-Acid glycoprotein (Schmid *et al.,* 1971)
	Transferrin (Charet and Montreuil, 1971)	Fibrinogen (Iwanaga *et al.,* 1968)
Pro		IgM (Hurst *et al.,* 1973)
Ser		IgG (Edelman *et al.,* 1969)
		IgM (Jouanneau *et al.,* 1970)
		Haptoglobin (Hew and Dixon, 1972)
Thr	IgG (Press and Hogg, 1970)	α_1-Acid glycoprotein (Schmid *et al.,* 1971)
Val	IgM (Putnam *et al.,* 1973)	Transferrin (Charet and Montreuil 1971)
	Ceruloplasmin (Rydén and Eaker, 1974)	

the formation of this bond, whereas proline alters the orientation of the peptide chain. A very unusual sequence, namely, Asn-Pro-Thr, has been reported for IgM glycopeptides (Hurst *et al.,* 1973), although this sequence does not match that of a corresponding IgM glycopeptide reported by Putnam *et al.* (1973). This sequence therefore needs to be confirmed before the above "rule" is said to be broken for plasma glycoproteins.

Although the sequence Asn-X-Ser/Thr is necessary for carbohydrate attachment, the converse does not follow, namely, that carbohydrate is always attached where there is that sequence (Shimizu *et al.,* 1971) and in fact only about 20% of such sequences are glycosylated (Hunt and Dayhoff, 1970). This is not necessarily the result of a deficiency of biosynthetic potential in certain cells because a species of ovalbumin has been isolated which contains two sequences consisting of Asn-Leu-Ser/Thr, only one of which is glycosylated (Wiseman *et al.,* 1972). It is likely that other factors are more important, such as the relationship of the tripeptide sequence to the surface of the glycoprotein molecule, or that the initial transferase, although requiring the tripeptide sequence, is highly specific and recognizes a larger area of the glycoprotein surface. The suggestion has been made (Jackson and Hirs, 1970) that the nature of the amino acid X influences the type of oligosaccharide unit that is biosynthesized on the adjacent asparagine. It was suggested that if X is apolar the unit is likely to be simple in type, whereas if X is polar, the unit is complex. There are so many exceptions to this suggestion that, although attractive from the biosynthetic point of view, it must be abandoned. Thus within IgM alone there are exceptions to both aspects of the "rule." Two glycopeptides were isolated from IgM (Ou) in which X was alanine in one and isoleucine in the other and yet both the adjacent oligosaccharide units were complex in type (Shimizu *et al.,* 1971; Putnam *et al.,* 1973). On the other hand, a glycopeptide was isolated from IgM (Ga) in which X was Ser and the adjacent unit was simple in type (Jouanneau *et al.,* 1970).

In proteoglycan biosynthesis, the O-glycosidically linked units require the tripeptide sequence Ser-Gly-Gly (Baker and Rodén, 1970). Such units are rare in plasma glycoproteins and therefore insufficient sequences are available to draw any conclusions. However, even in the few that have been published, no discernible pattern emerges. In rabbit IgG (Smyth and Utsumi, 1967) and human IgA1 (Frangione and Wolfenstein-Todel, 1972) there is a proline residue on the N-terminus adjacent to the carbohydrate-linked hydroxyamino acid. However, a glycine residue is present in a corresponding position in a heavy chain

(Zuc) disease protein (Frangione and Milstein, 1969). The three sequences are as follows[1]:

Rabbit IgG	Lys-Pro-Thr*-Cys-Pro
IgA 1	Thr-Pro-Ser*-Pro-Ser
Zuc	Gly-Gly-Ser*-Ser-Glu

The site of the oligosaccharide units within various glycoprotein molecules does not seem to follow any discernible pattern, but this may be because the three-dimensional (tertiary) structure of the molecules is not known. In immunoglobulins and in haptoglobin, carbohydrate is attached to one of the two types of polypeptide chains whereas in fibrinogen it is attached to two out of the three types of chains. There is similar variation in the distribution of oligosaccharide units within different polypeptide chains. In IgM heavy chain (Putnam *et al.*, 1973), four of the five units are reasonably spread out throughout the constant region. In contrast, although the single polypeptide chain of α_1-acid glycoprotein is approximately equal in length to that of the constant region, four out of the five units are found in a stretch of just 65 amino acids (see Fig. 7 of Chapter 4, Volume I). However, as mentioned before in discussing density of oligosaccharide units, this kind of information gives little idea of how the units are arranged three-dimensionally and it is possible that in both glycoproteins the units are evenly distributed over the protein surface.

V. Functions of the Carbohydrate Moiety in Plasma Glycoproteins

A number of theories have been advanced to explain the presence of carbohydrate in glycoproteins. While it is important in this respect, however, to distinguish between the various types of glycoprotein, only theories relevant to plasma glycoproteins are discussed in detail in this chapter.

Structural glycoproteins at the cell surface have been implicated in a number of processes involving the interaction of molecules with plasma membranes or of one cell with another. Such processes include cell recognition, cell adhesion, contact inhibition, and growth regulation (Cook and Stoddart, 1973).

Mucus glycoproteins consist of polypeptide chains to which are attached large numbers of oligosaccharide units that surround and shield

[1] * indicates carbohydrate attachment.

the protein core. The carbohydrate, therefore, must be the most important component in determining the physical, chemical, and biological properties of the molecules.

Plasma glycoproteins provide much more of a problem when attempts are made to assess the significance of the carbohydrate content and indeed to decide whether the carbohydrate has any function at all. For most glycoproteins that have some activity that is easily measured, such as enzymes, the presence or absence or modification of the oligosaccharide units usually has no effect on the activity, for example, in the two forms of ribonuclease (Plummer and Hirs, 1963, 1964). In a few cases, however, removal of some carbohydrate does appear to have an effect. Certain rabbit antibodies, but not all, lose complement-fixing and opsonic activities when the IgG is treated with an endoglycosidase (Williams *et al.,* 1973). There are also a number of examples where the removal of sialic acid has an apparent effect upon the biological properties of the glycoprotein and this effect will be discussed later. Nevertheless, it would still be correct to state that in the majority of plasma glycoproteins, the role, if any, of the carbohydrate is still unknown. It would certainly be energetically favorable to the cell to dispense with the mechanisms necessary for glycoprotein biosynthesis, and the fact that this type of molecule exists at all is a strong indication that the oligosaccharide units are biologically functional.

The survival and indeed widespread nature of glycoproteins could be explained on the basis of a general function or a specific function of the carbohydrate. However, it is unlikely that the carbohydrate fulfills some general function. For example, it is hard to imagine any general function or role which would be conferred by such a wide range of carbohydrate contents, varying from a few percent in IgG to 40% in α_1-acid glycoprotein. In addition, the carbohydrate contents of the various immunoglobulin classes tend to be quite characteristic. There is, for example, greater similarity between human IgG, IgA, and IgM on the one hand and the corresponding pig immunoglobulin classes on the other hand than there is among the individual human immunoglobulin classes (J. Bourne and J. Clamp, unpublished observation). This suggests that there is quite strong evolutionary pressure keeping the carbohydrate content characteristic of the class. Such observations not only support the idea that carbohydrate in glycoproteins is functional, but also suggest that the carbohydrate plays a specific or precise role rather than a general one. There may, of course, be a single function that is nevertheless specific in terms of that glycoprotein, or the oligosaccharide units may have evolved to play a number of quite different roles depending on the particular circumstances or upon the overall function of the protein.

For example, plasma glycoproteins in Antarctic fish have an effect on the depression of freezing point that is equivalent to an equal weight of sodium chloride (DeVries *et al.,* 1970). This is an extreme example of carbohydrate affecting the physicochemical properties of the entire molecule, but any oligosaccharide unit, because of its bulk and pronounced hydrophilic nature, must affect the tertiary structure and therefore properties of some portion of the glycoprotein. Thus it has been suggested (Shimizu *et al.,* 1971) that the carbohydrate in IgM acts as a spacer between subunits, thereby preventing steric interference between the multiple binding sites. The carbohydrate may also be necessary to prevent nonspecific adsorption in a similar way to the hydrophilic arms in affinity chromatography (O'Carra *et al.,* 1974).

Apart from any effect on glycoprotein structure, the oligosaccharide units may also facilitate interaction with cell membranes, either before release (export) from the cell or upon the final uptake (fate) by the appropriate peripheral cell.

Eylar (1965) first suggested that the process of glycosylation was associated with export of proteins from the synthesizing cell. For example, the carbohydrate might act as a recognition signal, enabling the cell to distinguish between those proteins destined for export and those that are to remain within the cell. Alternatively, it might be the process of synthesis that enables the distinction to be made. That is, the glycosyltransferases in the process of binding to the unfinished oligosaccharide unit, confine the glycoprotein to the cisternae of the endoplasmic reticulum and within the Golgi complex. However, there is evidence (Riordan *et al.,* 1974) that the binding site for asialoglycoproteins in Golgi membranes is separate from the sialyltransferase and galactosyltransferase activities.

There is some evidence in support of the export hypothesis. Thus myeloma cells containing IgA which is not being secreted from the cell are PAS negative, in contrast to those actively secreting IgA which are PAS positive (Hurez *et al.,* 1970). Small resting B lymphocytes, although synthesizing IgM, do not export this immunoglobulin which remains largely on the cell surface. This cell-bound IgM differs from normal plasma IgM in being monomeric and in containing only the core sugars, namely, mannose and *N*-acetylglucosamine (Melchers, 1972, 1974; Melchers and Andersson, 1973). On the other hand, the binding of immunoglobulin to cells may result not from a deliberate and exploited failure in the export process but because there are specific Fc receptors which anchor the protein molecule (Ramasamy *et al.,* 1974). For certain rabbit IgG antibodies, treatment with an endoglycosidase, which removes about half of the carbohydrate presumably from the Fc region (Williams *et al.,* 1973), prevents interaction between cells with Fc receptors and immunoglobulin-coated red blood cells. These two sets of observations on the relationship of carbohydrate to cell binding of immunoglobulins are difficult to reconcile although the former is concerned with monomeric IgM, whereas the latter is concerned with IgG.

Even if, in some cases, carbohydrate is associated with the export of certain glycoproteins, this cannot be true of the majority of glycoproteins and cannot therefore be a general function of the carbohydrate. Winterburn and Phelps (1972) have given a very careful rebuttal of this hypothesis and put forward the idea that the oligosaccharide units determine the extracellular fate of the protein molecule. The carbohydrate then would function as a means for coding for the "topographical location" of the target tissue within an organism. The oligosaccharide units would be admirably suited to carry out such a function. As mentioned in an earlier section, even relatively small numbers of monosaccharides when linked together can form a large number of structures. For example, an oligosaccharide unit containing 12 residues in exactly the same sequence can exist in over a million different isomeric forms by changes in the positions of linkage and so on. If the Winterburn and Phelps hypothesis is correct, then the "heterogeneity" of oligosaccharide units is not a haphazard consequence of the biosynthetic process but a precisely determined and necessary part of the procedure. Under this degree of control, the carbohydrate would provide a very efficient method of attaching a compact and specific homing device to a protein. This idea is in agreement with some views put forward about the carbohydrate in certain immunoglobulins. The immunoglobulin subclass IgA1 contains a stretch in the hinge region which is rich in proline, serine, and threonine and to which is attached one or more O-glycosidically linked oligosaccharide units. This stretch is very similar to that seen in mucus-type glycoproteins. It may be significant therefore that one of the main immunoglobulin components of exocrine secretions should itself possess a mucus-like stretch. This stretch may facilitate reversible binding to mucus membranes and act as a local concentration mechanism. The other immunoglobulin subclass present in exocrine secretions, namely, IgA2, does not possess this stretch and may function primarily free in the secretions themselves. These two subclasses are present in a number of species and presumably there is some evolutionary pressure maintaining their separate existences. A similar argument may well apply, for example, to the presence of simple and complex units in IgM. These again are present in a number of species and, in addition, the two types of unit are located in identical positions in different μ heavy chains (Shimizu *et al.,* 1971; Putnam *et al.,* 1973). Apart from possible roles for these units that have been mentioned previously, namely, effect on tertiary structure or any function as spacer units, the carbohydrate may facilitate binding of IgM to glycolipoprotein on cell surfaces (Shimizu *et al.*, 1971).

Up to now this discussion has been largely confined to the possibility that carbohydrate may determine the extracellular fate of protein molecules. Although not strictly relevant, it is nevertheless interesting that a similar function has been proposed for cell surface carbohydrate in determining the fate of small lymphocytes (Woodruff and Gesner, 1969). The migration of these cells can be modified by the removal of sialic acid residues from the cell surface by treatment with neuraminidase. After such treatment, many of the lymphocytes become trapped in the liver and there is a decrease in the selective accumulation of these cells in the lymph nodes and the spleen. In a similar way, incubation with neuraminidase and removal of sialic acid residues can have a significant effect on the biological properties of certain glycoproteins. Thus a factor is necessary for the release of carbohydrate from fibrinogen during clotting and this factor does not produce an insoluble clot from sialic acid-free fibrinogen (Chandrasekhar and Laki, 1964). The activities of certain hormones also appear to be dependent upon sialic acid content. This has been shown with follicle stimulating hormone (Gottschalk *et al.*, 1960) and with chorionic gonadotropin (Goverde *et al.*, 1968; Mori, 1969). These observations were originally interpreted as indicating that sialic acid residues were directly involved in the biological activities of the hormones. However, such findings can now be explained as part of a more general hypothesis as a result of the careful series of investigations by G. Ashwell and his co-workers (Ashwell, 1974). Studies with ceruloplasmin showed that if the glycoprotein was treated with neuraminidase and then returned to the body, virtually all the injected ceruloplasmin disappeared from the circulation within a few minutes (Morell *et al.*, 1968). Removal of sialic acid residues therefore has a profound effect upon the plasma survival time and although ceruloplasmin contains about 10 such residues, removal of only two is sufficient to affect the half-life (Van Den Hamer *et al.*, 1970) and metabolism (Gregoriadis *et al.*, 1970) of the glycoprotein. If the sialic acid residues are replaced on the desialized glycoprotein, the half-life tends to revert to normal (Hickman *et al.*, 1970). This effect does not appear to result from the presence of sialic acid directly inhibiting some elimination mechanism, but rather to be due to exposed galactose residues acting as the specific recognition signal for the process. Thus if the terminal galactose is either removed or modified in some way, for example, by treatment with galactose oxidase, then the half-life of the glycoprotein returns to that of the

original ceruloplasmin (Van Den Hamer *et al.*, 1970; Pricer and Ashwell, 1971).

Most of the original work described here was carried out on ceruloplasmin, but it is now clear that this elimination process is common to a
number of other plasma glycoproteins, including haptoglobin, fetuin,
α_1-acid glycoprotein, and α_2-macroglobulin (Morell *et al.*, 1971). It is
also the process by which chorionic gonadotropin and follicle stimulating
hormone are eliminated and this rapid removal from the circulation may
be the explanation for the apparent loss of biological activity when the
hormones are treated with neuraminidase.

Surprisingly, transferrin is an exception to the above list in that its
plasma survival time is not affected by the removal of sialic acid residues
(Morell *et al.*, 1971). There is some evidence that IgG and possibly
other immunoglobulins are subject to this elimination mechanism.

There is competitive inhibition of removal between the various sialic
acid-deficient glycoproteins that show this phenomenon (Morell *et al.*,
1971), suggesting that they all share a common binding site. This binding
site is in the plasma membranes of the parenchymal cells of the liver and
after binding, the glycoproteins eventually appear in the lysosomes. A
remarkable finding has been the dual role played by sialic acid (Ashwell,
1974). Thus the presence of sialic acid effectively blocks the binding of
glycoproteins to hepatic cells and yet sialic acid must be present on the
cell membrane for binding of the asialoglycoprotein to occur. Treatment
of the hepatic parenchymal cells with neuraminidase results in complete
loss of any binding activity.

There is no doubt that the elucidation of this mechanism has been one
of the fundamental discoveries of glycoprotein biochemistry. The simplest interpretation of these observations is that this elimination process
is a means whereby a proportion of glycoproteins are continually being
removed from the circulation as part of a turnover system. The system is
sophisticated in that it ignores recently synthesized glycoproteins possessing a full complement of sialic acid residues and tends to select
"time-expired" molecules that have been in the circulation for some time
and are more likely therefore to have lost the necessary number of sialic
acid residues. This implies that there is an additional mechanism causing
a slow loss of these residues. Possibly this loss could occur as a natural
process resulting from the lability of the glycosidic linkage together with
the acidic environment from the neighboring carboxyl group. Alternatively, the glycoproteins may come in contact with neuraminidases
either in low concentration in plasma (Warren and Spearing, 1960) or on
plasma membranes.

As with all the other theories that have been advanced to explain the
presence of carbohydrate in glycoproteins, this elimination mechanism is

not, on its own, sufficient to account for the diversity of carbohydrate in plasma glycoproteins. For example, both ceruloplasmin and α_1-acid glycoprotein are subject to this process and yet they show considerable qualitative and quantitative differences in their sugar content. On the other hand transferrin is not affected by this mechanism and yet quantitatively at least its carbohydrate content does not appear to be markedly different to that of ceruloplasmin. In addition, there are a number of plasma glycoproteins in which the sialic acid content is much less than that of galactose, which, unless it is blocked by fucose, is likely therefore to be in a terminal position. The extreme example of this is the sialic acid-free β_1-glycoprotein containing almost 8% galactose which, as its name implies, possesses no sialic acid at all and only 1% fucose. Finally, the elimination mechanism does not explain why simple oligosaccharide units are present in a number of plasma glycoproteins when these units do not possess either sialic acid or galactose.

A number of theories have been covered in this section which attempt to explain the presence of carbohydrate in glycoproteins. The relationship between some of these theories has been illustrated by fitting them into one or more places in the following scheme:

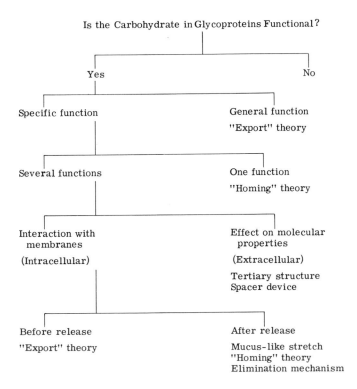

Obviously diagrams of this type have only a limited usefulness except for depicting some rather broad roles that carbohydrate might play. Most theories in this field are put forward with the intention of being all-embracing, for example, the "export" hypothesis of Eylar (1965). Although such theories are not tenable in an overall sense, they may still apply to a limited number of glycoproteins and therefore they appear in the scheme in more than one protein.

In summary, it can be said that no one theory appears to explain satisfactorily the presence of carbohydrate in plasma glycoproteins. It is likely that this type of protein molecule appeared early in evolution explaining the widespread occurrence of glycoproteins in nature. In addition, in the evolutionary time available, the carbohydrate may well have taken on a large number of roles, both general and specific, depending on the organism, the environment, and the properties and function of the protein component.

REFERENCES

Ashwell, G. (1974). *Biochem. Soc. Symp.* **40**, 117.
Baenziger, J., and Kornfeld, S. (1974a). *J. Biol. Chem.* **249**, 7260.
Baenziger, J., and Kornfeld, S. (1974b). *J. Biol. Chem.* **249**, 7270.
Baenziger, J., Kornfeld, S., and Kochwa, S. (1974a). *J. Biol. Chem.* **249**, 1889.
Baenziger, J., Kornfeld, S., and Kochwa, S. (1974b). *J. Biol. Chem.* **249**, 1897.
Baker, J. R., and Rodén, L. (1970). *Fed. Proc., Fed. Amer. Soc. Exp. Biol.* **29**, 338.
Beeley, J. G. (1971). *Biochim. Biophys. Acta* **230**, 595.
Beisswenger, P. J., and Spiro, R. G. (1970). *Science* **168**, 596.
Bierry, H. (1934). *C. R. Soc. Biol.* **116**, 702.
Blix, G. (1936). *Hoppe-Seyler's Z. Physiol. Chem.* **240**, 181.
Blix, G. (1938). *Skand. Arch. Physiol.* **80**, 46.
Blix, G. (1940). *Acta Physiol. Scand.* **1**, 29.
Blix, G., Gottschalk, A., and Klenk, E. (1957). *Nature (London)* **179**, 1088.
Bogdanov, V. P., Kaverzneva, E. D., and Andrejeva, A. P. (1962). *Biochim. Biophys. Acta* **65**, 168.
Bogdanov, V. P., Kaverzneva, E. D., and Andrejeva, A. P. (1964). *Biochim. Biophys. Acta* **83**, 69.
Bourrillon, R., Razafimahaleo, E., and Parnaudeau, M. A. (1968). *Biochim Biophys. Acta* **154**, 405.
Brown, W. V. Levy, R. I., and Fredrickson, D. S. (1970). *J. Biol. Chem.* **245**, 6588.
Bürgi, W., and Schmid, K. (1961). *J. Biol. Chem.* **236**, 1066.
Calcott, M. A., and Müller-Eberhard, H. J. (1972). *Biochemistry* **11**, 3443.
Chandrasekhar, N., and Laki, K. (1964). *Biochim. Biophys. Acta* **93**, 392.
Charet, P., and Montreuil, J. (1971). *C. R. Acad. Sci., Ser. D* **273**, 533.
Cheftel, R. I., Cloarec, L., Moretti, J., and Jayle, M.-F. (1965). *Bull. Soc. Chim. Biol.* **47**, 385.
Chipowsky, S., and McGuire, E. J. (1969). *Fed. Proc., Fed. Amer. Soc. Exp. Biol.* **28**, 606.
Clamp, J. R. (1974). *Biochem. Soc. Trans.* **2**, 64.

Clamp, J. R., and Johnson, I. (1972). *In* "Glycoproteins" (A. Gottschalk, ed.), 2nd ed., p. 612. Elsevier, Amsterdam.

Clamp, J. R., and Putnam, F. W. (1964). *J. Biol. Chem.* **239**, 3233.

Clamp, J. R., Dawson, G., Hough, L., and Khan, M. Y. (1966). *Carbohyd. Res.* **3**, 254.

Clamp, J. R., Dawson, G., and Spragg, B. P. (1967). *Biochem. J.* **106**, 16P.

Clamp, J. R., Dawson, G., and Franklin, E. C. (1968). *Biochem. J.* **110**, 385.

Clamp, J. R., Bhatti, T., and Chambers, R. (1972). *In* "Glycoproteins" (A. Gottschalk, ed.), 2nd ed., p. 300. Elsevier, Amsterdam.

Cook, G. M. W., and Stoddart, R. W. (1973). "Surface Carbohydrates of the Eukaryotic Cell." Academic Press, New York.

Cunningham, L. W., Nuenke, B. J., and Nuenke, R. B. (1957). *Biochim. Biophys. Acta* **26**, 660.

Dawson, G., and Clamp, J. R. (1967a). *Biochem. J.* **103**, 5P.

Dawson, G., and Clamp, J. R. (1967b). *Biochem. Biophys. Res. Commun.* **26**, 349.

Dawson, G., and Clamp, J. R. (1968). *Biochem. J.* **107**, 341.

DeVries, A. L., Komatsu, S. K., and Feeney, R. E. (1970). *J. Biol. Chem.* **245**, 2901.

Dische, Z. (1928). *Biochem. Z.* **201**, 74.

Dunn, J. T., and Spiro, R. (1967a). *J. Biol. Chem.* **242**, 5549.

Dunn, J. T., and Spiro, R. (1967b). *J. Biol. Chem.* **242**, 5556.

Edelman, G. M., Cunningham, B. A., Gall, W. E., Gottlieb, P. D., Rutishauser, U., and Waxdal, M. J. (1969). *Proc. Nat. Acad. Sci. U.S.* **63**, 78.

Eylar, E. H. (1962). *Biochem. Biophys. Res. Commun.* **8**, 195.

Eylar, E. H. (1965). *J. Theor. Biol.* **10**, 89.

Eylar, E. H., and Jeanloz, R. W. (1962a). *J. Biol. Chem.* **237**, 622.

Eylar, E. H., and Jeanloz, R. W. (1962b). *J. Biol. Chem.* **237**, 1021.

Fanger, M. W., and Smyth, D. G. (1972). *Biochem. J.* **127**, 757.

Fletcher, A. P., Marshall, R. D., and Neuberger, A. (1963). *Biochem. J.* **88**, 37P.

Frangione, B., and Milstein, C. (1969). *Nature (London)* **224**, 597.

Frangione, B., and Wolfenstein-Todel, C. (1972). *Proc. Nat. Acad. Sci. U.S.* **69**, 3673.

Gaffney, P. J. (1972). *Biochim. Biophys. Acta* **263**, 453.

Gerbeck, C. M., Bezkorovainy, A., and Rafelson, M. E. (1967). *Biochemistry* **6**, 403.

Gotto, A. M., Brown, W. V., Levy, R. I., Birnbaumer, M. E., and Fredrickson, D. S. (1972). *J. Clin. Invest.* **51**, 1486.

Gottschalk, A. (1972). *In* "Glycoproteins" (A. Gottschalk, ed.), 2nd ed., p. 24. Elsevier, Amsterdam.

Gottschalk, A., Whitten, W. K., and Graham, E. R. B. (1960). *Biochim. Biophys. Acta* **38**, 183.

Goverde, B. C., Veenkamp, F. J. N., and Homan, J. D. H. (1968). *Acta Endocrinol. (Copenhagen)* **59**, 105.

Gregoriadis, G., Morell, A. G., Sternlieb, I., and Scheinberg, I. H. (1970). *J. Biol. Chem.* **245**, 5833.

Haupt, H., and Heide, K. (1964). *Clin. Chim. Acta* **10**, 555.

Haupt, H., and Heide, K. (1965). *Clin. Chim. Acta* **12**, 419.

Haupt, H., and Heide, K. (1972). *Blut* **24**, 94.

Haupt, H., Heide, K., and Schwick, H. G. (1970). *Klin. Wochenschr.* **48**, 550.

Haupt, H., Baudner, S., Kranz, T., and Heimburger, N. (1971). *Eur. J. Biochem.* **23**, 242.

Haupt, H., Heimburger, N., Kranz, T., and Baudner, S. (1972). *Hoppe-Seyler's Z. Physiol. Chem.* **353**, 1841.

Heide, K., and Schwick, H. G. (1973). *Angew. Chem., Int. Ed. Engl.* **12**, 721.

Heimburger, N., and Haupt, H. (1965). *Clin. Chim. Acta* **12**, 116.

Heimburger, N., Haupt, H., Kranz, T., and Baudner, S. (1972). *Hoppe-Seyler's Z. Physiol. Chem.* **353,** 1133.

Hew, C. L., and Dixon, G. H. (1972). *In* "Atlas of Protein Sequence and Structure" (M. O. Dayhoff, ed.), Vol. 5, p. D315. Nat. Biomed. Res. Found., Washington, D.C.

Hewitt, L. F. (1934). *Biochem. J.* **28,** 2080.

Hickman, J., Ashwell, G., Morell, A. G., Van Den Hamer, G. J. A., and Scheinberg, I. H. (1970). *J. Biol. Chem.* **245,** 795.

Hickman, S., Kornfeld, R., Osterland, C. K., and Kornfeld, S. (1972). *J. Biol. Chem.* **247,** 2156.

Holtzmann, N. A., Naughton, M. A., Iber, F. L., and Gaumnitz, B. M. (1967). *J. Clin. Invest.* **46,** 993.

Hrkal, Z., and Müller-Eberhard, U. (1971). *Biochemistry* **10,** 1746.

Hughes, R. C. (1973). *Progr. Biophys. Mol. Biol.* **26,** 191.

Hughes, R. C., and Jeanloz, R. W. (1964a). *Biochemistry* **3,** 1535.

Hughes, R. C., and Jeanloz, R. W. (1964b). *Biochemistry* **3,** 1543.

Hughes, R. C., and Jeanloz, R. W. (1966). *Biochemistry* **5,** 253.

Hunt, L. T., and Dayhoff, M. O. (1970). *Biochem. Biophys. Res. Commun.* **39,** 757.

Hurez, D., Preud'homme, J.-L., and Seligmann, M. (1970). *J. Immunol.* **104,** 263.

Hurst, M. M., Niedermeier, W., Zikan, J., and Bennett, J. C. (1973). *J. Immunol.* **110,** 840.

Isemura, M., and Schmid, K. (1971). *Biochem. J.* **124,** 591.

Iwanaga, S., Blombäck, B., Grondahl. N. J., Hessel, B., and Wallen, P. (1968). *Biochim. Biophys. Acta* **160,** 280.

Iwasaki, T., and Schmid, K. (1970). *J. Biol. Chem.* **245,** 1814.

Jackson, R. L., and Hirs, C. H. W. (1970). *J. Biol. Chem.* **245,** 624.

Jamieson, G. A. (1964). *Biochem. Biophys. Res. Commun.* **17,** 775.

Jamieson, G. A. (1965a). *J. Biol. Chem.* **240,** 2019.

Jamieson, G. A. (1965b). *J. Biol. Chem.* **240,** 2914.

Jamieson, G. A. (1966). *Biochim. Biophys. Acta* **121,** 326.

Jamieson, G. A., Jett, M., and DeBernardo, S. L. (1971). *J. Biol. Chem.* **246,** 3686.

Jeanloz, R. W., and Closse, A. (1963). *Fed. Proc., Fed. Amer. Soc. Exp. Biol.* **22,** 538.

Jevons, F. R. (1958). *Nature (London)* **181,** 1346.

Johansen, P. G., Marshall, R. D., and Neuberger, A. (1958). *Nature (London)* **181,** 1345.

Johansen, P. G., Marshall, R. D., and Neuberger, A. (1961). *Biochem. J.* **78,** 518.

Johnson, I., and Clamp, J. R. (1971). *Biochem. J.* **123,** 739.

Jouanneau, J., Razafimahaleo, E., and Bourrillon, R. (1970). *Eur. J. Biochem.* **17,** 72.

Kamiyama, S., and Schmid, K. (1962a). *Biochim. Biophys. Acta* **58,** 80.

Kamiyama, S., and Schmid, K. (1962b). *Biochim. Biophys. Acta* **63,** 266.

Kaverzneva, E. D. (1966). *Chimia* **2,** 130.

Kennedy, J. F. (1974). *Biochem. Soc. Trans.* **2,** 54.

Kisiel, W., and Hanahan, D. J. (1973). *Biochim. Biophys. Acta* **304,** 103.

Klenk, E. (1941). *Hoppe-Seyler's Z. Physiol. Chem.* **268,** 50.

Kohno, M., and Yamashina, I. (1969). *Abstr. 42nd Meet. Jap. Biochem. Soc.* p. 621.

Kornfeld, R., Keller, J., Baenziger, J., and Kornfeld, S. (1971). *J. Biol. Chem.* **246,** 3259.

Krantz, M. J., Lee, Y. C., and Hung, P. P. (1974). *Nature (London)* **248,** 684.

Krawkow, N. (1897). *Arch. Gesamte Physiol. Menschen Tiere* **65,** 281.

Kühn, R., and Gauhe, A. (1965). *Chem. Ber.* **98,** 395.

Labat, J., and Schmid, K. (1969). *Experientia* **25,** 701.

Labat, J., Ishiguro, M., Fujisaki, Y., and Schmid, K. (1969). *J. Biol. Chem.* **244,** 4975.

Lanchantin, G. F., Hart, D. W., Friedmann, J. A., Saavedra, N. V., and Mehl, J. W. (1968). *J. Biol. Chem.* **243,** 5479.

Li, Y. T. (1966). *J. Biol. Chem.* **241,** 1010.

Lindahl, U., and Rodén, L. (1972). *In* "Glycoproteins" (A. Gottschalk, ed.), 2nd ed., p. 491. Elsevier, Amsterdam.

Makino, M., and Yamashina, I. (1966). *J. Biochem. (Tokyo)* **60,** 262.

Makino, M., Kojima, T., Ohgushi, T., and Yamashina, I. (1968). *J. Biochem. (Tokyo)* **63,** 186.

Margolis, S. (1969). *In* "Structural and Functional Aspects of Lipoproteins in Living Systems" (E. Tria and A. M. Scanu, eds.), p. 369. Academic Press, New York.

Margolis, S., and Langdon, R. G. (1966). *J. Biol. Chem.* **241,** 469.

Marks, G. S., Marshall, R. D., and Neuberger, A. (1962). *Biochem. J.* **85,** 15P.

Marks, G. S., Marshall, R. D., and Neuberger, A. (1963). *Biochem. J.* **87,** 274.

Marshall, R. D. (1972). *Annu. Rev. Biochem.* **41,** 673.

Marshall, W. E., and Kummerow, F. A. (1962). *Arch. Biochem. Biophys.* **98,** 271.

Marshall, W. E., and Porath, J. (1965). *J. Biol. Chem.* **240,** 209.

Melchers, F. (1972). *Biochemistry* **11,** 2204.

Melchers, F. (1974). *Biochem. Soc. Symp.* **40,** 73.

Melchers, F., and Andersson, J. (1973). *Transplant. Rev.* **14,** 76.

Mester, L., and Szabados, L. (1968). *Bull. Soc. Chim. Biol.* **50,** 2561.

Meyer, K. (1938). *Cold Spring Harbor Symp. Quant. Biol.* **6,** 91.

Meyer, K. (1945). *Advan. Protein Chem.* **2,** 249.

Montreuil, J., and Biserte, G. (1959). *Bull. Soc. Chim. Biol.* **41,** 959.

Moore, V., and Putnam, F. W. (1973). *Biochemistry* **12,** 2361.

Morell, A. G., Irvine, R. A., Sternlieb, I., Scheinberg, I. H., and Ashwell, G. (1968). *J. Biol. Chem.* **243,** 155.

Morell, A. G., Gregoriadis, G., Scheinberg, I. H., Hickman, J., and Ashwell, G. (1971). *J. Biol. Chem.* **246,** 1461.

Mori, K. F. (1969). *Endocrinology* **85,** 330.

Mörner, K. A. H. (1893). *Zentralbl. Physiol.* **1,** 581.

Muldoon, T. G., and Westphal, U. (1967). *J. Biol. Chem.* **242,** 5636.

Müller-Eberhard, H. J., Nilsson, U., and Aronsson, T. (1960). *J. Exp. Med.* **111,** 201.

Murakami, M., and Eylar, E. H. (1965). *J. Biol. Chem.* **240,** PC556.

Nishigaki, M., Muramatsu, T., and Kobata, A. (1974). *Biochem. Biophys. Res. Commun.* **59,** 638.

O'Carra, P., Barry, S., and Griffin, T. (1974). *FEBS (Fed. Eur. Biochem. Soc.) Lett.* **43,** 169.

Odin, L. (1955). *Acta Chem. Scand.* **9,** 714.

Pappenheimer, A. M., Lundgren, H. P., and Williams, J. W. (1940). *J. Exp. Med.* **71,** 247.

Pavy, F. W. (1893). *Proc. Roy. Soc.* **54,** 53.

Peterson, P. A. (1971). *J. Biol. Chem.* **246,** 34.

Plummer, T. H., and Hirs, C. H. W. (1963). *J. Biol. Chem.* **238,** 1396.

Plummer, T. H., and Hirs, C. H. W. (1964). *J. Biol. Chem.* **239,** 2530.

Plummer, T. H., Tarentino, A. L., and Maley, F. (1968). *J. Biol. Chem.* **243,** 5158.

Poortmans, J. R., Jeanloz, R. W., and Schmid, K. (1967). *Clin. Chim. Acta* **17,** 305.

Popenoe, E. A. (1958). *Fed. Proc., Fed. Amer. Soc. Exp. Biol.* **17,** 290.

Popenoe, E. A. (1959). *Biochim. Biophys. Acta* **32,** 584.

Press, E. M. and Hogg, N. M. (1970). *Biochem. J.* **117,** 641.

Pricer, W. E. and Ashwell, G. (1971). *J. Biol. Chem.* **246,** 4825.

Putnam, F. W., Florent, G., Paul, C., Shinoda, T., and Shimizu, A. (1973). *Science* **182,** 287.

Ramasamy, R., Munro, A., and Milstein, C. (1974). *Nature (London)* **249,** 573.

Razafimahaleo, E., Frenoy, J. P., and Bourrillon, R. (1969). *C. R. Acad. Sci., Ser. D* **269**, 1567.

Reid, K. B. M. (1974). *Biochem. J.* **141**, 189.

Reid, K. B. M., Lowe, D. M., and Porter, R. R. (1972). *Biochem. J.* **130**, 749.

Rimington, C. (1929). *Biochem. J.* **23**, 430.

Riordan, J. R., Mitchell, L., and Slavik, M. (1974). *Biochem. Biophys. Res. Commun.* **59**, 1973.

Robbins, K. C., Summaria, L., Elwyn, D., and Barlow, G. H. (1965). *J. Biol. Chem.* **240**, 541.

Roseman, S. (1970). *Chem. Phys. Lipids* **5**, 270.

Rosevear, J. W., and Smith, E. L. (1958). *J. Amer. Chem. Soc.* **80**, 250.

Roston, C. P. J., Caygill, J. C., and Jevons, F. R. (1965). *Biochem. J.* **97**, 43P.

Rothfus, J. A., and Smith, E. L. (1963). *J. Biol. Chem.* **238**, 1402.

Rydén, L. (1971). *Int. J. Protein Res.* **111**, 191.

Rydén, L., and Eaker, D. (1974). *Eur. J. Biochem.* **44**, 171.

Sato, T., Yosizawa, Z., Masubuchi, M., and Yamauchi, F. (1967). *Carbohyd. Res.* **5**, 387.

Scanu, A. (1966). *J. Lipid Res.* **7**, 295.

Scanu, A. (1969). *In* "Structural and Functional Aspects of Lipoproteins in Living Systems" (E. Tria and A. M. Scanu, eds.), p. 425. Academic Press, New York.

Schauer, R., Buscher, H.-P., and Casals-Stenzel, J. (1974). *Biochem. Soc. Symp.* **40**, 87.

Schmid, K., and Bürgi, W. (1961). *Biochim. Biophys. Acta* **47**, 440.

Schmid, K., Kamiyama, S., Pfister, V., Takahashi, S., and Binette, J. P. (1962). *Biochemistry* **1**, 959.

Schmid, K., Ishiguro, M., Emura, J., Isemura, S., Kaufmann, H., and Motoyama, T. (1971). *Biochem. Biophys. Res. Commun.* **42**, 280.

Schneider, S. L., and Slaunwhite, W. R. (1971). *Biochemistry* **10**, 2086.

Schultze, H. E., and Heremans, J. F. (1966). *In* "Molecular Biology of Human Proteins," Vol. 1, p. 176. Elsevier, Amsterdam.

Schultze, H. E., Heide, K., and Haupt, H. (1962). *Clin. Chim. Acta* **7**, 854.

Schwick, H. G., Haupt, H., and Heide, K. (1968). *Klin. Wochenschr.* **46**, 981.

Shimizu, A., Putnam, F. W., Paul, C., Clamp, J. R., and Johnson, I. (1971). *Nature (London), New Biol.* **231**, 73.

Smith, E. L., Greene, R. D., and Bartner, E. (1946). *J. Biol. Chem.* **164**, 359.

Smith, F., and Unrau, A. M. (1959). *Chem. Ind. (London)* **78**, 881.

Smyth, D., and Utsumi, S. (1967). *Nature (London)* **216**, 332.

Spik, G., and Montreuil, J. (1969). *Bull. Soc. Chim. Biol.* **51**, 1271.

Spik, G., Monsigny, M., and Montreuil, J. (1965a). *C. R. Acad. Sci.* **260**, 4282.

Spik, G., Monsigny, M., and Montreuil, J. (1965b). *C. R. Acad. Sci.* **261**, 1137.

Spiro, R. G. (1964). *J. Biol. Chem.* **239**, 567.

Spiro, R. G. (1967). *J. Biol. Chem.* **242**, 4813.

Spragg, B. P., and Clamp, J. R. (1969). *Biochem. J.* **114**, 57.

Stacey, M. (1943). *Chem Ind. (London)* **62**, 110.

Stacey, M. (1946). *Advan. Protein Chem.* **2**, 161.

Sterling, K., Hamada, S., Takemura, Y., Brenner, M. A., Newman, E. S., and Inada, M. (1971). *J. Clin. Invest.* **50**, 1758.

Tarentino, A. L., and Maley, F. (1969). *Arch. Biochem. Biophys.* **130**, 295.

Tarentino, A. L., and Maley, F. (1974). *J. Biol. Chem.* **249**, 811.

Van Den Hamer, C. J. A., Morell, A. G., Scheinberg, I. H., Hickman, J., and Ashwell, G. (1970). *J. Biol. Chem.* **245**, 4397.

Warren, L., and Spearing, C. W. (1960). *Biochem. Biophys. Res. Commun.* **3**, 489.

Watkins, W. M. (1966). *Science* **152**, 172.

Wagh, P. V., Bornstein, I., and Winzler, R. J. (1969). *J. Biol. Chem.* **244**, 658.

Willard, J. J. (1962). *Nature (London)* **194**, 1278.

Williams, R. C., Osterland, C. K., Margherita, S., Tokuda, S., and Messner, R. P. (1973). *J. Immunol.* **111**, 1690.

Winterburn, P. J., and Phelps, C. F. (1972). *Nature (London)* **236**, 147.

Winzler, R. J. (1958). *Chem. Biol. Mucopolysaccharides, Ciba Found. Symp. 1957* p. 245.

Wiseman, R. L., Fothergill, J. E., and Fothergill, L. A. (1972). *Biochem. J.* **127**, 775.

Woodruff, J. J., and Gesner, B. M. (1969). *J. Exp. Med.* **129**, 551.

Yamashina, I. (1956). *Acta Chem. Scand.* **10**, 1666.

Yamashina, I., and Makino, M. (1962). *J. Biochem. (Tokyo)* **51**, 359.

Yamashina, I., Ban-I, K., and Makino, M. (1963). *Biochim. Biophys. Acta* **78**, 382.

Yamashina, I., Makino, M., Ban-I, K., and Kojima, T. (1965). *J. Biochem. (Tokyo)* **58**, 168.

Yamauchi, T., Makino, M., and Yamashina, I. (1968). *J. Biochem. (Tokyo)* **64**, 683.

Yu, R. K., and Leeden, R. (1969). *J. Biol. Chem.* **244**, 1306.

Zanetti, C. U. (1897). *Ann. Chim. Med. Farmaceut. Farmacol. (Milan)* **26**, 529.

Zanetti, C. U. (1903). *Gazz. Chim. Ital.* **33**, 160.

5 / Tissue-Derived Plasma Enzymes

William H. Fishman and George J. Doellgast

I. Introduction

In the 15 years since the chapter "Plasma Enzymes" was included in the first edition of "The Plasma Proteins," there has grown an appreciation of the significance of enzymes present in plasma that extends well beyond the attempt to record and correlate elevated levels of enzymes with pathological states.

Implicit in this correlation is the concept that the enzymes which are measured in plasma originate in diseased tissues, and their elevation is representative of events occurring in a particular diseased tissue. However, we now know that abnormal levels of a particular plasma enzyme may not originate at all from pathological tissue but may persist in the blood because of a defect in the clearance of enzymes from the blood. Moreover, genetic and physiological factors can in combination result in abnormal plasma values in the absence of disease.

How should one view enzymes in plasma in relation to the plasma proteins? In the case of the latter, one can readily understand the separate roles in the plasma, for example, of albumin, of fibrinogen, and of immunoglobulins. These are, respectively, maintenance of the osmotic pressure of the blood, provision of the fibrin clot for control of bleeding, and the mounting of an immune response to a foreign agent. Even with regard to the polypeptide hormones, insulin and gonadotropin, their presence in minute amounts in plasma is essential for regulating biological processes which are mediated by these substances. However, plasma enzymes, *apart from those involved in blood clotting,* have no known function analogous to the functions associated with the examples presented.

The plasma enzymes do serve as indicators of the normality or lack of normality of the tissues from which they originated. Accordingly, it is for the purpose of emphasizing the *normal* as well as the pathological aspects of the phenomenon of enzyme secretion and clearance that we have entitled this chapter "Tissue-Derived Plasma Enzymes" and have excluded enzymes involved in the complement cascade and in blood coagulation. The latter are dealt with in Volume I, Chapter 8 and in this volume, Chapter 3 and Volume III, Chapter 7, respectively.

As defined above, "plasma" and "serum" are equivalent in the measurement of tissue-derived plasma enzymes.

As before, we are inclined in this treatise to view plasma enzymes first as proteins and then as biological catalysts. In this context, such proteins may be expected to be regulated by the same mechanisms which control the levels of other plasma proteins. What is new is the fact that with the aid of modern techniques of protein purification and characterization, it has now been possible to recognize certain of the plasma enzymes as being sialoglycoproteins, metalloproteins, etc. Moreover, the expectation that the heterogeneity of individual proteins as, for example, the hereditary hemoglobins could apply to plasma enzymes, has been amply realized by the demonstration of polymorphic forms of many enzymes.

One should note that increasing attention is now being paid to specific plasma enzyme deficiencies in connection with many genetic disorders. Thus in addition to the long-known hypophosphatasemia, a hereditary bone disease, one can now add a variety of missing enzymes from the glycogen cycle which characterize seven types of glycogenoses, a number of specific glycosidases lacking in the plasma of patients with a large variety of cerebrosidoses, and so on.

The questions considered earlier to be basic ones with regard to plasma enzymes still are relevant. We asked, "Where do they (plasma enzymes) come from and what is their fate? How does one measure activity in plasma and how does one identify and quantitate the tissue source of a plasma enzyme? What is a "normal" value? What is the nature of the immediate mechanism that governs the release of an enzyme from its intracytoplasmic location? Its tissue home? And how is this affected by physiological and pathological factors?"

The most significant contribution to a better understanding of the etiology and relevance of tissue-derived plasma enzymes has been the development of the field of isoenzymology. The existence of multiple forms of enzymes has been exploited to define, in some cases with a great degree of precision, the tissue origin of particular enzymes in plasma, the detection of variant forms that are representative of phenotypic differences in human populations, and the occurrence of isoenzymatic forms specific for embryonic tissues that are found in adults with cancer. The latter have been termed carcinoembryonic isoenzymes.

In this chapter, we therefore attempt to present the relevant information on the properties of tissue-derived plasma enzymes which permit their detection and differentiation in plasma, and briefly discuss some aspects of cellular metabolism and endocytosis of enzyme proteins by cells that bear upon the release of enzymes into plasma and the catabolism of plasma enzymes in different tissues.

Because of the broad scope of this chapter, it will be necessary to restrict ourselves to only the most cursory examination of the properties of individual enzymes. The normal levels of enzymes which are measured in human plasma are presented in Table I, and the reader is referred, where available, to more extensive reviews on individual enzymes for more detailed descriptions of their properties. For the same

TABLE I

Normal Levels of Plasma Enzymes in Man

Enzyme	pH	Activity Value	Activity S.D.[b]	Activity Range	Units[a]; reference
Acetylcholinesterase	7.65	1760		1390–2190	I.U.; (Sabine, 1940)
Acid phosphatase	4.9			0–6.7	I.U.; (Green et al., 1968)
Adenosine deaminase				0–33	I.U.; (Ellis et al., 1973)
Alcohol dehydrogenase	7.5			2160–13,700	I.U.; (Wolfson et al., 1958)
Aldolase	7.4	1.74	1.20		I.U.; (Berlet, 1968)
Alkaline phosphatase	9.8				
Children		15.23	6.11		King-Armstrong units; (Green et al., 1971)
Adults		6.36	2.11		
Amylase	7.1			18–75	Formazin turbidity units/min/ml; (Zinterhofer et al., 1973b)
Arginase	8.5	6.5	3.2		I.U.; (Adlung et al., 1971)
Arylsulfatase	6.05	52	14		pmoles/min/ml; (Geokas and Rinderknecht, 1973)
Catalase	6.8	690		420–950	See reference (Dille and Watkins, 1948)
Creatine phosphokinase	6.8			10–35	I.U.; (Swanson and Wilkinson, 1972)
	7.6			0–17	I.U.; (Winckers and Jacobs, 1973)
	9.0			0–21	I.U.; (Snehalatha et al., 1973)
Diaminopeptidases					
I	4.0	2.32	1.33		I.U.; (Vanha-Perttula and Kalliomäki, 1973)
II	5.0	6.9	4.4		I.U.; (Vanha-Perttula and Kalliomäki, 1973)
IV	7.8	12.1	1.7	8.7–16.8	I.U.; (Hopsu-Havu et al., 1970)
Dopamine β-hydroxylase	5.0	42.6	27.0	3–100	I.U.; (Nagatsu and Udenfriend, 1972)
β-Glucuronidase	4.5				
Adult					
female		0.392	0.123		I.U.; (Fishman, 1967)
male		0.525	0.142		

Enzyme	pH	Mean	S.D.	Normal range	Units; reference
Child					
female		0.571	0.302		
male		0.495	0.224		
Glut-oxaloacetic transaminase	7.4			6–25	I.U.; (Sax and Moore, 1970)
Glut-pyruvic transaminase	7.4			37–55	I.U.; (Lippi and Guidi, 1970)
γ-Glutamyl transpeptidase	7.4			37–52	I.U.; (Lippi and Guidi, 1970)
Males		13.08	7.60	5.17–37.33	I.U.; (Sweetin and Thomson, 1973a)
Females		7.49	3.52	2.75–18.75	
Glyceraldehyde-3-phosphate dehydrogenase		1.0			See reference (Hess, 1958)
Guanase	7.2	2.5			I.U.; (Ellis et al., 1973)
Isocitric dehydrogenase	8.2	4670			I.U.; (Sterkel et al., 1958)
Lactate dehydrogenase	7.0				I.U.; (McQueen et al., 1973)
Males		330.5	55		
Females		346.0	65		
Leucine naphthylamidase		29.4	8.0		I.U.; (Spiegel and Symington, 1972)
				24–78	I.U.; (Vanha-Perttula and Kalliomäki, 1973)
Lipase	8.8			0–110	I.U.; (Shihabi and Bishop, 1971)
				0–15	Formazin turbidity units/min/ml; (Zinterhofer et al., 1973)
Lysozyme	6.25			7–15	μg/ml of egg white lysozyme equivalents; (Zucker and Webb, 1972)
Malic dehydrogenase	7.5	13.2		8.7–18.9	See reference (Hess, 1958)
5'-Nucleotidase	7.0			3.2–11.6	I.U.; (Schwartz, 1972)
Ornithine carbamyltransferase	7.5			0.5–10.5	I.U.; (Ceriotti, 1973)
Pentose phosphate isomerase	7.4			11–30	I.U.; (Bruns and Neuhaus, 1955, 1956)
Phosphohexose isomerase	8.4	58.4		36.6–75.0	Bodansky units; (Griffith and Beck, 1967)
				20–90	I.U.; (Schwartz et al., 1971)
Phosphoglucomutase	7.5	46	17		See reference (Bodansky, 1957)
Pseudocholinesterase	7.6	1070	210	650–1490	I.U.; (Zapf and Coghlan, 1974)
(U-phenotype)		8440	1780		I.U.; (Dietz et al., 1973)

[a] I.U.-International Units; μmoles/min/liter plasma.
[b] S.D.-standard deviation.

reason, the section on differentiation of isoenzymes is restricted to a few relevant examples of isoenzymes that have been relatively well categorized, and the emphasis is placed on generally applicable methodology in preference to a detailed explication of the properties of all enzymes that are measurable in plasma.

There now seem to be some experimental approaches to the explanation of what determines how long a protein will persist in the circulation. Apparently, the state of the terminal sugar groups in glycoproteins can be the condition which governs their uptake or rejection by parenchymal liver cells. As a rule, desialylated glycoproteins with a galactose terminal group are avidly taken up by hepatic cells and catabolized in their lysosomes. Inasmuch as a number of plasma enzymes are sialoglycoproteins, these newly presented phenomena may well apply to them. This chapter has given us an opportunity to discuss some interesting possibilities in this connection.

Identity of Plasma Enzymes

It is reasonable to suggest that the plasma may contain under one condition or another every enzyme associated with living tissue. Many do not register activities measurable with the usual enzyme methods but this may be the result of the absence of technique with the requisite sensitivity and specificity.

The classification for enzymes has become more systematic with the introduction of the numerical terminology of the International Commission on Enzyme Nomenclature.

At the same time, there has been a movement toward standardizing the expression of enzyme activity in terms of International Units (micromoles of substrate disappearance or of product formation per minute per liter of plasma).

Recognition of the newer nomenclature and International Unitage is made, whenever possible, in the listing of plasma enzymes in Table I. In order to avoid an encyclopedic dimension, a selection has been made to reflect those plasma enzymes which are the subject of interest in current investigations. For others not listed, the reader is referred to relevant treatises in the literature such as Bergmeyer's "Methods of Enzymatic Analysis" (1965), Richterich's "Clinical Chemistry" (1969), Vesell's "Multiple Molecular Forms of Enzymes" (1968b), Fishman's "Phosphohydrolases, Their Biology, Biochemistry and Clinical Enzymology" (1969), Shugar's "Enzymes and Isoenzymes" (1970); Blume and Freiers' "Enzymology" (1974), and the annual volumes of the "Advances in Clinical Chemistry."

Schmidt *et al.* (1965) have proposed a functional classification of plasma enzymes which distinguishes mainly between cellular and secreted enzymes. Of the cellular enzymes, a subclass termed "general metabolic" includes lactate and malate dehydrogenases, aldolases, and a variety of aminotransferases. Another subclass, "organ-specific," refers to hepatic urea cycle enzymes, for example. In the case of the secreted enzymes, specific plasma enzymes derived from the formed elements of the blood include prothrombin and ceruloplasmin, while those derived from other organ sources are exemplified by the amylases and prostatic phosphatase. How does one define secretion? Is it the release of enzyme in zymogen granules without destruction of the secreting cell or is it a partial disintegration of the plasma membrane containing enzymes?

Tumor tissue is now recognized as a source of plasma enzymes which are not identical to those of adult normal tissues. Included in this category are fetal and placental isoenzymes which will be discussed in detail in Section VI. Examples of these are the placental alkaline phosphatases (known as Regan isoenzyme, Nagao isoenzyme, Regan variant) and pyruvate kinase.

II. Physical Characteristics of Tissue-Derived Plasma Enzymes

A. Multiple Forms (Isoenzymes)

In the earlier review for "Plasma Proteins," Fishman (1960) drew attention to the heterogeneity of enzymes that had the same catalytic function. By use of specific tartrate inhibition of prostatic acid phosphatase (Fishman and Lerner, 1953; Stolbach *et al.* 1958), by selective inhibition of alkaline phosphatase from rat tissues by different amino acids (Fishman, 1960), and by specific immunoprecipitation of dog intestinal alkaline phosphatase with antisera prepared against an intestinal extract (Schlamowitz, 1958), some evidence had begun to accumulate that already indicated the molecular heterogeneity of enzymes in a single individual.

The postulate that this heterogeneity was in fact due to a molecular heterogeneity of proteins that fulfilled the same catalytic function was technically difficult to ascertain. A promising approach was electrophoresis, which Meyer *et al.* (1946, 1947a,b, 1948) used in conjunction with measurements of specific activity and solubility to differentiate human pancreatic amylases, and which Wieland and Pfleiderer (1957) used to separate forms of LDH obtained from single tissues. The introduction of simplified methodology that could be used to routinely differentiate isoenzymes was not available, however, until Hunter and Markert (1957) demonstrated that esterases from different tissues could be separated into forms which differed in their electrophoretic mobility on starch gels. The enzyme was visualized on the gel by use of specific stains for esterases, which were familiar tools in the histochemistry laboratory prior to that time (see review by Burstone, 1964).

One difficulty in working with esterases was recognized by Markert and Møller (1959), in their classic paper on separation of lactate, malate, and isocitrate dehydrogenase isozymes; that was, that since esterases have a broad substrate specificity and a poorly defined specific function within the cell, it is difficult to conclude that the esterases which have been separated do in fact represent different protein species that perform the same catalytic function *in vivo*. The separation of electrophoretically distinct forms of the dehydrogenases resolved this question. In this case, the dehydrogenases did fulfill recognizable biochemical functions within the cell, and there were physically distinguishable forms of these enzymes within a single tissue.

This then defines isoenzymes. They are physically distinguishable proteins that have the same catalytic function and are present in their various forms in the same organism. Isoenzymes may be made up of families of isozymes as suggested recently by Fishman (1974).

The combination of electrophoretic resolution, specific localization of the separated enzymes by histochemical stains, and the use of organ-specific inhibitors was responsible for the rapid development of the field of isoenzymology.

The recognition of physically distinct enzymes having the same catalytic function has had considerable implications for the study of enzymes in plasma. Since distinct forms of enzymes are found to be present in different tissues, it is possible to identify the tissue of origin, in some cases, by the individual properties of the organ-derived enzymes.

B. Physical State

Since the enzymes found in plasma have been released from the tissues of origin, it has always been assumed that they are free in solution and not associated with other proteins or the membrane structure from which they may originate. In most cases, this assumption has not been challenged, and the enzymes in plasma have been presented as soluble single proteins. Several cases have now been documented, however, which contest this facile assumption.

Alkaline phosphatase, as considered in a recent review by Fishman

(1974), is known to be a plasma membrane-associated enzyme. It is frequently highly elevated in the serum of patients with various forms of liver and bone disease. Dymling (1966) demonstrated that there was a form of alkaline phosphatase in the serum of a patient with biliary occlusion that was excluded from Sephadex G-200. This form of alkaline phosphatase was recognized by clinical researchers as a variant form that had considerable potential in the study of different disease states. Dunne *et al.* (1967), Fennelly *et al.* (1969a,b), Hattori *et al.* (1967, 1969), and Akedo *et al.* (1967) documented the occurrence of high molecular weight variants of alkaline phosphatase in different disease states.

The origin of this high molecular weight form was first elucidated by Shinkai and Akedo (1972), who used Sepharose 4B, an agarose gel with a much higher exclusion limit than Sephadex G-200, to separate the alkaline phosphatase from other serum proteins. They showed the association of other membrane markers (ATPase, 5′-nucleotidase, leucine aminopeptidase, phospholipid) with the excluded fractions and demonstrated immunological similarity of the excluded fractions with plasma membrane of liver. Doellgast and Fishman (1975) demonstrated a similar form of alkaline phosphatase in ascites fluids from patients with ovarian cancer and showed the progressive increase in the relative amount of excluded alkaline phosphatase during the course of the disease.

This work has demonstrated that the form in which an enzyme is present in the bloodstream may be closely related to the physical state of the enzyme within the cell of origin. The correlation of disease state with amount of excluded alkaline phosphatase, in this instance, may be a quantitative rather than a qualitative phenomenon. It is at least conceivable that membrane fragments are frequently delivered into the bloodstream as a normal manifestation of tissue catabolism, and that the elevation in relative amounts of membrane fragments in certain states reflects excessive pathological tissue destruction.

Another example of anomalous physical states of enzymes in plasma is the association of lactate dehydrogenase in immune complexes with IgA and IgG (Ganrot, 1967; Kindmark, 1969; Biewenga and Thijs, 1970; Nagamine, 1972; Biewenga, 1972). Nagamine (1972) has interpreted this phenomenon as a variant in the normal mechanism of removal of LDH from the serum. It brings into view the formation of immune complexes as a possible mechanism of removal of plasma enzymes.

There is a common element that is apparent in both the presence of membrane-associated alkaline phosphatase and IgG-LDH immune complexes in serum; that is, the presence of enzymes in plasma reflects the metabolism of an entire organism. The concentrations and physical states of enzymes are thus dependent on events occuring in both the tissues from which they are released and those in which they are catabolized. This is implicit in the use of enzymes in serum diagnosis of disease states, so it is not surprising that unexpected behavior of enzymes should be observed in this complex metabolic interaction.

III. Measurement of Enzymes in Plasma — General Considerations

A. Enzyme Assay

With the evolution of plasma enzymology and the introduction of automated techniques for quantitation, it has been possible to control some of the variables pointed out earlier (Fishman, 1960), which are particular to plasma enzyme methodology. For example, the influence of plasma on the buffering capacity of the plasma digest is equalized by introducing an equivalent dilution of enzyme-inactivated serum into the serial dilutions of reference standards. Two such standards are employed, one of the chromogenic product and the other of a stable preparation of known activity. This has been the practice in this laboratory for acid and alkaline phosphatase (Green *et al.*, 1968; Cantor *et al.*, 1972). Reagents for "quality control" of a number of enzymes are available commercially.

Now with the development of immunological techniques such as radial immunodiffusion and radioimmunoassay, it is possible to measure the enzyme protein through its antigenic determinants. This would avoid many of the problems inherent in enzyme activity measurements, but would perhaps introduce different problems, such as the difficulty of distinguishing between active and inactive forms of the enzymes.

1. Sources of Variation in Measurement

Plasma and serum are obtained from blood, which contains a large number of enzyme-rich leukocytes and erythrocytes. Thus, the methods of collection and processing of blood are critical for the accurate determination of plasma enzyme levels. Tanaka and Valentine (1960) have found a 10,000 times greater arginase activity in leukocytes than in serum, Brydon and Roberts (1972) demonstrated an increase in aminotransferases, acid phosphatase, creatine phosphokinase, and lactate dehydrogenase in hemolyzed relative to unhemolyzed plasma, and Wolfson and Williams-Ashman (1957) reported 80-fold more isocitrate dehydrogenase and 450-fold more glucose-6-phosphate dehydrogenase in erythrocytes than in plasma.

Schwartz (1973a) has reviewed a number of factors that can influence the determination of enzymes in body fluids. The choice of anticoagulant for preparation of plasma is extremely important. Oxalate can inhibit LDH, acid phosphatase (Caraway, 1962), and amylase (McGeachin *et al.,* 1957). Heparin has been demonstrated to polymerize enzymes (Bergman *et al.,* 1971) and to inhibit acid phosphatase (Woodward, 1959), but to have distinct advantages over clotted serum for determination of LDH, malic dehydrogenase, aspartate aminotransferase, aldolase, and isocitrate dehydrogenase in rats (Korsrud and Trick, 1973).

Products of hemolysis can also inhibit enzymes, as documented for lipase (Yang and Biggs, 1971), and drugs can be inhibitory in serum enzyme determinations (Young *et al.* 1972), especially pseudocholinesterase (Dietz *et al.,* 1973; Zapf and Coghlan, 1974).

It is therefore clear that no determination of enzyme levels can be performed accurately unless the collection and processing of serum or plasma are carefully controlled. In addition, the handling of glassware and purity of reagents are clearly of the first importance, since traces of detergents and impurities in the reagents could add uncontrolled variables to the determination.

2. Substrate Specificity, pH Optimum, Normal Levels

As noted above, the field of isoenzymology has considerably broadened the scope of investigation of plasma enzymes, so that determination of total enzyme activity in plasma or serum is usually only a first step in the diagnosis of disease states. However, elevations in total activities of certain enzymes can still be useful in detection of disease states. Creatine phosphokinase can be used to diagnose myocardial infarction (Praetorius and Körtge, 1966) and muscular dystrophy (Pennington, 1971), 5'-nucleotidase can be used to diagnose hepatobiliary disorders (Bodansky and Schwartz, 1968), phosphohexose isomerase has been used to diagnose various types of cancer (Schwartz *et al.,* 1971; Ratliff *et al.,* 1970), and dopamine β-hydroxylase has been linked to hypertension (Schanberg *et al.,* 1974). Extremely low values of certain enzymes in plasma are diagnostic of genetic disorders, as will be discussed below.

A number of enzymes that have been determined in human serum or plasma are listed in Table I, with pH optima and range of normal values. An emphasis has been placed on choosing recent references, and using new developments in methodology where available.

B. Differentiation and Characterization of Isoenzymes

The potential of isoenzymes as a tool to study complex factors in genetics and metabolism in higher organisms has resulted in the development of a plethora of technology for precise characterization and quantitation of isoenzymes.

Basically, the efforts in this direction can be divided into two main thrusts, the elaboration of variations in the catalytic function of isoenzymes and the study of isoenzymes as distinct proteins. As an indication of the distinction between these two aspects of the study of isoenzymes, the approaches of utilizing methods which had been developed to separate enzyme proteins with great resolution revolutionized the field. Up to that time, the emphasis had been to utilize the catalytic function, which was the recognizable distinct feature of enzyme proteins, to elucidate variations. This broadening of perspective has resulted in the use of all the techniques that are available for separation of proteins and for determination of the structure of proteins for elucidation of isoenzymic variations.

In addition, methods for the study of catalytic activity and inhibition along with the use of specific immunological reagents have achieved a great deal of sophistication. The combination of these main thrusts has made the study of isoenzymes among the most versatile tools in mammalian biochemistry.

In this section, we will attempt to give a few examples of how this multidisciplinary approach has been applied to the elucidation of the properties of two specific types of isoenzymes: lactate dehydrogenase and alkaline phosphatase.

1. Lactate Dehydrogenase (LDH)

The early development of the study of lactate dehydrogenase isoenzymes has been reviewed by Markert (1968) and by Everse and Kaplan (1973). Vesell and Bearn (1957, 1958) and Sayre and Hill (1957) first demonstrated by serum fractionation the heterogeneity of lactic dehydrogenase. This was followed by a number of studies on species specificity of LDH isoenzymes (Haupt and Giersberg, 1958; Wieland *et al.*, 1959).

Markert and Møller (1959) developed the simple starch gel zymogram procedure for LDH isoenzyme differentiation, and this technique resulted in the identification of five isoenzymes that were present in body fluids and tissues. The initial hypothesis that these were conformational variants was disproved by Appella and Markert (1961), who demonstrated the presence of two types of subunits in LDH, each having one-fourth the molecular weight of the intact LDH molecule. These two types of subunits were demonstrated to differ in their amino acid composition and tryptic peptide maps (Markert, 1963a).

The postulate that grew from this work was that the tetrameric LDH molecule consisted of five combinations of the two subunits, designated A (M, LDH-5) and B (H, LDH-1).

The combinations would then be A_4, A_3B_1, A_2B_2, A_1B_3, and B_4, which could account for all the five isoenzymic forms. Markert (1963b) found that five isoenzymic forms could be produced by freezing and thawing equal amounts of the A_4 and B_4 types, thus producing the five isoenzymes in the expected proportions.

The biological individuality of the A and B subunits of LDH was first demonstrated by Shaw and Barto (1963) who found a mutant form of the B subunits in a strain of mice and showed that this form was inherited as a single autosomal codominant gene. The expected number of variants was found at each of the isozyme bands for a combination of four subunits. A similar pattern has been seen in human populations, with variations in the B subunit (Boyer, 1963; Vesell, 1965a,b) and in the A subunit (Nance *et al.,* 1963).

The biological significance of variations in the relative amounts of the different enzyme forms of LDH in different tissues is difficult to assess. Remarkable tissue specificity is especially notable in the occurrence of a unique form of LDH in sperm (Blanco and Zinkham, 1963), and the cell-type specific isoenzymic variation in rat liver (Berg and Blix, 1973).

Cancer cells have been demonstrated to have primarily the A subunit in mouse (Prasad *et al.,* 1972, 1973) and human (Fottrell *et al.,* 1974) cancers. An important functional role for LDH isoenzyme variations is clearly indicated by these observations (see Weinhouse, 1973; and Schapira, 1973), and yet a case has been reported (Kitamura *et al.* 1971) of the complete absence of the B subunit of LDH in the serum, saliva, leukocytes, erythrocytes, and platelets of an apparently normal elderly Japanese male. Markert (1968) has discussed some of the ambiguities in assigning biological significance to LDH isoenzyme variations.

2. Alkaline Phosphatase and the Regan Isoenzyme

Considerable variation in the catalytic properties of alkaline phosphatases from different organs was recognized by Bodansky as long ago as 1937. Much of the succeeding study of the catalytic properties of the alkaline phosphatases revealed striking organ differences in the inhibition of the alkaline phosphatases by a variety of inhibitors, as first reported in the previous review (Fishman, 1960). Subsequent studies on organ-specific inhibitions have been reviewed by Fishman (1974). Alkaline phosphatases differ from lactate dehydrogenase isoenzymes in several important respects: (1) they remain strongly associated with cell membranes after homogenization (Fishman and Lin, 1973); and (2) although the subunit structures of the different alkaline phosphatases have not been elucidated in detail, immunochemical characterizations (Fishman and Ghosh, 1967; Boyer, 1963; Sussman *et al.,* 1968; Pankovitch *et al.,* 1972) have indicated that no simple relationship of subunit hybrids can explain the heterogeneity of alkaline phosphatases.

There thus appears to be a marked organ specificity of alkaline phosphatase isoenzymes. As indicated by Fishman (1974), this specificity is largely responsible for the extensive interest in alkaline phosphatase isoenzymes. The assumption to date has been that if simple procedures could be developed to discriminate between the alkaline phosphatases arising from different tissues, then the identification of the organ from which an elevation in total serum alkaline phosphatase originates could be an invaluable aid in diagnosis and evaluation of therapy for a wide variety of human diseases.

Table II lists some of the properties of alkaline phosphatases from tissues which have been used in our laboratory to differentiate the tissue sources of human alkaline phosphatases in serum. It is clear from this table, that there are considerable differences among the different alkaline phosphatases from human tissues, with respect to all of the parameters that are routinely used in our laboratory for discrimination of these isoenzymes. By use of differential inhibition by phenylalanine and homoarginine, heat inactivation, starch gel electrophoresis, and reaction with appropriate antisera, it is possible to differentiate among intestinal, placental, bone, and liver types of alkaline phosphatase. The greatest ambiguity in the methodology still remains, however, in the facile discrimination between bone and liver alkaline phosphatases. Considerable effort has been expended in this direction (Fishman, 1974).

The alkaline phosphatase that originates from placenta, by virtue of its extraordinary heat stability (stable to heating at 65°C for 5 min) is the easiest enzyme to discriminate in serum, since the nonplacental forms are heat-inactivated.

Placental alkaline phosphatase has been examined for phenotypic differences in genetic studies (Beckman *et al.,* 1966, 1967, 1969; Beckman and Beckman, 1969; Beckman and Johannson, 1967; Harris, 1966) and recognition of its existence was largely responsible for the discovery of a placental-type alkaline phosphatase in sera of a cancer patient named Regan (Fishman *et al.,* 1968a,b), which has added the "Regan isoenzyme" to the list of carcinoembryonic antigens (W. H. Fishman *et al.,*

TABLE II

Properties of Alkaline Phosphatases of Liver, Bone, Intestine, and Placenta

	Alkaline phosphatase of				*References*
	Liver	*Bone*	*Intestine*	*Placenta*	
Inhibition by L-phenylalanine (%)	0–10	0–10	75	75	Fishman and Ghosh, 1967
Inhibition by L-homoarginine (%)	78	78	5	5	Lin and Fishman, 1972
Heat inactivation	50–70	90–100	50–60	0	Fishman and Ghosh, 1967
Anodal migration on starch gel (cm)	4.4–5.0	4.0–6.0	3.0	3.8–4.2	Fishman *et al.,* 1968a
Effect of pretreatment with neuraminidase	+	+	0	+	Robinson and Pierce, 1964 Fishman *et al.,* 1968
Reaction with dilute antisera to placental isoenzyme	0	0	0	+	Inglis *et al.,* 1971
Reaction with dilute antisera to liver isoenzyme	+	+	0	0	L. Fishman *et al.,* 1971
Reaction with dilute antisera to intestinal isoenzyme	0	0	+	0	Fishman *et al.,* 1972

1971) that have been identified in human embryonic tissue and in cancer tissue (Fishman, 1973).

The alkaline phosphatase isoenzymes differ from lactate dehydrogenase in one more important respect, and that is in the lack of a unique substrate specificity. Although, as noted above, much remains to be known about the tissue specificity of lactate dehydrogenase profiles, it is nevertheless clear that lactate dehydrogenase functions in the interconversion of pyruvate and lactate *in vivo*. If alkaline phosphatase is regarded as a pyrophosphatase (Fishman, 1974; Fernley, 1971), it would correspond to LDH in the biochemical uniqueness of substrate specificity. However, such a pyrophosphatase would still possess the ability to hydrolyze many monophosphoric acid esters, the characteristic which is identified with alkaline phosphatase.

A primary difference from LDH is the fact that alkaline phosphatase is an integral part of the plasma membrane, whose function remains as undefined as in the case of other cell membrane enzymes in this part of the cell (Fishman and Lin, 1973; Fishman, 1974), whereas LDH is not a plasma membrane enzyme.

C. Enzymes as Antigens and Immunological Quantitation

In recent years there has been a rapid increase in the number of studies that have adapted immunochemical methods to the study of enzymes. In a sense, the transition has been too gradual to identify a landmark in this development comparable to the use of starch gel zymograms by Markert and Møller (1959) in the development of isoenzymology, and yet it is extremely likely that the continuing development in this area will be eventually responsible for a radical restructuring of the field of isoenzymology. At this point, we would like to consider several relevant examples of the utility of this approach for the study of isoenzymes.

Lanzerotti and Gullino (1972a) demonstrated that antisera prepared against crude lysosomal preparations of rat mammary tumors could be used to quantitate the amount of β-galactosidase and acid phosphatase by a single radial immunodiffusion procedure coupled with specific enzyme stains, and used this tool to study the induction of lysosomal hydrolases during mammary tumor regression (Lanzerotti and Gullino, 1972b). Similarly, Cho-Chung and Gullino used radial immunodiffusion (1973a) and quantitative immunoprecipitation (1973b) to study change in acid ribonuclease and cathepsin during mammary tumor regression. These approaches were particularly significant, since they permitted the quantitation of the amount of enzyme protein as well as activity, thus allowing the authors to show new enzyme synthesis during the regression.

Similarly, Singer and Fishman (1974) used a modification of Lanzerotti and Gullino's technique developed by G. J. Doellgast (unpublished) to evaluate net synthesis of placental-type alkaline phosphatase in prednisolone-treated HeLa (TCRC-1) cell cultures.

Milisauskas and Rose (1972) prepared an antiserum specific for prostatic acid phosphatase by injection of an ammonium sulfate precipitate of urine from a patient with prostatic cancer into a monkey, and used a Laurell "rocket" immunoelectrophoresis technique coupled with specific staining for acid phosphatase to quantitate the prostatic acid phosphatase component. Similarly, these same authors (1973) used the "rocket" technique to quantitate the amounts of esterase, acid phosphatase, glucosaminidase, and β-glucuronidase in aging cell cultures.

Tedesco and Mellman (1971) and Tedesco (1972) found inactive protein that cross-reacted with antiserum to galactose-1-phosphate uridyltransferase in galactosemic patients, thereby identifying the lack of enzyme in this genetic disorder as a structural mutation. Robinson *et al.* (1974) and Carroll and Robinson (1974) used an immunological method to demonstrate a possible regulatory subunit of hexosaminidase, which they postulate is responsible for the Tay-Sachs disease variation in hexosaminidase (see below).

Recently, Holmes and Scopes (1974) have used immunological techniques to detect homologies among vertebrate lactate dehydrogenase isoenzymes, and Burd *et al.* (1973) have quantitated the amount of M-type lactate dehydrogenase by a simple inhibition procedure.

These serve to demonstrate the broad utility of immunological procedures for specific analysis of isoenzymes. Since radioimmunoassay is virtually the only immunoquantitation technique with the sensitivity to detect protein concentrations in the ranges normally found for enzymes in serum, it is very encouraging to find that the same sensitivity of determination of enzyme activity that permitted the development of the starch gel method can be used in development of methods alternative to RIA for enzyme protein quantitation. Perhaps this approach, as documented for galactosemic variants (Tedesco, 1972), could be used to identify new (and somewhat fragile) phenotypic variants in human serum, which Harris (1966) has pointed out must certainly exist for a variety of enzymes.

IV. Enzyme Variants and Genetic Diseases

A number of inherited genetic disorders have been linked to deficiencies in specific enzymes, and some of these can be detected in serum. Reviews on this subject have been published (Milunsky and Littlefield, 1972; Ganschow, 1973; Brady, 1970; O'Brien *et al.*, 1971; Sidbury, 1965; Hsia, 1970; Brady and Kolodny, 1972; Kirkman, 1972). In addition, benign genetic variants have been identified and used to discriminate genetic variants in human populations as noted above for dehydrogenase and placental alkaline phosphatase variants.

The most important application of ascertaining genetic variations in human populations is in the detection of heterozygotes for genetic diseases that result in mental retardation and early death. The best example of this is Tay-Sachs disease, which has been linked to a deficiency in hexosaminidase A (Okada and O'Brien, 1969) and for which serum determinations have been developed that can detect carriers (O'Brien *et al.*, 1970; Saifer and Rosenthal, 1973; Lowden *et al.*, 1973), and Sandhoff's disease (Sandhoff *et al.*, 1968), a variant of Tay-Sachs, that has a deficiency for hexosaminidase A and B and for which a serum test for heterozygotes has been developed (Suzuki *et al.*, 1973). Similarly, Fabry's disease (α-galactosidase deficiency) heterozygotes can be detected by serum assay (Desnick *et al.,* 1973), as can β-glucuronidase (Glaser and Sly, 1973) and α-fucosidase (Zielke *et al.,* 1972a,b: Borrone *et al.,* 1974) heterozygotes in mucopolysaccharidosis.

In general, heterozygotes for most inherited disorders are presently determined by measurement of enzyme activities in leukocytes, erythrocytes, and fibroblast cultures (Milunsky and Littlefield, 1972; Wagner *et al.,* 1971), which means a much greater expense and correspondingly less practicality for mass screening purposes. The special value of serum diagnosis in the cases mentioned above is their practicality.

Serum pseudocholinesterase variants provide a particularly interesting example of enzyme variants that normally do not have any deleterious effect on an individual, but can under certain circumstances produce alarming symptoms. Thus the enzyme acts on acetylcholine analogs, but not directly on acetylcholine itself. When the muscle relaxant, succinylcholine, is used in anesthesia, pseudocholinesterase rapidly hydrolyzes this drug, and so recovery of the patient from the effects of the anesthesia is extremely rapid. In a number of cases, however, paralysis resulted from the administration of the drug, lasting over a period of several days.

This clinical manifestation was related to the apparent absence of serum pseudocholinesterase, and so it became a routine procedure in most hospitals that administered succinylcholine for anesthesia to determine serum pseudocholinesterase levels. This has resulted in the identification of a large number of patients that have deficiencies in this enzyme, and careful genetic studies on this phenotype have been performed (Harris *et al.,* 1963; Kalow and Staron, 1957; Lehmann and Liddell, 1964; Dietz *et al.,* 1973).

Lehmann and Liddell (1964) have related the recognition of this enzyme deficiency by its clinical symptoms to the discovery of the sickle-cell defect in hemoglobin.

V. Normal Tissue Sources of Enzymes in Plasma

A given tissue compartment represents the collection of a number of cell populations properly arranged by a process of development to carry out the function of the organ. Enzymes may normally leave such organs by processes of (a) diffusion, (b) active secretion, (c) permeability change, and (d) shedding of structures such as the glycocalyx of plasma membranes.

One wonders why some enzymes are ubiquitous in their tissue distributions and others not. Examples of the former are β-glucuronidase, alkaline phosphatase, dipeptidases, glutamate-oxaloacetate transaminase, and glutamate-pyruvate transaminase. Nonubiquitous enzymes and their tissue sites are homogentisate oxidase, liver; acid phosphatase, prostate; glutamine synthetase, brain and liver; aldolase, skeletal muscle; and oxaloacetate transacetylase, heart.

It is no longer sufficient to attribute a plasma enzyme to a tissue origin but one is required to identify the particular cell type (since tissues are heterocellular) and, if possible, the individual cell organelle which is responsible. All of this has become feasible with the development of ultracentrifugation techniques for tissue homogenates and with advances in enzyme visualization at the level of the electron microscope (for example, refer to Shnitka and Seligman, 1971). Because of the fundamental importance of these considerations to our understanding of the significance of alterations in levels of individual plasma enzymes, an effort is made in the following to describe the present status of information.

In evaluating the enzyme complement of organelles of the cell, the investigator finds himself either measuring enzyme activities in extracts of subcellular fractions prepared from tissue homogenates or examining electron micrographs bearing evidence of enzyme sites in ultrathin sections of tissues or both. If the results from each technique support the same interpretation, he should be pleased.

The various subcellular fractions not only overlap with each other in their organelle composition but may be essentially heterogeneous.

In this connection, the "microsomes," which sediment at higher gravitational force than mitochondria and lysosomes, consist of membranous vesicles which have been pinched off during the process of homogenization from structures as diverse as plasma membrane, rough and smooth endoplasmic reticulum, Golgi apparatus, infolding basal membranes, and pinocytotic vesicles. It is possible to separate from this mixture vesicles of rough endoplasmic endothelium and smooth endoplasmic reticulum. However, the preparation of reasonably enriched fractions of endoplasmic reticulum, of plasma membrane, and of Golgi apparatus each requires an individual set of fractionations of the homogenates. The identification of a given organelle population is based most conveniently on the assay of "marker" enzymes.

We became familiar with some of the complexities of differentiating enzyme localization on the basis of centrifugation data alone in our study of the alkaline phosphatase component contained in the ascites fluids of patients with ovarian cancer that was excluded from Sepharose 4B (Doellgast and Fishman, 1975). Only 10% of the total alkaline phosphatase was precipitable by centrifugation of one fluid at 350,000 g_{max} for 2 hr, and yet over 60% of the total alkaline phosphatase was excluded from Sepharose 4B in this same fluid sample. After separation of the excluded fractions, the excluded enzyme could be pelleted upon centrifugation at 150,000 g_{max} for 1 hr. To this material was associated typical membrane "marker" enzymes such as 5'-nucleotidase and leucine aminopeptidase. This observation formed the basis for a protocol for preparation of membrane-derived alkaline phosphatase from a variety of human tissues (Doellgast and Fishman, 1975).

This same combination of methodology, i.e., a combination of differential centrifugation with chromatography of separated fractions, would probably be appropriate in cases where some question exists as to the secretion of "soluble" versus "membrane-bound" enzymes, as in the case of γ-glutamyltranspeptidase (Szewczuk, 1966).

A. Plasma Membrane

The suggested markers for the plasma membrane (Oseroff *et al.*, 1973) include ATPase, 5'-nucleotidase, aminopeptidase, sialidase, and phospholipase A. It follows that a change in the same direction of several of these enzymes in the plasma could reasonably be explained by alterations in circulating plasma membrane fragments.

The utility of serum γ-glutamyltranspeptidase as a sensitive indicator of liver dysfunction has been documented (Szczeklik *et al.*, 1961), which is supported by the absence of elevation of this enzyme in myocardial infarction (Cook and Carter, 1973).

The induction of microsomal enzymes by drugs and steroid hormones (Parke, 1971) has its counterpart in the increase in plasma γ-glutamyltranspeptidase in patients receiving enzyme-inducing drugs (Rosalki *et al.*, 1971). Damage to the microsomes has been favored for interpretation of this elevation (Rosalki *et al.*, 1971). The liberation of γ-glutamyltranspeptidase in cervical cancer has similarly been interpreted as release from granular structures (Wieczorek, 1972).

Interesting plasma membrane enzyme components are the various hydrolases associated with microvilli of the intestine (illustrated in Fig. 1) and of the placenta (Fishman and Ghosh, 1967). The microvillar alkaline phosphatase enters the circulation associated with chylomicrons via the intestinal lymph in proportion to the extent of fat absorption.

A view of the site of microvillar alkaline phosphatase in the bile canaliculi of hepatocytes is presented in Fig. 2. The microvilli project into the lumen of the bile canaliculi and, as a consequence of biliary obstruction, could disintegrate and enter the circulation.

In cancer cells as seen in Fig. 3, the plasma membrane enzymes are in contact with the extracellular fluid and one can visualize their ready access to the circulation.

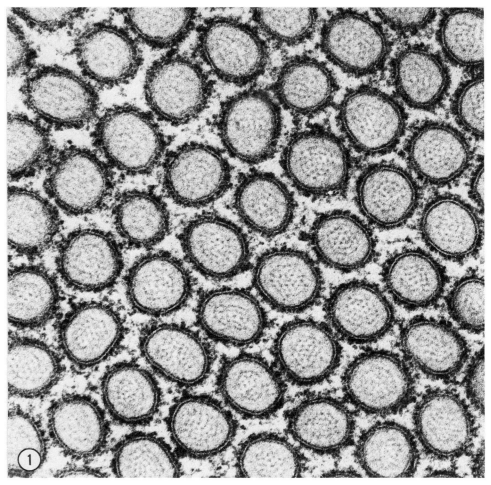

Fig. 1. Electron micrograph of alkaline phosphatase reaction in a cross section of the tips of the microvilli of an absorbing cell of the duodenum of adult male hamster. The electron dense lead reaction product is localized on the external leaflet of the double membrane, but some of it appears also on the internal leaflet. (Unpublished results, courtesy of Dr. J. S. Hugon.) ×135,000.

B. Lysosomes

The history of the concept of the lysosome has been reviewed by de Duve (1969). As a result of the careful work in his laboratory and elsewhere, the lysosome has come to be recognized as the source of most of the catabolic functions for digestion of ingested macromolecules (Gordon, 1969) and of macromolecules being degraded intracellularly

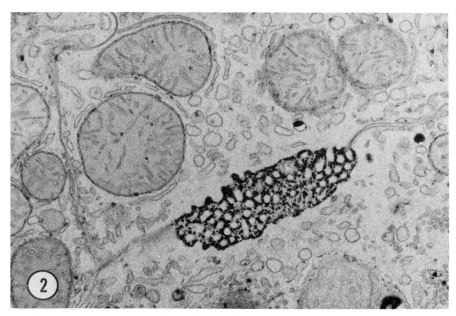

Fig. 2.   Electron micrograph of alkaline phosphatase reaction in a bile canaliculus of adult mouse liver. The reaction product is present on the microvilli and does not extend in the intercellular spaces beyond the terminal bar. (Unpublished results, courtesy of Dr. J. S. Hugon.) ×23,000.

(Ericsson, 1969). Consistent with this catabolic function, the lysosome contains all of the hydrolytic enzymes which are necessary to degrade macromolecules, including proteins (cathepsins, renin, and aminopeptidases), nucleic acids (ribonuclease and deoxyribonuclease), lipids (lipases and phospholipases), glycosyl bonds (glycosidases), phosphoric esters (acid phosphatases), carboxylic esters (esterases), and sulfuric esters (arylsulfatases) (Barrett, 1969).

Since the lysosome is maintained at an acid pH, it is not surprising that most of the hydrolytic enzymes associated with the lysosomes have been found to have acid pH optima. Thus, although both acid and alkaline phosphatases hydrolyze phosphoric esters, the differences in pH optima identify the acid phosphatases as originating primarily in the lysosomes. Figure 4 illustrates not only the acid phosphatase-rich lysosomes but also the extralysosomal sites on infolding membranes, so-called dual localization (Sasaki and Fishman, 1973).

Similarly, the difference between acid and neutral pH optima has been used to differentiate arylamidases of lysosomal and nonlysosomal origin (McDonald *et al.*, 1971; Vanha-Perttula and Kalliomäki, 1973).

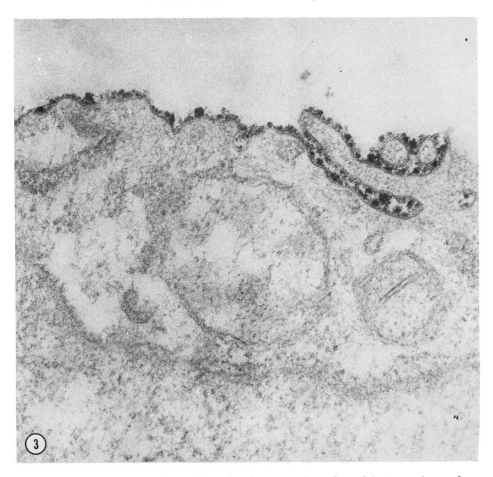

Fig. 3. Reaction product for alkaline phosphatase on the surface of the external part of the plasma membrane of a HeLa cell. (Unpublished results, courtesy of Dr. J. S. Hugon.) ×90,000.

In a sense, then, the difference in pH optima is one criterion which can both discriminate isoenzymes and indicate the intracellular organelle from which a particular isoenzyme originates.

The release of lysosomal enzymes in disease states has been extensively studied, largely with a view of determining the correlation of elevations in particular enzymes, such as β-glucuronidase (Fishman, 1967) and acid phosphatase (Bodansky, 1972; Yam, 1974) in disease. The diagnostic value of prostatic acid phosphatase in diagnosis of prostatic cancer (Green *et al.*, 1968) is an example of this application.

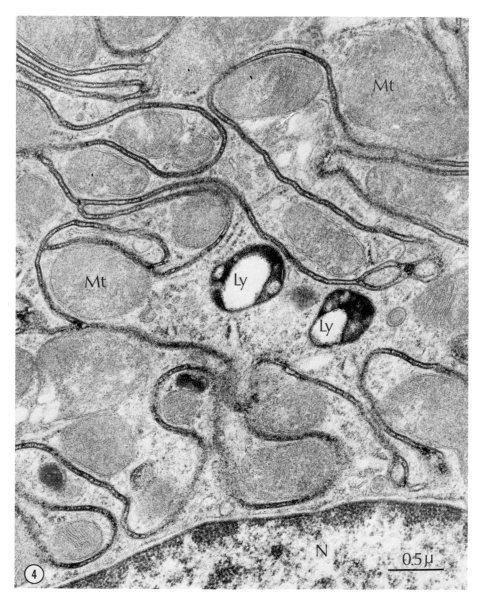

Fig. 4. Acid phosphatase in cytoplasm of an epithelial cell of a distal mouse renal tubule demonstrating tortuous infoldings of basal membranes and two lysosomes (Ly) in the center of the field (Smith-Fishman method). N, Nucleus; Mt, mitochondria. [Courtesy of Sasaki and Fishman (1973) and the *Journal of Histochemistry and Cytochemistry*.]

The recognition of a possible specialized role for acid hydrolases in pathological processes due to exocytosis (Dingle, 1969; Smith and Winkler, 1969) has been postulated. Thus, the possible involvement of lysosomal enzymes in the extracellular degradation of bone (Vaes, 1969) and connective tissue (Barrett, 1968; Weinstock and Iodice, 1969) has led to the study of the concentrations of hydrolytic enzymes in serum and synovial fluid of arthritics (Thomas, 1969; Kalliomäki and Vanha-Perttula, 1972) and in cerebrospinal fluid of motor neuron disease (Yates *et al.*, 1973).

Lysosomal storage diseases, as mentioned above, have been demonstrated to represent in some cases the absence of particular lysosomal enzymes. In some cases (O'Brien *et al.*, 1971; Zielke *et al.*, 1972a,b) the identification of the missing enzyme has been made by measurement of a number of lysosomal enzymes. A comparison of the activities of the different enzymes indicates the particular defect. The absence of hexosaminidase A in Tay-Sachs disease (see above) is an example of this principle.

C. Mitochondria

As yet, the mitochondrial enzymes have not been utilized as widely as the microsomal and lysosomal enzymes for interpretations of plasma enzyme alterations. One reason for this could be the special difficulties associated with study of mitochondrial functions (Roodyn, 1967). The frequent contamination of mitochondria with lysosomal and other subcellular organelles, for example, and the occurrence of most of the mitochondria-specific enzymes in soluble forms within the cell, complicates any precise identification of mitochondria-associated plasma enzymes that are elevated in particular disease states.

Succinic dehydrogenase and cytochrome oxidase, are the recognized marker enzymes associated with mitochondria (Shnitka and Seligman, 1971), but as yet measurement of these two enzymes in plasma has not received much attention.

Several other enzymes, such as malate dehydrogenase (Thorne, 1960; Skilleter *et al.*, 1970), isocitrate dehydrogenase (Criss, 1971), and aspartate aminotransferase (Nisselbaum and Bodansky, 1969), are recognized to have dual localizations.

D. Soluble

As noted above, a dual localization for many enzymes, including the dehydrogenases of the citric acid cycle and the transaminases, has been found. These enzymes are both soluble and mitochondria-associated, and so isoenzyme analysis and subcellular fractionation of each tissue would be necessary to differentiate the source of each tissue-derived enzyme. No such simplifying generalization as the acid pH optima of the lysosomal hydrolases is usable for mitochondrial enzymes, although cofactor specificity has been demonstrated for the dehydrogenases (Criss, 1971).

Perhaps the most widely studied soluble enzyme is lactate dehydrogenase. The general utility of this enzyme is indicated by the number of disease states that can be studied by elevations in specific LDH isoenzymes (Cawley, 1974). The release of LDH in myocardial infarction (Spooner and Goldberg, 1973) and in liver disorders (Nathan *et al.,* 1973) has been documented.

It is thus apparent that the use of soluble enzymes in clinical diagnosis has received wide application. The particular advantage of working with soluble enzymes is that they can be readily separated by electrophoresis, and are not complicated by association with other structures, which was found to be a complication in the study of alkaline phosphatases (see above).

E. "Other"

Specialized cells have been demonstrated to contain unique structures associated with them, and in some cases specific enzymatic functions are localized in these structures. Thus, the association of catalase and α-hydroxy acid oxidase with peroxisomes, of tyrosinase with melanosomes, and of acetylcholinesterase with motor endplates serves to identify these organelles in subcellular fractionation studies (Shnitka and Seligman, 1971).

A specialized enzyme that has received considerable attention recently is dopamine β-hydroxylase, due to the demonstration of low concentrations in the brains of schizophrenics (Wise and Stein, 1973), and the demonstration of increased plasma levels of this enzyme in torsion dystoma (Wooten *et al.,* 1972) and in hypertension (Schanberg *et al.,* 1974). De Potter *et al.,* (1970) have found β-hydroxylase in catecholamine storage vesicles.

The Golgi apparatus has received special attention as a functional organelle (Fleischer and Fleischer, 1971; Morré *et al.,* 1971). It has been recognized that it serves to transport vesicles for membrane flow from nuclear membranes or endoplasmic reticulum (Morré *et al.,* 1971). With Golgi apparatus are associated the specific markers, galactosyl transferase, thiamine pyrophosphatase, and nucleoside diphosphatase (Shnitka and Seligman, 1971). It should be recognized, from the example of a recent assignment of a role for this organelle, that localizations of enzymes and functions within cells are not as yet precisely delineated. It is reasonable to assume that, as subcellular fractionation of organelles achieves greater sophistication, the assignment of a precise pathological process by the levels of a particular enzyme in plasma may become feasible. Measurement of nuclear, mitochondrial, lysosomal, Golgi, and microsomal enzymes in plasma could prove rewarding in terms of a precise definition of pathological processes. At present, this approach has not been pursued, but the increasing amount of information about enzyme localization seems to make it likely that this approach will be fruitful.

VI. Tumor Tissue Sources of Enzymes in Plasma — Carcinoembryonic Isozymes

The tumor enzymes may be either identical to their counterparts in normal adult tissues or they may be products of the activation of embryonic, fetal, or placental genes.

With regard to the first category, one is reminded of the correlation of prostatic cancer with the L-tartrate-sensitive acid phosphatase of the prostate gland recently reviewed by Yam (1974). This enzyme does enrich the serum in many cases of prostatic cancer, its levels increasing with androgen administration and diminishing with estrogen therapy.

Also, although necrosis is a characteristic process in neoplasia, it produces enzyme phenomena which are not usually analogous to, say, LDH release in myocardial infarction. Thus, in the work of Lanzerotti and Gullino (1972b) and Cho-Chung and Gullino (1973a,b), the regression of experimental mammary tumors is associated with a *de novo* synthesis of acid hydrolases such as β-glucuronidase.

In connection with carcinoembryonic enzymes, these have the same biological significance in tumors as do α-fetoprotein and human chorionic gonadotropin. Namely, that activation of embryonic genes is a manifestation of cancer. Examples in experimental animals are the fetal forms of hexokinase, phosphorylase, pyruvate kinase, and aldolase, which have been studied extensively by Weinhouse (1973) and Schapira (1973) in a variety of rat hepatomas. On the other hand, in humans a family of placental type alkaline phosphatases has been studied most extensively, e.g., Regan isoenzyme (Fishman *et al.,* 1968a,b), Nagao isoenzyme (Nakayama *et al.,* 1970), and Regan variant (Warnock, 1968; Warnock and Reisman, 1969; Higashino *et al.,* 1972). Finally, it should be noted that nonplacental alkaline phosphatases have been found as tumor products (Timperley, 1968; Timperley and Warnes, 1970; Timperley *et al.* (1971).

In the light of this information, tumors should always be suspected in cancer patients as sources of plasma enzymes and it is also desirable to distinguish between embryonic and adult forms to improve interpretation.

VII. Turnover of Tissue Enzymes in Plasma

As has been pointed out in a review by Posen (1970), the interrelationship between release of enzymes into blood and the removal of enzymes from blood is a dynamic process, the steady state of which is measured as the "level" of a particular enzyme in plasma. In the study of enzyme levels in plasma, therefore, the actual measurement is the steady state level of enzyme, for which the separate rates of release and catabolism are relevant. We discuss below how pathological changes in the systems for either release or catabolism can affect the enzyme levels in plasma, and how a postulated mechanism for clearance of glycoproteins from plasma (the Ashwell-Morell hypothesis) can explain differences in rates of turnover of plasma alkaline phosphatases derived from different organs.

The process of turnover of plasma enzymes is therefore analogous to the turnover of other plasma proteins. To illustrate the importance of the separate rates of release and catabolism, therefore, it is appropriate to consider the two immunoglobulin classes, IgA and IgG. IgA is present in plasma at one-fifth the concentration of IgG, and yet its release into the plasma occurs at the same rate as IgG (Tomasi, 1968). IgA is therefore catabolized at a much higher rate than IgG, and so these two major plasma constituents differ greatly in their concentrations, due to a difference in their rates of degradation. A similar situation is found for LDH isoenzymes, as found by Boyd (1967a,b) and Bär and Ohlendorf (1970), and recently reviewed by Cawley (1974). Since the rate of disappearance of the "H" type (LDH-1) LDH isoenzyme species is much slower in plasma than the "M" type (LDH-5), a measurement of LDH isoenzymes in a normal individual results in the identification of a predominance of "H" subunit in plasma (Cawley, 1974).

There is one additional complication in the study of enzyme turnover as a measure of the separate rates of catabolism and release, and that is the marked instability of certain enzymes. Thus, it is known that most enzymes are more readily denatured in the absence of their specific substrates or cofactors and that enzymes such as acid phosphatase and bone alkaline phosphatase are thermolabile at 37°C. In order to obtain an accurate picture of enzyme turnover, it may therefore be necessary to use immunological quantitation methods for particular enzymes, which have been demonstrated (Kolb, 1974) to be capable of measuring the quantity of denatured enzyme protein in solution.

We here consider some relevant observations on the release of enzymes into plasma and the clearance and catabolism of enzymes from plasma, with a view to outlining various mechanisms which could account for these separate but interdependent phenomena. Most of the mechanisms which we consider have not, with the exception of release of lysosomal enzymes and catabolism of enzymes by lysosomes, been based upon studies of enzyme turnover. It must, therefore, be recognized that many of the conclusions which shall be reached are inferential and based upon turnover of other plasma proteins. We are still of the opinion that plasma enzymes can be expected to travel the same routes as do the nonenzymatic plasma proteins, and this view is the basis for the analogy which shall be drawn.

A. Factors Controlling Release of Tissue Enzymes into Plasma

Fifteen years ago, some of the following ideas were of interest in explaining the mechanism of enzyme release. Thus, physiological disintegration of erythrocytes and other blood cells as well as a high cellular turnover rate of intestinal mucosa were suggested by Hess (1958) as phenomena which could explain increases in serum lactate and malate dehydrogenases.

Also, the possibility that the presence of substrate may regulate enzyme activity within a tissue developed from the study earlier of Henley *et al.* (1958) who found the presence of alanine at pH 9.0 in the medium of liver slices promoted glutamate-pyruvate transaminase. Finally, anoxia which adversely affects permeability was found by Sibley (1958) to cause a greater release of aldolase from liver slices than from tumor cells. On the other hand, lack of glucose was associated with release of tumor aldolase, just as it caused an efflux of aldolase from diaphragm muscle as described by Zierler (1958).

1. Physiological

Intuitively, it is extremely difficult to accept the secretion of enzymes from intact cells as a normal physiological process when there is no recognizable function for those enzymes in the bloodstream. There are tissues which secrete enzymes as a normal part of their function [for example pancreatic exocrine cells (Jamieson, 1972)], but this type of functional role cannot explain the lactate dehydrogenase or alkaline phosphatase in the blood plasma.

The measurement of enzyme levels in normal subjects does compel the supposition, however, that the secretion of enzymes from tissues is a normal physiological process. Therefore physiological processes which could result in enzyme secretion remain to to be identified. Young (1974) has pointed out how difficult it is to obtain supporting data for any model system of enzyme secretion, principally because of the low levels of enzyme protein in the plasma (Hess and Raftopulo, 1957), which make accurate measurement of turnover by use of isotopic labeling techniques difficult.

It is for these reasons that studies on enzyme "turnover" in plasma have principally measured the rates of degradation of injected enzymes (Fleisher and Wakim, 1963a, b; Wakim and Fleisher, 1963a, b; Mahy *et al.*, 1965, 1967, Mahy and Rowson, 1965; Posen *et al.*, 1965; Saini and Posen, 1969). The assumption has been that the half-life ($t_{1/2}$) for disappearance of a large amount of injected enzyme represents the rate of removal and catabolism of that enzyme in the maintenance of the steady-state levels.

One of the features of enzyme catabolism that seems to argue against the utility of this assumption is that rates of removal are in general biphasic, with an initial fast rate and a secondary slow rate [exceptions to this have been documented (Fleisher and Wakim, 1963b)]. It is not possible therefore to accurately determine turnover rates of enzymes using this measure, since two constants are obtained. Overall rates and differences in rates of catabolism can, however, be compared by using the disappearance rates of injected enzymes, as was used in explaining the differences in levels of LDH isoenzymes in plasma (Cawley, 1974).

Stolbach *et al.* (1972) took advantage of the circumstances surrounding the removal of a Regan isoenzyme-rich lymphoma from the intestine of a patient to study the half-life in the serum of this placental-type alkaline phosphatase. As seen in Fig. 5, the decay followed an exponential course yielding a $t_{1/2}$ of 10 days.

From these observations, it is evident that the half-lives of enzymes in plasma cannot be determined as accurately as have the half-lives of the nonenzymatic plasma proteins (Schultze and Heremans, 1966; Winzler, 1968).

The release of enzymes is a consequence of cellular metabolism. That is, intracellular enzyme turnover, comprising both catabolic and anabolic pathways, is related to delivery of enzymes into the plasma.

Several comprehensive reviews have been written on protein turnover

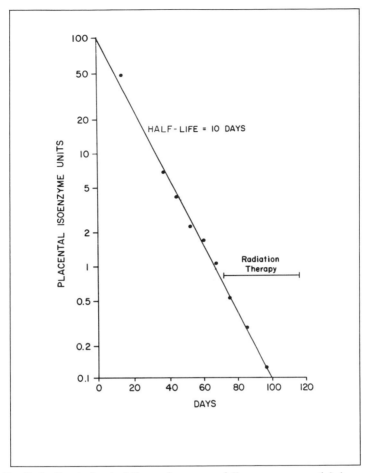

Fig. 5. Reduction in level of Regan isoenzyme follows an exponential decay pattern with a calculated half-life of approximately 10 days. Day 0 is the day of surgery. First serum determination for Regan isozyme obtained on day 13. [Courtesy of L. L. Stolbach *et al.* (1972) and the *Archives of Surgery.*]

(Schimke, 1969, 1973; Schimke and Dehlinger, 1971; Goldberg *et al.,* 1974). It is easily apparent from them that all intracellular proteins are turned over. As Schimke (1973) has pointed out, the life-span of hepatic cells is 160–400 days, but the proteins contained in these cells have half-lives of 4–5 days. Furthermore, the proteins of different subcellular compartments have different mean half-lives (Arias *et al.,* 1969).

Individual enzymes are degraded at different rates (Schimke, 1973), and the rates of synthesis and degradation can be separately altered by selective treatments (Schimke *et al.*, 1965). Circadian and diurnal rhythms have been demonstrated to affect the levels of specific enzymes (Hopkins *et al.*, 1973), as have hormone treatments (Fishman, 1965; Wicks *et al.*, 1974; Jefferson *et al.*, 1974) and a wide variety of other physiological factors, including work and food deprivation (Goldberg *et al.*, 1974) and administration of drugs (Ideo *et al.*, 1971; Kuntzman, 1969).

It is, therefore, easy to recognize that this wide variety of factors which can influence enzyme turnover within a cell, and the inheritance of variations in enzyme activity, which Paigen and Felton (1971) and Ganschow (1973) have demonstrated in inbred mouse strains, all affect the levels of specific enzymes within a given tissue. The sum of all of these factors constitutes the level of a particular enzyme in a given cell at a given time. Clearly, the intracellular concentrations of enzymes must affect the amount of enzyme which can be released.

The release of enzymes from cells has been most actively studied for lysosomal enzymes (Dingle, 1969), principally because of the possible direct relevance of this phenomenon to extracellular digestion in bone resorption (Vaes, 1969) and connective tissue catabolism (Barrett, 1968). The secretion of lysosomal hydrolases has been demonstrated to be affected by vitamins A and E (Roels, 1969) and by parathyroid hormone (Vaes, 1969).

Most of these studies have been performed in organ cultures, which have the advantage (Dingle, 1969) of a precise definition of the medium of the cells, but it is difficult to draw firm conclusions based on such studies purporting relevance to secretion of enzymes into plasma, except that the process has been demonstrated to be associated with viable cells (Dingle, 1969), so that it is not necessary to prove the feasibility of secretion of enzyme from viable, rather than dead cells. Relatively fewer studies have been performed on the secretion of tissue enzymes into the blood plasma in normal individuals.

In this connection, the rapid release of intestinal alkaline phosphatase upon fat ingestion (Keiding, 1964, 1966) represents a recognizable benign release of a particular isoenzyme into serum, whose level of elevation was proportional to the degree of stimulation (i.e., fat intake) (Inglis *et al.*, 1967) and was correlated to blood group type (Walker *et al.*, 1971).

Pregnancy results in a logarithmic increase in placental-type alkaline phosphatase (Fishman *et al.*, 1973) and in considerable increase of amine oxidase which is kinetically identical to placental-type (Bardsley *et al.*, 1974) and of oxytocinase (Chapman *et al.*, 1973; Usategui-Gomez *et al.,* 1973). The identification of placenta-derived enzymes has achieved special significance recently, due largely to the demonstration of a specific utility of placental-type alkaline phosphatase as a manifestation of certain cancers (Fishman, 1973) (see Section VI).

The effect on muscle enzymes in anoxia of excised muscles (Zierler, 1958) has been confirmed for increases in serum enzymes in intact animals after hypoxia (Highman and Atland, 1960) and for creatine kinase after muscular activity in humans (Griffiths, 1966) and dogs (Sweetin and Thomson, 1973b). Sweetin and Thomson (1973b) have suggested the active retention of enzymes in cells, with release of these enzymes being caused by a reduction in the ATP available.

2. Pathological

The interest in plasma enzymes is largely due to their potential as indices of pathological changes; and the measurement of elevations in particular disease states is used in diagnosis of disease states and response to therapy. In short, then, most of the literature on plasma enzymes deals with pathological alteration in release of enzymes, and therefore it is impossible to adequately review the full scope of this subject. The reader is referred to reviews on enzymes in cancer by Schwartz (1973b) and Schapira (1973), on acid phosphatase by Bodansky (1972) and Yam (1974), and on alkaline phosphatase by Fishman (1974).

The increase in plasma levels of liver-type alkaline phosphatase has been found to be caused by an increased rate of release of liver-type alkaline phosphatase in hepatobiliary disorders (Fishman, 1974), which in some cases has been identified with an increase in the intracellular levels of enzyme (Righetti and Kaplan, 1974; Kryszewski *et al.,* 1973; Moss *et al.,* 1974) and associated with elevations in other enzymes (Kryszewski *et al.,* 1973). Similarly, pathological alterations in bone (Fishman, 1974) have resulted in increased secretion of bone-type alkaline phosphatase.

In pancreatitis, pancreatic enzymes have been found to be secreted in excess amounts into the bloodstream (Edmondson *et al.,* 1952; Vogel and Zieve, 1963; Patt *et al.,* 1966).

It has been known for some time that myocardial infarction results in a rapid and significant rise in a number of serum enzymes (La Due *et al.,* 1954; Kattus *et al.,* 1957), which in the case of LDH has been identified with the isoenzyme-1, which has greater specificity for reduction of α-hydroxybutyrate (Rosalki and Wilkinson, 1964). This fact is frequently used to diagnose myocardial infarction by the definition of "α-hydroxybutyrate dehydrogenase" (Spooner and Goldberg, 1973). Similarly, methods are still being developed to discriminate the LDH-5 isoenzyme (Nathan *et al.*, 1973), which is of significance in liver disorders (Cawley, 1974).

In diabetes, almost all enzymes can be elevated, depending on the state of the disease. Belfiore *et al.* (1973) have considered the clinical significance of each of several categories of enzymes which can be elevated in different stages of diabetes.

Hypothermia, or reduction in body temperature, has been found to have associated with it elevation of a number of serum enzymes (MacLean *et al.*, 1974).

In summary, then, a wide variety of pathological changes can alter the levels of plasma enzymes. Although the cellular mechanism for this release is not known in any one case, the organ source can frequently be defined with some precision.

B. Factors Controlling Removal of Tissue-Derived Enzymes from Plasma

It is still our view that plasma enzymes can be expected to travel the same routes of degradation and removal as do the nonenzymatic plasma proteins. It should be understood however that the rate of disappearance of enzyme activity need not necessarily be the same as the rate of clearance of enzyme protein from the circulation. A lack of such a parallelism would be expected in the case of a particularly fragile enzyme whose active site would be preferentially disturbed in the circulation. Thus, it is known that enzymes are more readily denatured in the absence of their specific substrate or cofactors and that enzymes such as acid phosphatase and bone alkaline phosphatase are thermolabile at 37°C. The examination of such a situation calls for the use of both enzymatic and immunological techniques.

1. Physiological

In contrast to the measurement of factors affecting release of tissue enzymes into plasma, the removal of and catabolism of plasma enzymes have been extensively studied. In this case, the study of enzyme activity provides a certain advantage in that relatively small amounts of an enzyme protein (with a high turnover number of a chromogenic substrate) can be injected into an animal, and its disappearance from the plasma can be measured over an extended period of time. In this sense, en-

TABLE III

Disappearance Rates of Three Enzymes

Enzyme	Fast phase $t_{1/2}$ (hr)	Slow phase $t_{1/2}$ (hr)
Glutamic-pyruvate transaminase	$17\frac{1}{2} \pm 1.1$	60.9 ± 2.9
Glutamic-oxaloacetate transaminase I	4.0 ± 0.15	11.8 ± 0.29
Glutamic-oxaloacetate transaminase II	0.85 ± 0.12	[a]

[a] Rate of removal increased after 2 hours (Fleisher and Wakim, 1963b).

zymes have distinct advantages over proteins without measurable catalytic activity in that no radioisotope methodology is required.

Thus Fleisher and Wakim (1963a,b) and Wakim and Fleisher (1963a,b) studied the disappearance of pyruvate-glutamate and glutamic-oxaloacetate transaminases I and II injected into dogs, and found that the disappearance rates of these functionally related enzymes differed considerably. The results are shown in Table III.

Clearly, these enzymes, which are very closely related in their catalytic activities, are not similarly recognized by the systems for removal of enzymes from plasma. The same situation applies to LDH-1 and LDH-5 (*vide infra*).

A similar difference has been observed among the alkaline phosphatase isoenzymes in humans. Thus, some 10 years ago, Posen *et al.* (1965) injected placental alkaline phosphatase intravenously into humans and found that it was, like albumin, distributed within the intravascular compartment. Its half-life is approximately 7 days corresponding to that of ^{131}I-albumin. This enzyme is very sturdy as indicated by its unusual heat stability (McMaster *et al.*, 1964).

Posen (1967) contrasted this experience with placental alkaline phosphatase with the failure of intestinal phosphatase of equivalent activity entering the circulation via the thoracic duct to increase serum alkaline phosphatase more than 25% as observed by Langman and his co-workers in 1966, who studied the influence of diet on intestinal alkaline phosphatase in the serum of individuals differing in blood group type and secretor status. The half-life of intestinal alkaline phosphatase was presumed to be very much shorter than the half-life of placental alkaline phosphatase. Moreover, individuals possessing blood groups O and B and who were secretors showed a higher serum "intestinal" alkaline phosphatase.

Earlier studies have described a rather rapid disappearance from the circulation (1–24 hr) of enzymes such as aldolase (Warburg and Christian, 1943; Sibley, 1958), isocitric dehydrogenase (Wolfson *et al.*, 1958), β-glucuronidase (Fishman, 1960), acid phosphatase (Huggins, 1947), and lactic acid dehydrogenase (Wroblewski and La Due, 1955). A recent compilation of the half-lives of additional enzymes such as amylase, creatine phosphokinase, γ-glutamyltranspeptidase, lipase, leucine aminopeptidase, and malate dehydrogenase has been made by Young (1974).

All the data obtained prove that there are a wide variety of rates of removal of different enzymes from the plasma and point to considerable specificity for this process.

2. Pathological

The study of enzyme removal from plasma has identified a number of modifiers of this system, and has to some extent identified the principal tissues responsible for removal of some enzymes. Thus, zymosan, which affects the reticuloendothelial system, was found to reduce the clearance of enzymes from the plasma of dogs (Wakim and Fleisher, 1963b). Similarly, Mahy *et al.*, (1965,1967) found that stilbesterol and thorotrast, which also affect the reticuloendothelial system, diminish the plasma clearance of several enzymes in mice.

One of the most interesting findings in the area of pathological effects on plasma clearance of enzymes was the discovery by Riley *et al.* (1960) of a transmissible agent, which was associated with neoplasms, that caused a marked increase in the levels of lactate dehydrogenase (Riley *et al.*, 1960), and of isocitrate and malate dehydrogenase, phosphohexose isomerase, and glutamic-oxaloacetate transaminase, but not of alkaline phosphatase or aldolase (Notkins *et al.*, 1963).

Mahy *et al.* (1964) demonstrated that the increase in plasma enzyme levels did not occur in animals infected with Friend, Moloney, and polyoma viruses. It was therefore clear that the mechanism of action of the Riley virus was specific for this virus and was not a general effect of viruses.

Next, Mahy and Rowson (1965) investigated the specificity of clearance of injected LDH isoenzymes LDH-1 and LDH-5 from plasma of mice infected with the Riley virus and postulated that the reduced rate of clearance of LDH-5 accounted for the specific elevation of this isoenzyme in plasma of mice infected with Riley virus. Mahy *et al.* further demonstrated (1965, 1967) that substances which affected the reticuloendothelial system had an effect similar to the Riley virus on the elevation of LDH levels in mice.

The action of the Riley virus was particularly interesting, in that it identified an effect on one type of tissue that caused an alteration of the removal of some enzymes from plasma, but not of others (Notkins *et al.*, 1963; Mahy and Rowson, 1965). It was clear from this work that the removal of enzymes involves a variety of tissues, and that considerable specificity exists in the removal of enzymes from plasma.

3. The Ashwell-Morell Hypothesis of the Regulation of Serum Glycoprotein Levels

Considerable specificity at the plasma membrane has been demonstrated for the uptake of immunoglobulins (Waldmann *et al.*, 1971; Waldmann and Jones, 1973) and of serum glycoproteins (Ashwell and Morell, 1974). It has become recognized from these studies that binding of molecules to the plasma membranes of the receptor cells accounts for the specific uptake.

Ashwell and Morell (1974) have worked extensively on the uptake of plasma glycoproteins by rat livers following the injection of pure isotopically labeled glycoproteins.

The hypothesis advanced by these authors is that terminal sialic acid residues on glycoproteins are responsible for their continued maintenance in the circulation. It arose out of their first observation of the disappearance within 10 min of radioactive asialoceruloplasmin after its injection into rabbits in face of the half-life of 56 hr characteristic of sialoceruloplasmin (Morell *et al.*, 1966). The asialoceruloplasmin now has a terminal galactose residue which was found to be an essential factor in its rapid elimination from the circulation.

Next it was shown that coincident with the disappearance of the radioactive asialoceruloplasmin from the circulation there was an almost exclusive uptake of the labeled glycoprotein in the parenchymal, but not the Kupffer cells of the liver (Morell *et al.*, 1968). Similar results were obtained in rats with the demonstration that the labeled asialoceruloplasmin concentrated in the lysosomes of the hepatocytes and there underwent hydrolysis.

The phenomenon appears to be a general one with a single exception, transferrin. Thus, desialylated macroglobulin, thyroglobulin, haptoglobin, fetuin, orosomucoid (Morell *et al.*, 1971), and human chorionic gonadotrophin (Vaitukaitis *et al.*, 1971) all disappeared rapidly from the plasma after injection. It was further established that sialic acid must be present in hepatocyte plasma membranes in order for the liver to accomplish the uptake of the desialylated glycoprotein. One could suggest that this is a circumstance in which the participation of a plasma membrane sialyltransferase to accomplish the connection to plasma membrane seems tailor-made.

Of some interest in this system for a specific uptake of glycoproteins at the plasma membrane, beginning with glycoproteins that have terminal sialic acid residues removed, is the demonstration that the prior biosynthesis of glycoproteins proceeds by addition of sugar residues after assembly of the polypeptide chain, with addition of sialic acid to *N*-acetylgalactosamine or *N*-acetylneuraminic acid just prior to secretion of the protein (Gottschalk, 1973). This provides a recognizable link between the secretion and uptake of this class of glycoproteins.

The studies of Ashwell's group did not include investigations on plasma enzymes, and so any suggestions as to the contribution of this postulated mechanism to plasma enzyme uptake by hepatic cells must of necessity be inferential but relevant, since a number of plasma enzymes are known to be sialoglycoproteins (certain alkaline phosphatases, β-glucuronidase, ribonuclease, etc.).

It was of particular interest that Morell *et al.* (1968) found that none of the asialoceruloplasmin was taken up by the reticuloendothelial system, in view of the demonstrations of Fleisher and Wakim (1963a,b), Wakim and Fleisher (1963a,b), and Mahy *et al.* (1965, 1967) that the reticuloendothelial system accounts for a considerable portion of the removal rate of a number of enzymes from plasma. Excluded from this group that is affected by selective inhibition of the reticuloendothelial system was the serum alkaline phosphatase (Notkins *et al.*, 1963).

In this connection, the alkaline phosphatases (see Table II) are known to have terminal sialic acid residues, with the exception of intestinal alkaline phosphatase. Upon injection of rat intestinal alkaline phosphatase into rats (Saini and Posen, 1969), the alkaline phosphatase disappeared within a few hours in contrast to an interval of many days for placental sialoalkaline phosphatase in humans. Posen (1970) and Fishman (1974) have pointed out, however, that no firm evidence as to the rate of removal of intestinal enzyme has been obtained in the normal individual except in the case of injected enzyme.

Although the evidence is not conclusive with respect to the normal turnover of intestinal alkaline phosphatase, it is clear that the catabolic rate of injected intestinal phosphatase is extremely fast, and this may be due to its demonstrated deficiency in terminal sialic acid residues.

It is possible therefore that the desialylated alkaline phosphatases could be specifically catabolized in the parenchymal hepatocyte rather than by the reticuloendothelial system, which appears to be the site of catabolism of the dehydrogenases, phosphohexose isomerase, and glutamic-oxaloacetate transaminase (Notkins *et al.,* 1963; Mahy *et al.,* 1964). It follows that the possibility must be recognized that lysosomes of liver cells may contain in addition to their endogenously produced acid hydrolases, a number of desialylated glycoprotein enzymes which are losing activity due to intralysosomal digestion.

4. Intracellular Sites of Enzyme Catabolism

The concept of the lysosome, as developed in great detail in the three-volume series edited by Dingle and Fell (1969), has provided a rational approach to the catabolism of proteins removed from serum.

Thus, as cited by Maunsbach (1969), lysosomes are the catabolic sites for the sialoglycoprotein horseradish peroxidase in kidney cells. Similarly, Ashwell's group (Gregoriadis *et al.,* 1970) have demonstrated the specific lysosomal catabolism of isotope-labeled glycoprotein taken up by rat liver cells.

Indeed, the active process of endocytosis (Jacques, 1969) could in large measure account for the removal of enzymes from plasma, and perturbation of this system can account then for the changes in plasma levels induced by selective inhibitors of enzyme removal from plasma (Wakim and Fleisher, 1963b; Mahy *et al.,* 1965). These inhibitors have been found to be localized in the lysosomes after being taken up (Bowers, 1969).

Thus, the connection between plasma enzymes and tissue enzymes becomes apparent. Discharge of enzymes by exocytosis or a failure in active retention becomes reflected in an elevated level of plasma enzymes, and the active processes of endocytosis and lysosomal catabolism can account for the removal from plasma, with substances limiting this process also being inhibitory toward removal of enzymes from plasma. A connection between exocytosis and endocytosis, as suggested by Verity (1973), suggests that uptake and exocytic secretion are closely related.

VIII. Discussion and Summary

The center of gravity of this universe of tissue-derived enzymes found in plasma is widely considered in terms of organ-specific isoenzymes. In the recognition of polymorphic forms of enzymes has come the realization that these may differ considerably according to tissue origin, in electrophoretic migration, and in subtle enzymatic properties while still retaining the same catalytic function. Slightly different arrays of antigenic determinants in each tissue's isoenzymes offers the opportunity to prepare specific antisera in other animals. These antisera can be employed as reagents to identify the individual tissue isoenzymes and to quantitate them through appropriate immunoassay techniques.

The ability to recognize the tissue "marker" isoenzyme is now expected to extend to the particular organelle of specific cells which generate this product. This expectation is now being realized in part by the discovery of multienzyme complexes in plasma and body fluids which have the characteristics of plasma membrane fragments as well as the presence in plasma of the familiar lysosomal acid hydrolases.

Clearly, a pattern of isoenzymes characteristic of an organelle of a given cell is more readily interpreted than is the behavior of a single enzyme. One can predict, therefore, that more attention will be paid to establishing what may be termed "fingerprint" isoenzyme patterns in serum.

Today, most investigators are giving even greater attention to the physiological factors which operate to control the release of tissue enzymes into plasma and their removal. In fact, it is the genome which determines (a) whether a given enzyme is produced in the organism to begin with and (b) whether it will express an abnormal or normal level in the plasma. An appreciation of these variables can do much to explain an abnormal plasma isoenzyme value in the absence of recognizable pathology.

Quantitative differences in plasma isoenzymes have been recognized in the case of the carcinoembryonic isoenzymes which are often the products of cancer cells and are not normally seen in adult life. The activation of embryonic genes residing in the genome of somatic cells is being accepted as a manifestation of neoplasia that has a real potential for evaluating the state of malignancy of a cell. The embryonic gene products may include individual isoenzymes as described in the text, polypeptide hormones such as HCG and ACTH, or fetal proteins such as α-fetoprotein.

In a cancer patient one can expect both tumor tissue and normal tissue to be contributors to the pool of plasma enzymes. Of relevance, of course, is the necessity to distinguish between the isoenzymes of tumor and nontumor origin. The examples given of LDH and alkaline phosphatase illustrate the dimensions of this phenomenon and the experimental approaches to its investigation.

Next, there are some indications of the existence of hitherto unrecognized routes of isoenzyme disappearance from the blood plasma. In one of these, it would appear that the nature of the terminal carbohydrate units of glycoproteins determines whether or not the glycoprotein isoenzyme is taken up by the parenchymal hepatocytes or by the reticuloendothelial system or not at all. The experimental findings of Ashwell and Morell (1974) on sialoglycoproteins and the control of their disappearance rate from plasma encourage similar studies on enzyme sialoglycoproteins.

Also, there is evidence of the formation of immune-isoenzyme complexes *in vivo*. If these have lost the catalytic activity of the enzyme, it has to all intensive purposes disappeared from the plasma.

Finally, in retrospect the advance of knowledge in the area of plasma enzymes during the past 15 years presages an even greater acceleration in the improvement of our understanding of their significance and of our ability to utilize this information in the management of disease.

ACKNOWLEDGMENTS

Experimental studies from this laboratory referred to in this chapter were aided by grants-in-aid (CA-12924, CA-13332) from the National Cancer Institute, National Institutes of Health, Public Health Service, Bethesda, Maryland. William H. Fishman is the recipient of Career Research Award (K6-18453) and George J. Doellgast holds a PHS Research Fellowship (5 F 22 CA-00064-02).

Our sincere thanks are expressed to Professor J. S. Hugon, University of Sherbrooke, Quebec, for providing the electron micrographs shown in Figs. 1, 2, and 3.

REFERENCES

Adlung, J., Lorentz, K., and Grajikowske, H. (1971). *Z. Klin. Chem. Klin. Biochem.* **9**, 411.

Akedo, H., Shinkai, K., Horiuchi, N., and Omori, K. (1967). *Annu. Rep. Cent. Adult Dis., Osaka* **7**, 1.

Appella, E., and Markert, L. (1961). *Biochem. Biophys. Res. Commun.* **6**, 171.

Arias, I., Doyle, D., and Schimke, R. T. (1969). *J. Biol. Chem.* **244**, 3303.

Ashwell, G., and Morell, A. G. (1974). "Advances in Enzymology" (A. Meister, ed.), Vol. 41, p. 99. Wiley & Sons, New York.

Bär, U., and Ohlendorf, S. (1970). *Klin. Wochenschr.* **48**, 776.

Bardsley, W. G., Crabbe, M. J. C., and Scott, I. V. (1974). *Biochem. J.* **139**, 169.

Barrett, A. J. (1968). *Compr. Biochem.* **26B**, 435.

Barrett, A. J. (1969). *In* "Lysosomes in Biology and Pathology" (J. T. Dingle and H. B. Fell, eds.), Vol. 2, p. 245. North Holland Publ., Amsterdam.

Beckman, G., and Beckman, L. (1969). *Hum. Hered.* **19**, 524.

Beckman, G., and Johannson, E. O. (1967). *Acta Genet. Med. Gemellol.* **17**, 413.

Beckman, L., Bjorling, G., and Christodoulou, C. (1966). *Acta Genet. Med. Gemellol.* **16**, 59.

Beckman, L., Beckman, G., Christodoulou, C., and Ifekwumigwe, A. (1967). *Acta Genet. Med. Gemellol.* **17,** 406.

Beckman, L., Beckman, G., and Mi, M. P. (1969). *Hum. Hered.* **19,** 258.

Belfiore, F., LoVecchio, L., and Napoli, E. (1973). *Clin. Chem.* **19,** 447.

Berg, T., and Blix, A. S. (1973). *Nature (London), New Biol.* **245,** 239.

Bergman, H., Carlstrom, A., Gustavsson, I., and Lindsten, J. (1971). *Scand. J. Clin. Lab. Invest.* **27,** 341.

Bergmeyer, H. U., ed. (1965). "Methods of Enzymatic Analysis." Academic Press, New York.

Berlet, H. H. (1968). *Z. Klin. Chem. Klin. Biochem.* **6,** 145.

Biewenga, J. (1972). *Clin. Chim. Acta* **40,** 407.

Biewenga, J., and Thijs, L. G. (1970). *Clin. Chim. Acta* **27,** 293.

Blanco, A., and Zinkham, W. H. (1963). *Science* **139,** 601.

Blume, P., and Freier, E. F. (1974). "Enzymology in the Practice of Laboratory Medicine." Academic Press, New York.

Bodansky, O. (1937). *J. Biol. Chem.* **118,** 341.

Bodansky, O. (1957). *Cancer* **10,** 859.

Bodansky, O. (1972). *Advan. Clin. Chem.* **15,** 43.

Bodansky, O., and Schwartz, M. K. (1968). *Advan. Clin. Chem.* **11,** 277.

Borrone, C., Gatti, R., Trias, X., and Durand, P. (1974). *J. Pediat.* **84,** 727.

Bowers, W. E. (1969). *In* "Lysosomes in Biology and Pathology" (J. T. Dingle and H. B. Fell, eds.), Vol. 1, p. 167. North-Holland Publ., Amsterdam.

Boyd, J. W. (1967a). *Biochim. Biophys. Acta* **132,** 221.

Boyd, J. W. (1967b). *Biochim. Biophys. Acta* **146,** 590.

Boyer, S. H. (1963). *Ann. N.Y. Acad. Sci.* **103,** 938.

Boyer, S. H., Fainer, D. C., and Watson-Williams, E. J. (1963). *Science* **141,** 642.

Brady, R. O. (1970). *Clin. Chem.* **16,** 811.

Brady, R. O., and Kolodny, E. H. (1972). *Progr. Med. Genet.* **8,** 225.

Bruns, F., and Neuhaus, J. (1955). *Biochem. Z.* **326,** 242.

Bruns, F., and Neuhaus, J. (1956). *Naturwissenschaften* **8,** 180.

Brydon, W. G., and Roberts, L. B. (1972). *Clin. Chim. Acta* **41,** 435.

Burd, J. F., Usategui-Gomez, M., Fernandez de Castro, A., Mhartre, N. S., and Yeager, F. M. (1973). *Clin. Chim. Acta* **46,** 205.

Burstone, M. S. (1964). *In* "Cytology and Cell Physiology" (G. H. Bourne, ed.), 3rd ed., Chapter 5, p. 181. Academic Press, New York.

Cantor, F., Green, S., Stolbach, L. L., and Fishman, W. H. (1972). *Clin. Chem.* **18,** 391.

Caraway, W. T. (1962). *Amer. J. Clin. Pathol.* **37,** 445.

Carroll, M., and Robinson, D. (1974). *Biochem. J.* **137,** 217.

Cawley, L. P. (1974). *In* "Enzymology in the Practice of Laboratory Medicine" (P. Blume and E. F. Freier, eds.), p. 323. Academic Press, New York.

Ceriotti, G. (1973). *Clin. Chim. Acta* **47,** 97.

Chapman, L., Burrows-Peakin, R., Jowett, T. P., Rege, V. P., and Silk, E. (1973). *Clin. Chim. Acta* **47,** 89.

Cho-Chung, Y. S., and Gullino, P. M. (1973a). *J. Biol. Chem.* **248,** 4743.

Cho-Chung, Y. S., and Gullino, P. M. (1973b). *J. Biol. Chem.* **248,** 4750.

Cook, V. P., and Carter, N. K. (1973). *Clin. Chem.* **19,** 774.

Criss, W. E. (1971). *Cancer Res.* **31,** 1523.

de Duve, C. (1969). *In* "Lysosomes in Biology and Pathology" (J. T. Dingle and H. B. Fell, eds.), Vol. 1, p. 1. North-Holland Publ., Amsterdam.

De Potter, W. P., Smith, A. D., and Schaepdryver, A. F. (1970). *Tissue & Cell* **2**, 529.

Desnick, R. J., Allen, K. Y., Desnick, S. J., Raman, M. K., Bernlohr, R. W., and Krivit, W. (1973). *J. Lab. Clin. Med.* **81**, 157.

Dietz, A. A., Rubinstein, H. M., and Lubrano, T. (1973). *Clin. Chem.* **19**, 1309.

Dille, R. S., and Watkins, C. H. (1948). *J. Lab. Clin. Med.* **33**, 480.

Dingle, J. T. (1969). *In* "Lysosomes in Biology and Pathology" (J. T. Dingle and H. B. Fell, eds.), Vol. 2, p. 421. North-Holland Publ., Amsterdam.

Dingle, J. T., and Fell, H. B., eds. (1969). "Lysosomes in Biology and Pathology," 3 vols. North-Holland Publ., Amsterdam.

Doellgast, G. J., and Fishman, W. H. (1975). *In* "Isozymes. I – Molecular Structure" (C. L. Markert, ed.), p. 293. Academic Press, New York.

Dunne, J., Fennelly, J. J., and McGeeney, K. (1967). *Cancer* **20**, 71.

Dymling, J. F. (1966). *Scand. J. Clin. Lab. Invest.* **18**, 129.

Edmondson, H. A., Berne, C. J., Homann, R. E., and Wertman, M. (1952). *Amer. J. Med.* **12**, 34.

Ellis, G., Spooner, R. J., and Goldberg, D. M. (1973). *Clin. Chim. Acta* **47**, 75.

Ericsson, J. L. E. (1969). *In* "Lysosomes in Biology and Pathology" (J. T. Dingle and H. B. Fell, eds.), Vol. 3, p. 89. North-Holland Publ., Amsterdam.

Everse, J., and Kaplan, N. O. (1973). *Advan. Enzymol.* **37**, 61.

Fennelly, J. J., Dunne, J., McGeeney, K., Chong, L., and Fitzgerald, M. X. (1969a). *Ann. N.Y. Acad. Sci.* **166**, 794.

Fennelly, J. J., Fitzgerald, M. X., and McGeeney, K. (1969b). *Gut* **10**, 45.

Fernley, H. N. (1971). *In* "The Enzymes" (P. D. Boyer, ed.), 3rd ed., Vol. 4, p. 417. Academic Press, New York.

Fishman, L., Inglis, N. R., and Fishman, W. H. (1971). *Clin. Chim. Acta* **34**, 393.

Fishman, L., Inglis, N. R., and Fishman, W. H. (1972). *Clin. Chim. Acta* **38**, 75.

Fishman, W. H. (1960). *In* "The Plasma Proteins" (F. W. Putnam, ed.), Vol. 2, Chapter 12, p. 59. Academic Press, New York.

Fishman, W. H. (1965). *Methods Horm. Res.* **4**, 273.

Fishman, W. H. (1967). *Methods Biochem. Anal.* **15**, 77.

Fishman, W. H. (1969). *Ann. N.Y. Acad. Sci.* **166**, 365–819.

Fishman, W. H. (1973). *Advan. Enzyme Regul.* **11**, 293. Pergamon Press.

Fishman, W. H. (1974). *Amer. J. Med.* **56**, 617.

Fishman, W. H., and Ghosh, N. K. (1967). *Advan. Clin. Chem.* **10**, 255.

Fishman, W. H., and Lerner, F. (1953). *J. Biol. Chem.* **200**, 89.

Fishman, W. H., and Lin, C. W. (1973). *In* "Metabolic Conjugation and Metabolic Hydrolysis" (W. H. Fishman, ed.), Vol. 3, p. 387. Academic Press, New York.

Fishman, W. H., Inglis, N. R., Stolbach, L. L., and Krant, M. J. (1968a). *Cancer Res.* **28**, 150.

Fishman, W. H., Inglis, N. R., Green, S., Anstiss, C. L., Ghosh, N. K., Reif, A. E., Rustigian, R., Krant, M. J., and Stolbach, L. L. (1968b). *Nature (London)* **219**, 679.

Fishman, W. H., Inglis, N. R., and Green, S. (1971). *Cancer Res.* **31**, 1054.

Fishman, W. H., Anstiss, C. L., Pirnik, M. P., and Driscoll, S. G. (1973). *Amer. J. Clin. Pathol.* **60**, 353.

Fleischer, B., and Fleischer, S. (1971). *In* "Biomembranes" (L. A. Manson, ed.), p. 75. Plenum, New York.

Fleisher, G. A., and Wakim, K. G. (1963a). *J. Lab. Clin. Med.* **61**, 76.

Fleisher, G. A., and Wakim, K. G. (1963b). *J. Lab. Clin. Med.* **61**, 98.

Fottrell, P. F., Spellman, C. M., and O'Dwyer, E. M. (1974). *Cancer Res.* **34**, 979.

Ganrot, P. O. (1967). *Experientia* **23**, 593.

Ganschow, R. (1973). *In* "Metabolic Conjugation and Metabolic Hydrolysis" (W. H. Fishman, ed.), Vol. 3, p. 189. Academic Press, New York.

Geokas, M. C., and Rinderknecht, H. (1973). *Clin. Chim. Acta* **46**, 27.

Glaser, J. H., and Sly, W. S. (1973). *J. Lab. Clin. Med.* **82**, 969.

Goldberg, A. L., Howell, E. M., Li, J. B., Martel, S. B., and Prouty, W. F. (1974). *Fed. Proc. Fed. Amer. Soc. Exp. Biol.* **33**, 1112.

Gordon, A. H. (1969). *In* "Lysosomes in Biology and Pathology" (J. T. Dingle and H. B. Fell, eds.), Vol. 3, p. 89. North-Holland Publ., Amsterdam.

Gottschalk, A. (1973). *Z. Naturforsch. C* **28**, 94.

Green, S., Giovanello, T. J., Cote, R. A., and Fishman, W. H. (1968). *Automat. Anal. Chem., Technicon Symp.* **1**, 563.

Green, S., Anstiss, C. L., and Fishman, W. H. (1971). *Enzymologia* **41**, 9.

Gregoriadis, G., Morell, A. G., Sternlieb, I., and Scheinberg, I. H. (1970). *J. Biol. Chem.* **245**, 5833.

Griffith, M. M., and Beck, J. C. (1967). *Cancer* **16**, 1032.

Griffiths, P. D. (1966). *Clin. Chim. Acta* **13**, 413.

Harris, H. (1966). *Cancer Res.* **26**, 2054.

Harris, H., Hopkinson, D. A., Robson, E. B., and Whittaker, M. (1963). *Ann. Hum. Genet.* **26**, 359.

Hattori, N., Hattori, K., and Arai, M. M. (1967). *Proc. Jap. Cancer Ass.* p. 31.

Hattori, N., Murayama, H., and Arima, M. (1969). *Acta Hepatol.* **10**, 40.

Haupt, F., and Giersberg, H. (1958). *Naturwissenschaften* **45**, 268.

Henley, K. S., Wiggins, H. S., Pollard, H. M., and Dullaert, E. (1958). *Ann. N.Y. Acad. Sci.* **75**, 270.

Hess, B. (1958). *Ann. N.Y. Acad. Sci.* **75**, 292.

Hess, B., and Raftopulo, R. (1957). *Deut. Arch. Klin. Med.* **204**, 97.

Higashino, K., Hashinotsume, M., Kang, K. Y., Takahashi, Y., and Yamamura, Y. (1972). *Clin. Chim. Acta* **40**, 67.

Highman, B., and Atland, P. D. (1960). *Amer. J. Physiol.* **199**, 981.

Holmes, R. S., and Scopes, R. K. (1974). *Eur. J. Biochem.* **43**, 167.

Hopkins, H. A., Bonney, R. J., Walker, P. R., Yager, J. D., and Potter, V. R. (1973). *Advan. Enzyme Regul.* **11**, 169.

Hopsu-Havu, V. K., Jansen, C. J., and Järvinen, M. (1970). *Clin. Chim. Acta* **28**, 25.

Hsia, D. Y.-Y. (1970). *Progr. Med. Genet.* **7**, 29.

Huggins, C. (1947). *Harvey Lect.* **42**, 148.

Hunter, R. L., and Markert, C. L. (1957). *Science* **125**, 1294.

Ideo, G., DeFranchis, R., Del Ninno, E., and Dioguardi, N. (1971). *Lancet* **2**, 825.

Inglis, N. R., Krant, M. J., and Fishman, W. H. (1967). *Proc. Soc. Exp. Biol. Med.* **124**, 699.

Inglis, N. R., Guzek, D., Kirley, S., Green, S., and Fishman, W. H. (1971). *Clin. Chim. Acta* **33**, 287.

Jacques, P. J. (1969). *In* "Lysosomes in Biology and Pathology" (J. T. Dingle and H. B. Fell, eds.), Vol. 2, p. 395. North-Holland Publ., Amsterdam.

Jamieson, J. D. (1972). *Curr. Top. Membranes Transp.* **3**, 273.

Jefferson, L. S., Rannels, D. E., Munger, B. L., and Morgan, H. E. (1974). *Fed. Proc., Fed. Amer. Soc. Exp. Biol.* **33**, 1098.

Kalliomäki, J. L., and Vanha-Perttula, J. (1972). *Scand. J. Rheumatol.* **1**, 21.

Kalow, W., and Staron, N. (1957). *Can. J. Biochem. Physiol.* **35**, 1305.

Kattus, A. A., Watanabe, R., and Semenson, C. (1957). *Circulation* **15**, 502.

Keiding, N. R. (1964). *Clin. Sci.* **26,** 291.

Keiding, N. R. (1966). *Scand. J. Clin. Lab. Invest.* **18,** 134.

Kindmark, C.-O. (1969). *Scand. J. Clin. Lab. Invest.* **24,** 49.

Kirkman, H. N. (1972). *Progr. Med. Genet.* **8,** 125.

Kitamura, M., Iijima, N., Hashimoto, F., and Hiratsuka, A. (1971). *Clin. Chim. Acta* **34,** 419.

Kolb, H. J. (1974). *Eur. J. Biochem.* **43,** 145.

Korsrud, G. O., and Trick, K. D. (1973). *Clin. Chim. Acta* **48,** 311.

Kryszewski, A. J., Neale, G., Whitfield, J. B., and Moss, D. W. (1973). *Clin. Chim. Acta* **47,** 175.

Kuntzman, R. (1969). *Annu. Rev. Pharmacol.* **9,** 21.

La Due, J. S., Wróblewski, F., and Karmen, A. (1954). *Science* **120,** 497.

Langman, M. J. S., Leuthold, E., Robson, E. B., Harris, J., Luffman, J. E., and Harris, H. (1966). *Nature (London),* **212,** 41.

Lanzerotti, R. H., and Gullino, P. M. (1972a). *Anal. Biochem.* **50,** 344.

Lanzerotti, R. H., and Gullino, P. M. (1972b). *Cancer Res.* **32,** 2679.

Lehmann, H., and Liddell, J. (1964). *Progr. Med. Genet.* **3,** 75.

Lin, C.-W., and Fishman, W. H. (1972). *J. Biol. Chem.* **247,** 3082.

Lippi, U., and Guidi, G. (1970). *Clin. Chim. Acta* **28,** 431.

Lowden, I. A., Skomorowski, M. A., Henderson, F., and Kaback, M. (1973). *Clin. Chem.* **19,** 1345.

McDonald, J. K., Callahan, P. X., Ellis, S., and Smith, R. E. (1971). *In* "Tissue Proteinases" (A. J. Barrett and J. T. Dingle, eds.), p. 69. North-Holland Publ., Amsterdam.

McGeachin, R. L., Daugherty, H. K., Haryan, L. A., and Potter, B. A. (1957). *Clin. Chim. Acta* **2,** 75.

MacLean, D., Murison, J., and Griffiths, P. D. (1974). *Clin. Chim. Acta* **52,** 197.

McMaster, Y., Tennant, R., Clubb, J. S., Neale, F. C., and Posen, S. (1964). *J. Obstet. Gynaecol. Brit. Commonw.* **71,** 735.

McQueen, M. J., Watson, M. E., and Griffin, D. (1973). *Clin. Chim. Acta* **46,** 5.

Mahy, B. W. J., and Rowson, K. E. K. (1965). *Science* **149,** 756.

Mahy, B. W. J., Rowson, K. E. K., and Salaman, M. H. (1964). *Virology* **23,** 528.

Mahy, B. W. J., Rowson, K. E. K., Parr, C. W., and Salaman, M. H. (1965). *J. Exp. Med.* **122,** 967.

Mahy, B. W. J., Rowson, K. E. K., and Parr, C. W. (1967). *J. Exp. Med.* **125,** 277.

Markert, C. L. (1963a). *In* "Cytodifferentiation and Macromolecular Synthesis" (M. Locke, ed.), p. 65. Academic Press, New York.

Markert, C. L. (1963b). *Science* **140,** 1329.

Markert, C. L. (1968). *Ann. N.Y. Acad. Sci.* **151,** 14.

Markert, C. L., and Møller, F. (1959). *Proc. Nat. Acad. Sci. U.S.* **45,** 753.

Maunsbach, A. B. (1969). *In* "Lysosomes in Biology and Pathology" (J. T. Dingle and H. B. Fell, eds.), Vol. 1, p. 115. North-Holland Publ., Amsterdam.

Meyer, K. H., Fischer, E. H., and Bernfeld, P. (1946). *Experientia* **2,** 362.

Meyer, K. H., Fischer, E. H., and Bernfeld, P. (1947a). *Experientia* **3,** 106.

Meyer, K. H., Fischer, E. H., and Bernfeld, P. (1947b). *Helv. Chim. Acta* **30,** 64.

Meyer, K. H., Fischer, E. H., Bernfeld, P., and Duckert, F. (1948). *Arch. Biochem.* **18,** 203.

Milisauskas, V., and Rose, N. R. (1972). *Clin. Chem.* **18,** 1529.

Milisauskas, V., and Rose, N. R. (1973). *Exp. Cell Res.* **81,** 279.

Milunsky, A., and Littlefield, J. W. (1972). *Annu. Rev. Med.* **23,** 57.

Morell, A. G., VanDen Hamer, C. J. A., Scheinberg, I. H., and Ashwell, G. A. (1966). *J. Biol. Chem.* **241**, 3745.

Morell, A. G., Irvine, R. A., Sternlieb, I., Scheinberg, I. H., and Ashwell, G. (1968). *J. Biol. Chem.* **243**, 155.

Morell, A. G., Gregoriadis, G., Scheinberg, I. H., Hickman, J., and Ashwell, G. A. (1971). *J. Biol. Chem.* **246**, 1461.

Morré, D. J., Franke, W. W., Deumling, B., Nyquist, S. E., and Ovtracht, L. (1971). *In* "Biomembranes" (L. A. Manson, ed.), p. 95. Plenum, New York.

Moss, D. W., Panov, E. Y., and Whitaker, K. B. (1974). *Clin. Chim. Acta* **51**, 41.

Nagamine, M. (1972). *Clin. Chim. Acta* **36**, 139.

Nagatsu, T., and Udenfriend, S. (1972). *Clin. Chem.* **18**, 980.

Nakayama, T., Yoshida, M., and Kitamura, M. (1970). *Clin. Chim. Acta* **30**, 546.

Nance, W. E., Claflin, A., and Smithies, O. (1963). *Science* **142**, 1075.

Nathan, L. E., Feldbruegge, D., and Westgard, J. O. (1973). *Clin. Chem.* **19**, 1036.

Nisselbaum, J. S., and Bodansky, O. (1969). *Cancer Res.* **29**, 360.

Notkins, A. L., Greenfield, R. E., Marshall, D., and Bane, L. (1963). *J. Exp. Med.* **117**, 185.

O'Brien, J. S., Chen, A., and Fillerup, D. L. (1970). *N. Engl. J. Med.* **283**, 15.

O'Brien, J. S., Okada, S., Ho, M. W., Fillerup, D. L., Veath, M. L., and Adams, K. (1971). *Fed. Proc., Fed. Amer. Soc. Exp. Biol.* **30**, 956.

Okada, S., and O'Brien, J. S. (1969). *Science* **165**, 698.

Oseroff, A. R., Robbins, P. W., and Burger, M. M. (1973). *Annu. Rev. Biochem.* **42**, 647.

Paigen, K., and Felton, J. (1971). *In* "Drugs and Cell Regulation" (E. Mihich, ed.), p. 185. Academic Press, New York.

Pankovitch, A. M., Sclamberg, E. L., and Stevens, J. (1972). *Int. Arch. Allergy Appl. Immunol.* **43**, 401.

Parke, D. V. (1971). *In* "Effects of Drugs on Cellular Control Mechanisms" (B. R. Rabin and R. B. Freedman, eds.), p. 69. Macmillan, New York.

Patt, H. H., Kramer, S. P., Woel, G., Zeitung, D., and Seligman, A. M. (1966). *Arch. Surg. (Chicago)* **92**, 718.

Pennington, R. J. (1971). *Advan. Clin. Chem.* **14**, 409.

Posen, S. (1967). *Ann. Intern. Med.* **67**, 183.

Posen, S. (1970). *Clin. Chem.* **16**, 71.

Posen, S., Clubb, J. S., Neale, F. C., and Hotchkiss, D. (1965). *J. Lab. Clin. Med.* **65**, 530.

Praetorius, F., and Körtge, P. (1966). *Angiology* **17**, 640.

Prasad, R., Prasad, N., and Tevethia, S. S. (1972). *Science* **178**, 70.

Prasad, R., Prasad, N., and Prasad, K. N. (1973). *Science* **181**, 450.

Ratliff, C. R., Hall, F. W., Culp, J. W., and Gevedon, R. E. (1970). *Clin. Chem.* **16**, 527.

Richterich, R. (1969). "Clinical Chemistry." Karger, Basel.

Righetti, A. B. B., and Kaplan, M. M. (1974). *Proc. Soc. Exp. Biol. Med.* **145**, 726.

Riley, V., Lilly, F., Huerto, E., and Bardell, D. (1960). *Science* **132**, 545.

Robinson, D., Carroll, M., and Stirling, J. L. (1974). *Nature (London)* **243**, 415.

Robinson, J. C., and Pierce, J. E. (1964). *Nature (London)* **204**, 472.

Roels, O. A. (1969). *In* "Lysosomes in Biology and Pathology" (J. T. Dingle and H. B. Fell, eds.), Vol. 1, p. 254. North-Holland Publ., Amsterdam.

Roodyn, D. B. (1967). *In* "Enzyme Cytology" (D. B. Roodyn, ed.), p. 103. Academic Press, New York.

Rosalki, S. B., and Wilkinson, J. H. (1964). *J. Amer. Med. Ass.* **189**, 61.

Rosalki, S. B., Tarlow, D., and Rau, D. (1971). *Lancet* **2**, 376.

Sabine, J. C. (1940). *J. Clin. Invest.* **19**, 833.

Saifer, A., and Rosenthal, A. L. (1973). *Clin. Chim. Acta* **43**, 417.
Saini, P. K., and Posen, S. (1969). *Biochim. Biophys. Acta* **177**, 42.
Sandhoff, K., Andreae, U., and Jatzkewitz, H. (1968). *Life Sci.* **7**, 283.
Sasaki, M., and Fishman, W. H. (1973). *J. Histochem. Cytochem.* **21**, 653.
Sax, S. M., and Moore, J. J. (1970). *Stand. Methods Clin. Chem.* **6**, 149.
Sayre, F. W., and Hill, B. R. (1957). *Proc. Soc. Exp. Biol. Med.* **96**, 695.
Schanberg, S. M., Stone, R. A., Kirshner, N., Gunnells, J. C., and Robinson, R. R. (1974). *Science* **183**, 523.
Schimke, R. T. (1969). *Curr. Top. Cell. Regul.,* **1**, 77.
Schimke, R. T. (1973). *Advan. Enzymol.* **37**, 135.
Schimke, R. T., and Dehlinger, P. J. (1971). *In* "Drugs and Cell Regulation" (E. Mihich, ed.), p. 121. Academic Press, New York.
Schimke, R. T., Sweeney, E. W., and Berlin, C. M. (1965). *J. Biol. Chem.* **240**, 322.
Schlamowitz, M. (1958). *Ann. N.Y. Acad. Sci.* **75**, 373.
Schmidt, E., Schmidt, F. W., Horn, H. D., and Gerlach, U. (1965). *In* "Methods of Enzymatic Analysis" (H. U. Bergmeyer, ed.), p. 651. Academic Press, New York.
Schultze, H. E., and Heremans, J. F. (1966). *In* "Molecular Biology of Human Proteins," Vol. I, p. 173. Elsevier, Amsterdam.
Schwartz, M. K. (1972). *Stand. Methods Clin. Chem.* **7**, 1–7.
Schwartz, M. K. (1973a). *Advan. Clin. Chem.* **16**, 1.
Schwartz, M. K. (1973b). *Clin. Chem.* **19**, 11.
Schwartz, M. K., Bethune, V. G., Bachi, B. L., and Woodbridge, J. E. (1971). *Clin. Chem.* **17**, 656.
Searcy, R. L. (1969). *In* "Diagnostic Biochemistry," p. 84. McGraw-Hill, New York.
Schapira, F. (1973). *Advan. Cancer Res.* **18**, 77.
Shaw, C. R., and Barto, E. (1963). *Proc. Nat. Acad. Sci. U.S.* **50**, 211.
Shihabi, Z. K., and Bishop, C. (1971). *Clin. Chem.* **17**, 1150.
Shinkai, K., and Akedo, H. (1972). *Cancer Res.* **32**, 2307.
Shnitka, T. K., and Seligman, A. M. (1971). *Annu. Rev. Biochem.* **40**, 375.
Shugar, D., ed. (1970). "Enzymes and Isoenzymes." Academic Press, New York.
Sibley, J. A. (1958). *Ann. N.Y. Acad. Sci.* **75**, 339.
Sidbury, J. B. (1965). *Prog. Med. Genet.* **4**, 32.
Singer, R. M., and Fishman, W. H. (1975). *In* "Isozymes. III. Developmental Biology" (C. L. Markert, ed.), p. 753. Academic Press, New York.
Skilleter, D. N., Lee, N. M., and Kun, E. (1970). *Eur. J. Biochem.* **12**, 533.
Smith, A. D., and Winkler, H. (1969). *In* "Lysosomes in Biology and Pathology" (J. T. Dingle and H. B. Fells, eds.), Vol. 1, p. 155. North-Holland Publ., Amsterdam.
Snehalatha, C., Valmikinathan, K., Srinivas, K., and Jagannathan, K. (1973). *Clin. Chim. Acta* **44**, 229.
Spiegel, H. E., and Symington, J. A. (1972). *Stand. Methods Clin. Chem.* **7**, 43.
Spooner, R. J., and Goldberg, D. M. (1973). *Clin. Chem.* **19**, 1387.
Sterkel, R. L., Spencer, J. A., Wolfson, S. K., and Williams-Ashman, H. G. (1958). *J. Lab. Clin. Med.* **52**, 176.
Stolbach, L. L., Nisselbaum, J., and Fishman, W. H. (1958). *Amer. J. Clin. Pathol.* **29**, 379.
Stolbach, L. L., Skillman, J., and Goodman, R. (1972). *Arch Surg. (Chicago)* **105**, 491.
Sussman, H. H., Small, P. A., and Cottove, E. (1968). *J. Biol. Chem.* **243**, 160.
Suzuki, Y., Koizumi, Y., Togari, H., and Ogaro, Y. (1973). *Clin. Chim. Acta* **48**, 153.
Swanson, J. R., and Wilkinson, J. H. (1972). *Stand. Methods Clin. Chem.* **7**, 33.
Sweetin, J. C., and Thomson, W. H. S. (1973a). *Clin. Chim. Acta* **48**, 49.

Sweetin, J. C., and Thomson, W. H. S. (1973b). *Clin. Chim. Acta* **48**, 403.
Szczeklik, E., Orlowski, M., and Szewczuk, A. (1961). *Gastroenterology* **41**, 353.
Szewczuk, A. (1966). *Clin. Chim. Acta* **14**, 608.
Tanaka, K. R., and Valentine, W. N. (1960). *J. Lab. Clin. Med.* **56**, 754.
Tedesco, T. A., and Mellman, W. J. (1971). *Science* **172**, 727.
Tedesco, T. A. (1972). *J. Biol. Chem.* **247**, 6631.
Thomas, D. P. P. (1969). *In* "Lysosomes in Biology and Pathology" (J. T. Dingle and H. B. Fell, eds.), Vol. 2, p. 87. North-Holland Publ., Amsterdam.
Thorne, C. J. R. (1960). *Biochim. Biophys. Acta* **42**, 175.
Timperley, W. R. (1968). *Lancet* **2**, 356.
Timperley, W. R., and Warnes, T. (1970). *Cancer,* **26**, 100.
Timperley, W. R., Turner, P., and Davies, S. (1971). *J. Pathol.* **103**, 257.
Tomasi, T. P. (1968). *N. Engl. J. Med.* **279**, 1327.
Usategui-Gomez, M., Tarbulton, F., Yeager, A., and Fernandez de Castro, A. (1973). *Clin. Chim. Acta* **47**, 409.
Vaes, G. (1969). *In* "Lysosomes in Biology and Pathology" (J. T. Dingle and H. B. Fell, eds.), Vol. 1, p. 217. North-Holland Publ., Amsterdam.
Vaitukaitis, J. L., Sherins, R., Ross, G. T., Hickman, J., and Ashwell, G. A. (1971). *Endocrinology* **89**, 1356.
Vanha-Perttula, J., and Kalliomäki, J. L. (1973). *Clin. Chim. Acta* **44**, 249.
Verity, M. A. (1973). *In* "Metabolic Conjugation and Metabolic Hydrolysis" (W. H. Fishman, ed.), Vol. 3, p. 241, Academic Press, New York.
Vesell, E. S., and Bearn, A. G. (1957). *Proc. Soc. Exp. Biol. Med.* **94**, 96.
Vesell, E. S., and Bearn, A. G. (1958). *J. Clin. Invest.* **37**, 672.
Vesell, E. S. (1965a). *Progr. Med. Genet.* **4**, 128.
Vesell, E. S. (1965b). *Science* **148**, 1103.
Vesell, E. S. (1968). *Ann. N.Y. Acad. Sci.* **151**, 1.
Vogel, N. C., and Zieve, L. (1963). *Clin. Chem.* **9**, 168.
Wagner, R., Huijing, F., and Porter, E. (1971). *Amer. J. Med.* **51**, 685.
Wakim, K. G., and Fleisher, G. A. (1963a). *J. Lab. Clin. Med.* **61**, 86.
Wakim, K. G., and Fleisher, G. A. (1963b). *J. Lab. Clin. Med.* **61**, 107.
Waldmann, T. A., and Jones, E. A. (1973). "Protein Turnover." *Ciba Found. Symp.* **9**, 5.
Waldmann, T. A., Strober, W., and Blaese, R. M. (1971). *Progr. Immunol.* **1**, 891.
Walker, B. A., Eze, L. C., Tweedie, M. C. K., and Price-Evans, D. A. (1971). *Clin. Chim. Acta* **35**, 433.
Warburg, O., and Christian, W. (1943). *Biochem. Z.* **314**, 149 and 399.
Warnock, M. L. (1968). *Proc. Soc. Exp. Biol. Med.* **129**, 768.
Warnock, M. L., and Reisman, R. (1969). *Clin. Chim. Acta* **24**, 5.
Weinhouse, S. (1973). *Fed. Proc. Fed. Amer. Soc. Exp. Biol.* **32**, 2162.
Weinstock, I. M., and Iodice, A. A. (1969). *In* "Lysosomes in Biology and Pathology" (J. T. Dingle and H. B. Fell, eds.), Vol. 1, p. 450. North-Holland Publ., Elsevier.
Wicks, W. D., Barnett, C. A., and McKibbin, J. B. (1974). *Fed. Proc., Fed. Amer. Soc. Exp. Biol.* **33**, 1105.
Wieczorek, E. (1972). *Clin. Chim. Acta* **37**, 203.
Wieland, T., and Pfleiderer, G. (1957). *Biochem. Z.* **329**, 112.
Wieland, T., Pfleiderer, G., Haupt, I., and Wörner, W. (1959). *Biochem. J.* **332**, 1.
Winckers, P. L. M., and Jacobs, P. (1973). *Clin. Chim. Acta* **45**, 317.
Winzler, R. J. (1968). *In* "Biochemistry of Glycoproteins and Related Substances" (E. Rossi and E. Stoll, eds.), Part II, p. 226. Karger, Basel.

Wise, C. D., and Stein, L. (1973). *Science* **181**, 344.

Wolfson, S. K., and Williams-Ashman, H. G. (1957). *Proc. Soc. Exp. Biol. Med.* **96**, 231.

Wolfson, S. K., Spencer, J. A., Sterkerl, R. L., and Williams-Ashman, H. G. (1958). *Ann. N.Y. Acad. Sci.* **75**, 260.

Woodward, H. Q. (1959). *Amer. J. Med.* **27**, 902.

Wooten, G. F., Eldridge, R., Axelrod, J., and Stern, R. S. (1972). *N. Engl. J. Med.* **288**, 284.

Wroblewski, F., and La Due, J. S. (1955). *Proc. Soc. Exp. Biol. Med.* **90**, 210.

Yam, L. T. (1974). *Amer. J. Med.* **56**, 604.

Yang, J. S., and Biggs, H. G. (1971). *Clin. Chem.* **17**, 512.

Yates, C. M., Wilson, H., and Davidson, D. (1973). *Clin. Chim. Acta* **47**, 397.

Young, D. (1974). *In* "Enzymology in the Practice of Laboratory Medicine" (P. Blume and E. F. Freier, eds.), p. 253. Academic Press.

Young, D. S., Thomas, D. W., Friedman, R. B., and Pestaner, L. C. (1972). *Clin. Chem.* **18**, 1041.

Zapf, P. W., and Coghlan, C. M. (1974). *Clin. Chim. Acta* **44**, 237.

Zielke, K., Okada, S., and O'Brien, J. (1972a). *J. Lab. Clin. Med.* **79**, 164.

Zielke, K., Veath, M. L., and O'Brien, J. (1972b). *J. Exp. Med.* **136**, 197.

Zierler, K. L. (1958). *Ann. N.Y. Acad. Sci.* **75**, 227.

Zinterhofer, L., Wardlaw, S., Jatlow, P., and Seligson, D. (1973a). *Clin. Chim. Acta* **43**, 5.

Zinterhofer, L., Wardlaw, S., Jatlow, P., and Seligson, D. (1973b). *Clin. Chim. Acta* **44**, 173.

Zucker, S., and Webb, A. M. (1972). *Stand. Methods Clin. Chem.* **7**, 9.

6 / Fetal and Neonatal Development of Human Plasma Proteins

David Gitlin and Jonathan D. Gitlin

I. Introduction

All proteins which are found in the plasma of normal human adults are present in the plasma of the normal embryo as early as 6 weeks of gestation. Certainly the concentrations of these proteins in the early conceptus are not those of the adult, and not all are actually products of the embryo at this stage of development. Some of the proteins found in embryonic and fetal plasma are primarily maternal in origin, their appearance in the conceptus being largely the result of transfer from the mother across the placenta. But most plasma proteins are, in fact, actually synthesized by the embryo beginning at or before 5.5 weeks of gestation, albeit in relatively minute amounts at first. The concentrations of some proteins remain at but a fraction of their adult levels during all intrauterine life, but fetal synthesis of others increases as term approaches, so that the plasma levels of these may reach or even exceed adult concentrations by the time of delivery. Obviously, the synthesis of those proteins which appear in neonatal plasma at levels less than are present in the adult must increase to reach adult rates at some point in time postnatally. On the other hand, some proteins which gain adult levels by the time of delivery may not be sustained at these levels during the neonatal period; their concentrations fall after delivery and then regain adult levels at some later period. Most proteins are synthesized by the adult at rates greater than in the fetus. There are some, however, which the fetus produces at a rate greater than does the adult; one such protein, for example, reaches a concentration in the fetus that is at least 100,000 times greater than that seen in the normal adult.

It is with these kaleidoscopic changes that take place in the plasma concentrations of different proteins that this chapter is concerned. It may be helpful, therefore, to first review briefly some of the metabolic mechanisms that actually determine or regulate the concentration of a given protein in the plasma.

II. Plasma Protein Kinetics

A. Synthesis, Distribution, and Degradation

1. Effects of Synthesis and Degradation on Plasma Concentration

The plasma concentration of any protein is, of course, a reflection of the balance attained between the rate at which the protein is synthesized, the distribution of the protein in the body fluids and the rate at which the protein is degraded. During much of adult life, the plasma levels of most proteins remain relatively steady, and during this steady state, the amount of a specific protein that is degraded per unit time is equal to the amount of the protein that is synthesized in the same period of time. The rate of degradation of a plasma protein is dependent upon the total body pool of the protein as expressed in the simple relationship:

$$D = 0.693 \; P/t_{\frac{1}{2}} \qquad (1)$$

where D is the amount of protein degraded per unit time, P is the total exchangeable body pool of the protein and $t_{\frac{1}{2}}$ is the half-life of the protein or the time that is required for the degradation of half of the protein molecules which are present in the body pool at any given moment. It is clear from this equation that the *fractional* rate of degradation of a protein, D/P, is inversely proportional to the half-life of the protein.

For some plasma proteins such as fibrinogen, IgM or IgA, the fractional rate of degradation, and therefore, the half-life of the protein as well, remains relatively constant over a wide range of plasma levels. If the synthesis of such a protein increases, the amount of protein being degraded per unit time, D, will initially be less than the amount of protein being synthesized. Under these circumstances, the body pool of the protein must increase, and since D is proportional to P, the body pool will continue to increase until D, the rate of degradation, again equals the rate of synthesis. Conversely, if the protein's rate of synthesis decreases, its rate of degradation will initially be greater than the rate of synthesis, and the body pool will fall until once again the rate of degradation equals the rate of synthesis. In such instances, the increase or decrease in protein synthesis is followed by a corresponding increase or decrease in the body pool of the protein which in turn results in a concomitant increase or decrease in the protein's rate of degradation. On the other hand, a change in a protein's rate of degradation is not usually accompanied by a change in its rate of synthesis. Therefore, a change in the normal rate of degradation will be accompanied by an *inverse* change in the size of the body pool: an increase or decrease in the amount of protein being degraded decreases or increases, respectively, the size of the body pool; this, in turn, results in a decrease or increase, respectively, in the protein's rate of degradation until it again equals the rate of synthesis. Since the amount of a given protein that is present in the plasma represents from 40 to 80% of its total exchangeable body pool, it is apparent that a change in the size of the body pool means a change in the plasma concentration of the protein. As with the total body pool, then, an increase in the plasma concentration of a protein may be due to either an increase in the protein's rate of synthesis *or* a decrease in its rate of degradation. Conversely, a decrease in the plasma concentration of a protein can result from either a decrease in synthesis *or* an increase in the rate of degradation. Short-term changes in the rates of synthesis or degradation may not have any obvious immediate effects on the plasma concentrations of those proteins which have relatively long half-lives. On the other hand, short-term changes in synthesis, release into the circulation, degradation, or loss from the body can result in dramatic changes in the plasma concentrations of such proteins as growth hormone or insulin which have half-lives that measure in minutes.

The half-lives of some proteins, such as IgG, tend to vary in an *inverse* direction to their plasma concentrations (Solomon *et al.*, 1963). A marked increase in IgG synthesis resulting in an increased plasma IgG concentration, for example, may result in a decrease in the half-life of IgG. The resulting increase in the fractional rate of degradation under these circumstances would serve to diminish the impact that the increased IgG synthesis would otherwise have had on the plasma IgG concentration. Conversely, very low plasma levels of IgG due to decreased synthesis may be accompanied by a decrease in the fractional rate of IgG degradation.

The half-lives of still other proteins, such as haptoglobin, transferrin, and possibly IgD, seem to change in the same direction as their plasma concentrations, the half-life increasing with an increase in serum concentration and decreasing with a decrease in serum concentration (Rogentine *et al.*, 1966; Freeman, 1965). If unaccompanied by a concomitantly *greater* increase in synthesis, the change in half-life in the latter instances can be a cause of the change in serum concentration and not vice versa.

Obviously, the plasma concentration of a protein will be affected by contributions of the protein to, and losses from, the plasma compartment other than through endogenous synthesis and degradation. The administration of exogenous protein can behave as newly synthesized protein, and losses of protein from the body, as in nephrosis (Gitlin *et al.*, 1956) or through hemorrhage, add to the losses incurred through catabolism.

Throughout this discussion, synthesis has been taken to indicate synthesis followed by release of the protein into the exchangeable body pool of that protein. It may be pointed out that synthesis followed by storage is the normal sequence for some proteins, particularly protein hormones, release being a subsequent event; in these instances, any effect on plasma concentration occurs, of course, only upon release of the protein into the exchangeable body pool of that protein.

2. Distribution of Plasma Proteins in Body Fluids

The body pool of a plasma protein can be divided into two major compartments, the intravascular or plasma compartment and the extravascular-extracellular compartment. The extravascular-extracellular space consists of many different anatomical areas which differ in relative size and in the rate at which a protein may enter or leave the interstitial fluid in that area. Mathematical models which more or less accurately reflect the kinetics of distribution for many plasma proteins in the body pool have been described, and such models divide the body pool into three or more theoretical spaces. It must be emphasized, however, that subdivisions of the extravascular compartment in such models are defined mathematically, not anatomically (Donato *et al.*, 1966).

For most proteins, such as albumin or IgG, the vascular or plasma compartment contains approximately 40 to 50% of the total body pool of the protein. At least half of the body pool of that protein is, therefore, extravascular. Since the total volume of interstitial fluid is normally about 4 times the plasma volume, the average concentration of the protein in interstitial fluid is approximately one-fourth the concentration of the protein in plasma. It should be apparent, however, that the concentration of a given protein in interstitial fluid will vary from one anatomical site to another, depending upon such factors as protein diffusion, hydrostatic pressures, and bulk fluid flow in each area. A useful term which conveniently disregards such differences in local interstitial fluid concentrations is the "volume of distribution"; this may be defined as the volume which the total body pool of the protein would occupy, *if* the concentration of that protein in all body fluids were uniform and equal to the concentration in plasma. The volume of distribution obviously has no anatomical equivalent, but

$$P = CV_\mathrm{d} = Dt_{\frac{1}{2}}/0.693 \qquad (2)$$

where P is the body pool of the protein, C is the plasma concentration, V_d is the volume of distribution and $t_{\frac{1}{2}}$ is the protein's half-life.

Some proteins, such as fibrinogen and IgM, are found primarily in the plasma compartment, although as much as 20 to 30% of the total body pool for each of these proteins may be present extravascularly (Takeda, 1966; Rogentine *et al.*, 1966). Some proteins may be bound with great avidity by certain tissues, the binding being both specific and reversible, so that not all of the extravascular protein may be found in the interstitial fluids (Gitlin and Gitlin, 1973): insulin, for example, is strongly bound by cell membrane receptors in the placenta (Buse *et al.*, 1962; Gitlin *et al.*, 1965).

Thus, there is a circulation of plasma macromolecules within the body that takes place outside of the vascular system. Plasma proteins and protein hormones entering the vascular system after synthesis, either directly or indirectly, may soon pass from the vascular system into the extravascular-extracellular fluids. For a given protein such as albumin, approximately half of the protein present in the vascular system at any given moment will be in the extravascular-extracellular compartment 24 hr later. Needless to state, in the same period of time an equal amount of the protein is returned to the vascular system from the interstitial fluids, a feat accomplished largely through lymphatic flow. The fraction of the total body protein pool that is present in the interstitial fluids may be reduced drastically by conditions which increase lymphatic flow, such as increased intracapillary hydrostatic pressure or decreased plasma colloid osmotic pressure. Such conditions will lead to an expansion of the extravascular-extracellular space, but the greater flow of water into this space compared to the diffusion of protein from the vascular compartment results in a decreased concentration of protein in the interstitial fluid and an increased lymphatic return to the plasma. Conversely, conditions which increase the permeability of the blood vessel wall to plasma protein, such as vasculitis or anoxia, can result in increased concentrations of the proteins in interstitial fluid.

B. Maternofetal Exchange

The plasma concentration of a given protein in the conceptus is governed not only by fetal synthesis and degradation, but also by the *net* exchange of the protein between mother and fetus (Gitlin *et al.*, 1964a). The net exchange of a protein is the difference between the amount which passes from mother to conceptus and the amount which crosses from conceptus to mother, or

$$N = C_m V_{mf} - C_f V_{fm} \tag{3}$$

where N is the net maternofetal transfer rate, C_m and C_f are the amounts of the protein present per unit volume of maternal and fetal plasma respectively, V_{mf} is the volume that would be occupied by the protein transferred from mother to fetus per unit time, if it had the same protein concentration as in maternal plasma, and V_{fm} is the volume that would be occupied by the protein transferred from fetus to mother per unit time, if it had the same protein concentration as in fetal plasma. In other words, the clearance of a protein from the mother due to transfer to the conceptus can be expressed either as the amount of the protein transferred per unit time, $C_m V_{mf}$, or as the volume of maternal plasma cleared per unit time, V_{mf}. Similarly, the amount of the protein cleared from the conceptus per unit time due to transfer to the mother is $C_f V_{fm}$, and the volume of fetal plasma cleared per unit time is V_{fm}. When the concentrations of the protein in maternal and fetal plasma remain steady, during that period of time, the amount of the protein synthesized by the fetus, S_f, plus the amount transferred from mother to fetus, $C_m V_{mf}$, is equal to the amount of the protein degraded by the fetus, D_f, plus the amount transferred from fetus to mother, $C_f V_{fm}$, or

$$S_f + C_m V_{mf} = D_f + C_f V_{fm} \tag{4}$$

and $$C_m V_{mf} - C_f V_{fm} = N = D_f - S_f \tag{5}$$

When the amount of protein which passes from fetus to mother equals the amount which passes from mother to fetus in the same period of time, N is then zero, and the rate of fetal degradation of the protein becomes equal to the rate of fetal synthesis, or $D_f = S_f$. It should also be noted from Eq. (5) that when fetal synthesis of a specific protein is nil, the net maternofetal transfer rate is equal to the fetal degradation rate, or $N = D_f$.

Similarly, in the steady state, the amount of a protein synthesized by the mother, S_m, plus the amount transferred from the conceptus, $C_f V_{fm}$, is equal to the amount of the protein degraded by the mother, D_m, plus the amount transferred from mother to fetus, $C_m V_{mf}$, or

$$S_m + C_f V_{fm} = D_m + C_m V_{mf} \tag{6}$$

and $$C_f V_{fm} - C_m V_{mf} = N = D_m - S_m \tag{7}$$

When N is zero, then $D_m = S_m$.

In the special case where fetal synthesis of two different proteins is nil and the net maternofetal transfer rates of the two proteins are equal, then it can be seen from Eq. (5) that the degradation rate of one protein, D_{f_1}, equals the degradation rate of the other, D_{f_2}. Since the volume of distribution of a protein, V_d, equals $C_f k V$ where V is the plasma volume, then from Eq. (2)

$$D_{f_1} = D_{f_2} = C_{f_1} k_1 V_1 / t_{\frac{1}{2}1} = C_{f_2} k_2 V_2 / t_{\frac{1}{2}2} \tag{8}$$

In the same conceptus, of course, $V_1 = V_2$ and

$$C_{f_1}/C_{f_2} = k_3 t_{\frac{1}{2}1}/t_{\frac{1}{2}2} \tag{9}$$

Thus, if two radiolabeled proteins pass from mother to fetus at the same net rate but differ in the rates at which they are degraded in the fetus, their fetal plasma concentrations will be related to each other as are their half-lives.

III. Maternofetal Transfer of Specific Proteins

The transfer of macromolecules from mother to fetus can take place either directly via the placenta or indirectly via amniotic fluid. As was noted earlier, the plasma concentration of a protein is dependent in part upon the net maternofetal transfer rate of the protein. Therefore, the relative rates at which specific proteins traverse each of these pathways, and the transport mechanisms involved, must be considered in the development of plasma protein concentrations in the conceptus.

A. Amniotic Fluid Protein Exchange

1. Turnover of Amniotic Fluid Protein

In the normal conceptus at or near term not yet disturbed by the uterine contractions which attend labor, an average of 63% of a given protein in amniotic fluid is turned over per day regardless of the molecular size of the protein (Gitlin *et al.,* 1972a). About 85 to 90% of this turnover is attributable to fetal deglutition: each day, the fetus swallows a volume of amniotic fluid, which, on the average, equals a bit more than half of the amniotic fluid present in the amniotic space. Obviously, all elements in amniotic fluid, whether dissolved or merely suspended, are ingested at the same fractional rate (Pritchard, 1965; Gitlin *et al.,* 1972a). Approximately 10 to 15% of the total amount of a given protein turned over in amniotic fluid per day leaves the amniotic space by mechanisms other than fetal swallowing, most likely by diffusion. Interestingly, fetal swallowing of amniotic fluid increases during labor to a mean of 78% of the amniotic fluid volume per day, and the daily clearance of protein increases to 90% of the total in amniotic fluid (Gitlin *et al.,* 1972a).

The amount of amniotic fluid ingested by the fetus tends to vary directly with the amniotic fluid volume (Fig. 1): the larger the amniotic

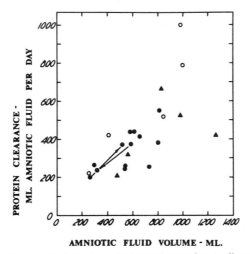

AMNIOTIC FLUID VOLUME - ML.

Fig. 1. Volume of amniotic fluid cleared of protein per day (ordinate) in relation to amniotic fluid volume (abscissa). Arrows connect values obtained in 2 patients studied 5 days apart; arrow points to second value. Open circles indicate conceptuses subsequently delivered vaginally, and solid circles indicate those delivered by hysterotokotomy. Solid triangles represent values calculated from data obtained by Pritchard (1965) using labeled erythrocytes. From Gitlin *et al.* (1972a).

fluid volume, the more amniotic fluid is swallowed, and conversely, the smaller the amniotic fluid volume, the less is the amount of amniotic fluid swallowed (Gitlin *et al.,* 1972a). Thus, the *fraction* of the total amniotic fluid that is ingested per day by the fetus tends to remain relatively constant. Such changes in fetal deglutition, whatever the mechanisms that control it, do tend to stabilize amniotic fluid volume by acting in an inverse direction to any net changes in amniotic fluid water exchange. However, amniotic fluid volume *will* vary directly with the net water change, much as the body pool of a protein varies directly with protein synthesis in the face of a constant fractional rate of protein degradation. Amniotic fluid volume is not necessarily constant even from day to day: increases of 100% in amniotic fluid volume and decreases as much as 50% have been recorded near term in as short a period as 5 days, apparently due to normal changes in the net exchange of water in the amniotic space. Changes in amniotic fluid volume can also occur, of course, if the fractional rate of amniotic fluid removal due to fetal deglutition changes, all other factors remaining equal. As was noted earlier, amniotic fluid is swallowed at a greater rate during labor than before the onset of labor, and it is entirely possible that short-term alterations in the fractional rate of deglutition may occur normally throughout labor. The mechanisms which regulate the rate of deglutition are not known, but clearly deglutition begins before the second trimester of gestation, the fractional rate being similar to or somewhat less than that observed near term. Even at term there is normally a fairly wide difference in the fractional rate of fetal deglutition from one fetus to the next.

2. Sources and Fate of Amniotic Fluid Protein

During the steady state, the amount of fluid entering the amniotic space equals the amount of fluid leaving the space. The fetus at or near term swallows an average of approximately 300 ml of amniotic fluid per day, the volume swallowed daily by individual fetuses being from 200 to 760 ml. Extrapolating data obtained in rhesus monkey fetuses, Chez et al. (1964) suggested that the human fetus at term produces approximately 400 ml of urine per day. Ultrasonic measurements of the fetal urinary bladder in utero suggest that the human fetus at 30 weeks' gestation produces an average of 250 ml of urine per day, and that urine production increases linearly with gestational age to an average of approximately 650 ml per day at 40 weeks (Wladimiroff and Campbell, 1974). Thus, the volume of urine produced by the fetus either is equal to or is more than the volume of amniotic fluid swallowed by the fetus. Even early in gestation, it is likely that the amniotic fluid swallowed can be replaced to a large extent by fetal urination. Although it has been generally assumed that the fetus does not urinate until the middle of the second trimester of gestation, this conclusion is based upon the observation that urea and other solutes in amniotic fluid begin to rise sharply at that time. However, it appears that the embryonic kidney cannot concentrate urea, and consequently urine entering the amniotic sac during early development will not alter the amniotic fluid urea level. Urine is found in the bladder of the human embryo at least as early as 9 weeks of gestation and perhaps even earlier (Gitlin and Boesman, 1966).

Normal embryonic and fetal urine contains a number of plasma proteins including α-fetoprotein, albumin, transferrin, and IgG among others. The amounts of protein passed into amniotic fluid by this route, however, are not large. Near term, fetal urine contributes less than 5% of the albumin turned over in amniotic fluid per day and less than 2% of the daily turnover of transferrin. Although almost 25% of the IgG cleared from amniotic fluid daily can be supplied via fetal urine, virtually all of this IgG comes indirectly from the mother via the placenta and not from fetal synthesis. On the other hand, serum α-fetoprotein is almost entirely a product of the conceptus, and the concentration of α-fetoprotein in amniotic fluid can be a guide to the antenatal diagnosis of such anomalies as open neural tube defects, e.g., anencephaly and spina bifida (Brock and Sutcliffe, 1972; Allan *et al.*, 1973). The amount of α-fetoprotein which passes into amniotic fluid by way of fetal urine normally is equal to the amniotic fluid clearance of this protein. Although the α-fetoprotein present in amniotic fluid is entirely, or almost entirely, of fetal origin, the other plasma proteins are of both fetal and maternal origin (Gitlin *et al.*, 1972a). At least 95% of the amniotic fluid proteins at or near term, however, are directly or indirectly of maternal origin (Gitlin *et al.*, 1972a), in accord with earlier conclusions of Derrington and Soothill (1961) and Ruoslahti *et al.* (1966). Approximately 95% of the albumin and 98% of the transferrin turned over per day in amniotic fluid, for example, come directly from the mother, as well as virtually all of the IgA. About 75% of the IgG present in amniotic fluid comes directly from the mother and almost all of the remainder is maternal IgG which reaches amniotic fluid indirectly via the fetus. It must be emphasized that the contribution of the conceptus to amniotic fluid is dependent in part upon the concentration of the protein in the plasma of the conceptus; therefore, early in development, e.g., before 16 to 20 weeks of gestation, the amount of a given protein in amniotic fluid which comes from the conceptus may be much *less* and that coming from the mother correspondingly *more* than at term, the major exception being α-fetoprotein (cf. Section V, E). In accord with the maternal origins of the bulk of amniotic fluid protein, the phenotypes of amniotic fluid transferrin, haptoglobin, Gc globulin, and a number of other proteins are largely those of the mother (Seppälä *et al.*, 1966). For proteins from 20,000 daltons in molecular weight to those of at least 165,000 daltons, the ratio of the concentration of a protein in amniotic fluid to that in maternal serum is inversely proportional to the square root of the protein's molecular weight (Nencioni *et al.*, 1970; Gitlin, 1974). Thus, these proteins seem to be transferred from mother to amniotic fluid by diffusion rather than by an active transport process, and this transfer takes place directly across the fetal membranes, i.e., the chorion and amnion, surrounding the amniotic space. The fetal membranes may be relatively more permeable to proteins smaller than 20,000 daltons in weight, but both IgM and the β-lipoproteins are excluded from amniotic fluid, the molecular weights of these proteins being 950,000 and a million or more daltons, respectively. Thus, the size distribution of "pores" in the fetal membranes seems to be skewed.

As was noted above, only 10 to 15% of the protein turnover in amniotic fluid clears through diffusion, at least in part via the fetal membranes, and about 85 to 90% is removed by fetal swallowing. Virtually all of the protein swallowed is hydrolyzed in the fetal gastrointestinal tract. Less than 0.1% of a tracer dose of labeled protein injected into the amniotic fluid near term can be found in the plasma and interstitial fluids of the conceptus from 3 hr to 13 days later (Gitlin et al., 1972a). Thus, there is little absorption of intact protein from amniotic fluid by the conceptus, whether via the gastrointestinal tract, skin, umbilical cord, or lungs. The average daily clearance of soluble protein from amniotic fluid in nonparturient women at term is 0.24 gm per kilogram of fetal weight and during labor it is 0.30 gm per kilogram of fetal weight. The average amount swallowed by the conceptus daily, therefore, is 0.19 gm and 0.24 gm per kilogram of fetal weight in nonparturient and parturient women, respectively (Gitlin et al., 1972a). Approximately 50% of this protein is albumin and an additional 15% consists of transferrin and IgG. Since over 95% of the soluble protein in amniotic fluid is of maternal origin, the protein swallowed by the conceptus is not simply recycled fetal protein, and provides about 10 to 15% of the minimum daily protein amino acid requirement near term.

B. The Placenta

Almost all of the plasma protein that is exchanged between maternal and fetal circulations does so by crossing the placenta. At first glance it appears as if placental selectivity in the transfer of plasma proteins were entirely unrelated to molecular size, and in some instances it is not. For example, IgG which has a molecular weight of 165,000 daltons passes from mother to fetus much more rapidly than does serum albumin which has a molecular weight less than half that of IgG; α_1-acid glycoprotein which has a molecular weight two-thirds that of albumin traverses the placenta more rapidly than does albumin, but growth hormone which has a molecular weight only a third that of albumin does not pass at all! However, as soon as it is recognized that maternofetal transfer of proteins involves several different mechanisms, patterns do evolve from the chaos.

1. A First-Order Process

When tracer doses of α_1-acid glycoprotein, albumin, transferrin, fibrinogen, α_2-macroglobulin, and IgM were given to pregnant women intravenously, each of the labeled proteins was subsequently detected in the cord blood of the infant at the time of delivery, which occurred from a few hours to 33 days after the injection of the tracer (Gitlin et al., 1964a). The concentrations of these labeled proteins in cord plasma, C_f, relative to their concentrations in maternal plasma, C_m, at delivery, or

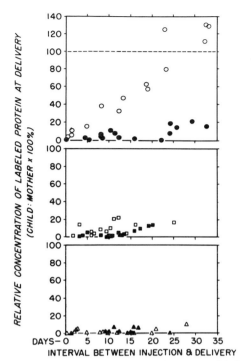

Fig. 2. Concentration of specific labeled protein in plasma of infant at birth relative to maternal plasma concentration at that time, C_f/C_m, as a function of the time elapsed between injection of labeled protein in mother and delivery. Each symbol represents an individual mother and her infant: IgG = ○; albumin = ●; α_1-acid glycoprotein = □; transferrin = ■; fibrinogen = △; α_2-macroglobulin and IgM = ▲. Adapted from Gitlin *et al.* (1964a).

C_f/C_m, are shown in Fig. 2. It was observed that C_f/C_m for each of the proteins increased, although at different rates, in direct proportion to the length of time that had elapsed between the injection and delivery. The average increase in C_f/C_m per unit time was found to be inversely proportional to the square root of the molecular weight of the protein at all levels of C_m (Table I). The transfer of these proteins from mother to fetus thus not only appeared to be a first order process, but this process also seemed to be related to diffusion. As will be seen in Section III,B, 2,a, the amount of human albumin transferred across the maternofetal barrier in mice is also directly proportional to the maternal serum concentration of this protein. Even IgG, which is transported from mother to fetus in a rather complex manner, crosses the placenta at least in part by a first-order mechanism. The plasma immunoglobulin IgE also seems

TABLE I

The Relationship between the Rate of Maternofetal Transfer and the Reciprocal of the Square Root of the Molecular Weight for Some Radioiodinated Plasma Proteins in the Pregnant Woman at Term

Protein	Average half-life of protein in mother (days)	MW	$MW^{-1/2}$	Change in fetal:maternal plasma concentration per day; or $(\Delta C_f/C_m)/\div t$	$\dfrac{(\Delta C_f/C_m)/\div t}{MW^{-1/2}}$
α_1-Acid glycoprotein	3.8	44,000	0.0047	0.0069	1.5
Albumin	14.5	68,000	0.0038	0.0057	1.5
Transferrin	12.0	90,000	0.0033	0.0051	1.5
Fibrinogen	2.5	341,000	0.0017	≤ 0.0026	≤ 1.5
IgM	8.0	800,000	0.0011	< 0.0020	< 1.82

to cross the placenta by a first-order mechanism, which may or may not be diffusion (Miller *et al.,* 1973a).

The data suggest that the first-order process whereby these and other proteins cross the placenta *may* be diffusion, but other mechanisms are also possible. It will be shown (Section III,B,2,e) that proteins are selectively bound by receptors present on cell membranes isolated from the placenta and that transplacental transfer of a protein seems to be related to the degree of this binding. Hence, one also could postulate an active transport mechanism rather than a passive one, the process being first-order at the maternal protein concentrations being studied. It certainly would be easier to explain the impermeability of the placenta to proteins such as growth hormone (cf. Section III,B,3), if the transfer process involved a receptor–carrier mechanism rather than simple diffusion.

It must be emphasized that the maternofetal transfer rate for albumin, α_1-acid glycoprotein, transferrin, and other proteins which traverse the placenta by this mechanism may vary widely from one pregnant woman to the next. As can be seen in Figs. 2 and 3, for example, in some instances very little albumin indeed passes from mother to fetus.

2. Active Transport

As can be seen in Fig. 2, the transfer of IgG from mother to fetus near term is much more efficient than is the maternofetal transfer of any of the other proteins studied. Although α_1-acid glycoprotein, albumin, and transferrin are smaller in molecular weight than IgG, they pass the

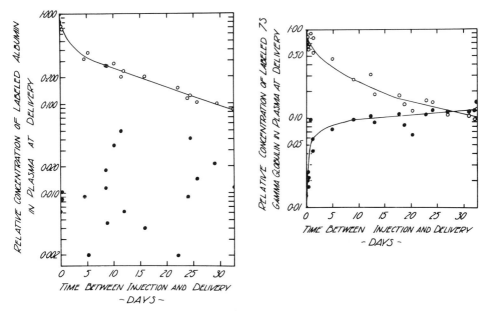

Fig. 3. The disappearance of radiolabeled albumin and IgG from the plasma of pregnant women (○), and the concentrations of these proteins in the plasma of their infants at delivery (●). From Gitlin *et al.* (1964a).

placenta much *less* readily than does IgG. This selectivity in the permeability of the placenta to IgG obviously cannot be attributed to diffusion.

a. THE MATERNOFETAL TRANSPORT OF HUMAN IgG.   In the pregnant mouse as in the pregnant woman, human IgG is transferred from mother to fetus much more readily than human albumin. The mechanisms which determine this selective permeability of the maternofetal barrier to IgG were investigated in the pregnant mouse near term by giving the mothers various amounts of both labeled human IgG and labeled human albumin intravenously (Gitlin and Koch, 1968). The concentrations of these proteins in the fetus, or C_f, relative to the maternal serum concentrations, C_m, were determined 24 hr later. As shown in Fig. 4, the relative fetal concentration, C_f/C_m, of human albumin remained relatively constant at all maternal levels attained with this protein; i.e., the concentration of human albumin found in the fetus was proportional to the maternal serum concentration (Fig. 5, upper graph). This first-order relation between the amount of albumin transferred from mother to fetus and the maternal serum concentration of albumin is, of course, compatible with diffusion being the principal process involved in the transfer.

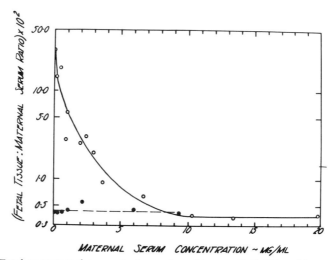

Fig. 4. Fetal to maternal concentration ratios of human IgG (○) and human albumin (●) in pregnant mice at different maternal serum levels 24 hr after injection of the protein into the mother; each circle is the average for 3 to 4 pregnant mice and their litters. From Gitlin and Koch (1968).

The concentration of human IgG found in the fetus relative to the maternal serum concentration of human IgG, C_f/C_m, in contrast to C_f/C_m for albumin, first decreased rapidly and then became constant as the maternal human IgG concentration was increased (Fig. 4). The changes in the fetal *concentration* of human IgG, C_f, proved to be quite complex (Fig. 5, upper graph): as the maternal serum concentration of the protein was increased to 2 mg per ml, the fetal human IgG concentration also increased, but at a much more rapid rate than the relative increase in the maternal level. When the maternal level of human IgG was further increased, the fetal concentration actually decreased as the maternal concentration approached 8 mg per milliliter and finally increased in direct proportion to the maternal level at maternal concentrations above 8 mg per milliliter. If the first-order process represented by the linear relationship between fetal and maternal concentrations at maternal levels above 8 mg per milliliter is subtracted from the overall changes in fetal concentration, the lower graph in Fig. 5 is obtained. Analysis of the latter suggests that the mechanism responsible for this type of transfer is probably a carrier or receptor-mediated process which is inhibited by its own substrate or "receptee," human IgG, at maternal human IgG levels above 2 mg per milliliter. The data also indicate that the first molecule of IgG which becomes attached to the transport system is bound more strongly than is the second IgG molecule. Thus, human IgG is trans-

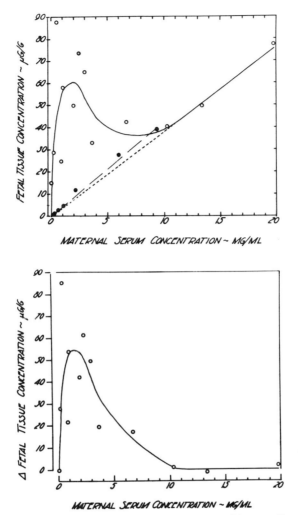

Fig. 5. Upper graph: Concentrations of human IgG (○) and human albumin (●) in the mouse fetus at different maternal levels 24 hr after intravenous injection into the mother. The solid line was calculated from the smoothed curve for the fetal to maternal IgG ratios shown in Fig. 4; the short dashed line is an extrapolation to zero of the first-order relation for IgG seen at higher maternal levels. Lower graph: The relation between maternal and fetal IgG concentrations when the first-order function for IgG transfer is subtracted from the total transfer curve. From Gitlin and Koch (1968).

ported from mother to fetus at term by at least two different mechanisms: one of these is a first-order process, possibly diffusion; the second is an active process which is mediated by a receptor or carrier which is inhibitable by human IgG.

At low maternal IgG concentrations, the active transport system involving the receptor–carrier mechanism is the more efficient, but at high maternal IgG levels, this system is inhibited and the first-order process predominates. The obvious consequence of such a dual process for maternofetal IgG transfer is a stabilization of fetal levels of IgG over relatively wide ranges in maternal IgG concentrations. The role of the active transport system would certainly enhance infant survival in the face of low IgG levels in the mother.

b. Transport binding sites on the IgG molecule.　When labeled Fab fragments and labeled Fc fragments obtained from human IgG by papain hydrolysis and labeled IgG light chains (cf. Chapter 1, Volume III) were given intravenously to pregnant women at term, each was found to cross the placenta (Gitlin *et al.,* 1964a). The half-life of the Fab fragment in the pregnant women was only 0.3 days, whereas the half-life of the Fc fragment was 4.0 days. As we noted for Eq. (9) in Section II, B, when 2 tracer proteins which cross from mother to fetus have different half-lives, their relative concentrations in the fetus during the steady state will differ as do their half-lives, all else being equal. If it can be assumed that the half-life of a given tracer protein in the mother is the same as that in the fetus, then the protein will disappear from the fetus at the same fractional rate as in the mother. Establishing the concentrations of tracer proteins in the fetus as fractions of the maternal levels, or C_f/C_m, not only corrects for differences in the amounts of the proteins given to the same or different individuals, but also corrects in part for differences in the fractional rates of disappearance of different tracers in the same or different individuals. As shown in Fig. 6, the rate of increase in C_f/C_m for the Fab fragment and for the IgG light chains after injection into the mother was similar to that for the Fc fragment but greater than that observed for intact IgG. It would appear, therefore, that the Fab fragment and the Fc fragment are transported from mother to fetus at similar rates and that both fragments may be more efficiently transported than the intact IgG molecule (Gitlin *et al.,* 1964b). Part of this greater transport of the fragments as compared to the intact molecule may be due to increased diffusion rates, since the fragments are each only a third the size of the parent molecule. However, it is clear that there are several sites responsible for the active transport of IgG across the human placenta, and that they are present in different areas of the IgG molecule.

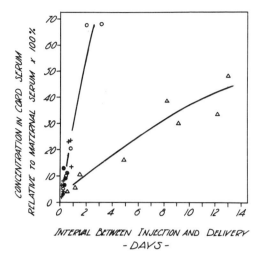

Fig. 6. Concentrations of IgG (△), Fab fragment (●), Fc fragment (○), and light chains (+) in plasma of infant at birth relative to mother's plasma concentration at that time. From Gitlin *et al.* (1964b).

In studying the relative maternofetal transport rates of rabbit Fab and Fc fragments and intact rabbit IgG in rabbits, Brambell and his colleagues (1960) placed these proteins in the uterine lumen of the pregnant doe and measured the amounts present in the fetus 24 hr later. The fetal serum concentration of the Fab fragment was found to be only a sixth to a tenth of that attained by the Fc fragment, and the latter was only a fourth of the fetal serum concentration reached by intact IgG. Interestingly, the relative fetal concentrations for rabbit IgG and its fragments in the rabbit are virtually the same as those obtained after maternofetal transfer of human IgG and its fragments in the human fetus: the fetal concentrations of Fab fragment in the human fetus were a fourth to a tenth those for Fc fragment, and the latter were only a fourth to three-fourths the levels found for IgG. When the rabbit data are considered in the light of Eq. (9), it would appear that in the rabbit, as in humans, the maternofetal transport of IgG is related to several sites in different portions of the IgG molecule.

c. MATURATION OF ACTIVE TRANSPORT SYSTEMS. The selective permeability of the human placenta to IgG which is manifest at term apparently is not present during early gestation. Passage of IgG from mother to conceptus does occur at least as early as the sixth week of embryonic development, and most likely earlier as well, but the transmission process involved is certainly neither particularly selective nor very active. The concentration of IgG in embryonic serum at this stage of development relative to that in maternal serum suggests instead that diffusion may be the principal, if not the sole, mechanism responsible for this transfer. At 12 to 16 weeks of gestation, labeled IgG has been shown to traverse the placenta (Dancis *et al.,* 1961), and at this stage the placenta is still not selective in its permeability to IgG as compared to albumin. At approximately 22 weeks of gestation, however, the fetal serum concentration of IgG rises sharply without a concomitant increase in fetal IgG synthesis (Gitlin and Biasucci, 1969a); approximately maternal levels are reached by 26 weeks of gestation (cf. Section V,N,5 and Fig. 18).

This relatively rapid change in the permeability of the placenta was investigated in the mouse, using radiolabeled human albumin and human IgG as tracers (Morphis and Gitlin, 1970). The labeled proteins were injected intravenously in pregnant mice at different stages of gestation, and their concentrations in the conceptus and in the maternal serum were determined 24 hr later. It was found (Fig. 7) that the fetal to maternal concentration for labeled IgG, C_f/C_m, increased abruptly, approximately 100-fold, between 11 and 15 days of gestation, much like the rapid increase observed in IgG levels in the human conceptus between 22 and 26 weeks of gestation. On the other hand, the fetal concentration of albumin relative to that in the mother, C_{fa}/C_{ma} remained constant until

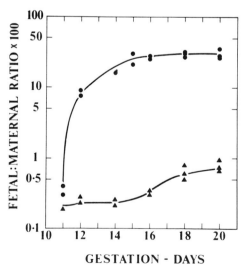

Fig. 7. Fetal tissue to maternal serum concentration ratios for human IgG (●) and human albumin (▲) in pregnant mice 24 hours after intravenous injection into the mother. From Morphis and Gitlin (1970).

after 14 days of gestation, and then increased only 4-fold between 14 days and term, with most of the increase occurring after 16 days of gestation (Fig. 7). As was noted in Section III,B,2,a, human albumin is transferred from mother to fetus in the pregnant mouse near term by a first-order process, and human IgG is transported by two processes, one of which, as for albumin, is first-order and the other is an active receptor or carrier-mediated mechanism. The relative amount of IgG transferred from mother to fetus by the first-order process alone, or C'_f/C'_m, is proportional, of course, to the relative amount of albumin transferred, C_{fa}/C_{ma}, and $(C'_f/C'_m) < (C_{fa}/C_{ma})$. The difference between C_f/C_m for IgG and C_{fa}/C_{ma} for albumin in Fig. 7, therefore, represents the minimum relative amount of IgG transferred from mother to fetus by the active transport system. It is easily seen that almost all of the abrupt increase in the transfer of IgG was attributable to a rapid maturation or a derepression of a specific active transport system and was not due to a general or nonspecific increase in the permeability of the placenta to macromolecules.

d. MULTIPLE TRANSPORT SYSTEMS. In the pregnant mouse at least, there is not just one system for the active transport of human IgG across the maternofetal barrier but several, each with different specificities and each inhibitable by the IgG it transports (Gitlin and Morphis, 1969). Mouse IgG, for example, is transferred from mother to conceptus with kinetics similar to that for human IgG, but the active transport component for mouse IgG is already markedly inhibited at normal maternal levels of mouse IgG, leaving only the first-order process operating. Thus, in the normal pregnant mouse near term, the maternofetal transfer of mouse IgG is like that of human albumin, the amount transferred to the fetus being proportional to the maternal serum concentration of the protein. At low maternal mouse IgG levels, however, such as are found in certain pathogen-free mice, transport of mouse IgG is much greater than at normal mouse IgG concentrations. The maternofetal transfer of bovine IgG in the mouse is similar to the transfer of mouse IgG, and bovine IgG can replace mouse IgG in the inhibiting effects of increased maternal IgG levels on either mouse or bovine IgG transport. While mouse IgG and bovine IgG can each affect the transport of the other, both have only a relatively small effect on the maternofetal transfer of either human, rabbit, guinea pig, or porcine IgG. On the other hand, each of the latter 4 immunoglobulins can inhibit the maternofetal transfer of not only itself, but also any of the other three and both mouse and bovine IgG as well. Thus, at least two different systems exist in the maternofetal barrier for the active transport of IgG: one transports both mouse and bovine IgG, and is inhibited by these as well as by human, rabbit, guinea pig, and porcine IgG; the other transports human, guinea pig, and porcine IgG and is readily inhibited by these, but is much less affected by either mouse or bovine IgG.

It must be emphasized that in species where there is relatively poor transport of IgG from mother to conceptus, this apparent lack of transfer may be due to specific inhibition of the active IgG transport system at *normal* maternal levels of IgG for the species and not due to the absence of such a system. This certainly is the case in the pregnant mouse near term and may be true as well for other species such as the guinea pig.

It was noted in Section III,B,2,b, that both the IgG Fab fragment, which consists of one light chain and part of one heavy chain, and the IgG Fc fragment, which consists of part of each of the two heavy chains, are actively transported across the human placenta. The fragments are both actively transported from mother to fetus in the mouse also, although in this species the Fab fragment is transferred somewhat less well than is the Fc fragment. The light chains of IgG are also transported across the placenta in both humans (Fig. 6) and mice by an active process. It is entirely possible that each of the sites on the IgG molecule is transported across the maternofetal barrier by a single receptor–carrier system having several binding specificities, each for different sites on the IgG molecule. It is also possible, however, that there are several receptor–carrier systems, each with binding sites of limited specificity. In the latter case, heavy chains and light chains would be mediated by different systems and in the former case, both would be transported by the same system. In fact, there are actually different receptors for different sites on the IgG molecule, and probably different transcellular transport systems as well, as is shown below.

e. SPECIFIC CELL MEMBRANE RECEPTORS AND ACTIVE TRANSPORT. The suckling murine intestine, like the human or murine placenta, is selectively permeable to IgG. To explain the preferential transport of proteins across such tissue barriers, Brambell (1966) suggested that proteins are selectively bound by cell receptors present on the cell membrane. During pinocytosis, the bound proteins would be enfolded intracellularly as the cell membrane invaginates to engulf a portion of the environmental fluid together with the protein present in that fluid. The bound proteins presumably would be protected from intracellular hydrolysis, whereas the free proteins would not. The amount of protein transported by this mechanism would then be proportional to the degree of binding. It has recently been found by Jones and Waldmann (1972) that cell membranes prepared from suckling rat intestines actually do selectively bind IgG.

A study of protein binding by cell membranes prepared from human, rat, and mouse placentas and from rat and mouse intestines confirms the presence of cell membrane receptors which specifically bind different proteins with different degrees of avidity (Gitlin and Gitlin, 1973). In fact, the avidity and specificity of protein binding by the cell membranes from each of these tissues paralleled to a remarkable degree the degree and specificity of protein transport across them (Gitlin and Gitlin, 1973). For example, the relative net transplacental transfer rates for human IgG, IgG light chains, and human albumin are similar to the relative binding avidities of the proteins to human placental cell membranes. The binding of human IgG, bovine IgG and human albumin to rat placental cell membranes and of human IgG and IgG light chains to mouse placental cell membranes parallel the relative maternofetal transfer of these proteins in the respective species. Just as the maternofetal transport of labeled human IgG, bovine IgG, and IgG light chains is inhibitable with human IgG, so is the binding of these labeled proteins inhibitable with human IgG. However, some proteins are bound relatively more avidly than would be suggested by their relative rates of maternofetal transport. For example, human growth hormone does not cross the placenta (cf. Section III,B,3) and albumin does; yet, human growth hormone is bound by placental cell membranes somewhat better than is albumin. Both human IgG and human insulin are bound by the placenta of 7 to 8 weeks of gestation as avidly as they are bound by the term placenta; yet, human IgG traverses the placenta at 7 to 8 weeks' gestation relatively poorly and only by diffusion, and human insulin apparently does not pass at all. At term both proteins pass the placenta quite actively. The binding of a protein without a corresponding degree of maternofetal transport would indicate either that the placental receptors are different in function as well as in specificity, or that maternofetal transport involved mechanisms other than, or in addition to, receptor binding, or both.

Proteins between 20,000 and 165,000 daltons in molecular weight traverse the human chorion and amnion (cf. Section III,B,1) at rates which are inversely proportional to the square roots of the molecular weights of the proteins. These membranes, however, bind human IgG, insulin, and albumin, among others, to the same extent as does human term placenta; i.e., the binding of insulin is about 1.5 times that of IgG which, in turn, is bound about 15 to 30 times as avidly as albumin. Obviously, the binding of these three proteins by fetal membranes is not determined by their molecular weights, an observation which is in accord with the concept that protein transport is not determined solely by cell membrane receptors.

It is interesting, but not surprising, that fetal membranes should bind proteins with the same specificity and avidity as does the fetal portion of the placenta, since the chorionic layer of the fetal membranes and the placenta are extensions of each other. The binding of these proteins by cell membranes from *other* tissues is quite different than that observed with the placenta. Human IgG is bound by suckling murine intestine, for example, about 8 to 12 times as avidly as it is bound by the murine or human placenta; the transfer of IgG across the murine suckling intestine is faster than is the transfer of IgG across the placenta. Human IgG light chains, however, are also bound by suckling murine intestine, albeit only a fifth as avidly as human IgG, but little or none of the protein crosses the intestine into the circulation intact.

The mouse transplacental transport system for human IgG *in vivo* is not only saturable, but it is also completely inhibitable by IgG (Gitlin and Koch, 1968). The murine transintestinal transport system for human IgG is also saturable *in vivo,* although not inhibitable by IgG. The binding of human IgG by cell membranes from these tissues is not saturated at IgG levels which easily saturate the transport systems *in vivo.* The data again indicate that the transport system *in vivo* is not entirely represented by the cell membrane receptor *in vitro.*

It seems, therefore, that the active transport of proteins across such organs as the placenta or suckling intestine involves at least two different factors (Gitlin and Gitlin, 1973). One of these, the selective binding of proteins by specific cell membrane receptors, may be an essential first step in the transport process, but binding of the protein does not of itself ensure completion of the transfer. A second specific factor or mechanism in addition to, or other than, cell membrane receptors must be involved to ensure that the bound protein is actually transferred.

3. The Placenta as an Impermeable Barrier

For some proteins, the placenta is an impermeable barrier. Human growth hormone, for example, does not cross from mother to fetus at any stage of development, and human insulin, which readily passes the placenta at or near term, does not do so at all during early gestation. Yet proteins such as α_1-acid glycoprotein, albumin, transferrin, and even some of the immunoglobulins, among others, traverse the placenta by a first-order process which appears to be related to the molecular weight of the protein (Section III,B,1). If the latter process is truly diffusion, it is difficult to understand how the placenta can be impermeable to growth hormone, when it is permeable to proteins at least 2 to 10 times as large. It is possible, therefore, that the first-order process whereby some proteins cross the placenta, despite the obvious relation between rate of transfer and molecular weight, may not be simple diffusion and could be a receptor-mediated mechanism. The fact that the binding of growth hormone by placental cell membranes is twice that of albumin does not, of course, rule out a receptor-mediated mechanism operating with first-order kinetics. As indicated earlier (Section III,B,2,e), different receptors may have different functions, and not all of the protein bound may reach the fetal circulation.

4. Directional Transfer across the Placenta

The permeability of the placenta to a protein is not necessarily the same in both directions; i.e., the fractional rate of transfer of a protein from fetus to mother, V_{fm}, may not be the same as the fractional rate of transfer from mother to fetus, V_{mf}. An example of directional transfer is seen in the maternofetal exchange of IgG at term. The plasma concentration of IgG in the fetus at term, C_f, is approximately equal to, and often exceeds, that of the mother, C_m. Rewriting Eq. (4):

$$C_m V_{mf} = C_f [V_{fm} + (D_f/C_f) - (S_f/C_f)]$$

and since $C_m = C_f$, this becomes

$$V_{mf} = V_{fm} + (D_f/C_f) - (S_f/C_f)$$

The rate of IgG synthesis by the fetus at term is but 1% or less of the rate of degradation, and therefore $V_{mf} > V_{fm}$. Thus, the placenta transfers IgG from mother to fetus more efficiently than from fetus to mother.

IV. Ontogeny and Plasma Protein Synthesis

As discussed in Section II,A,1, the concentration of a given protein in plasma is dependent, for the most part, upon the rate at which the protein is synthesized and the rate at which it is degraded. Therefore, if the concentration of a protein in the serum of the neonate is either sustained or increased during the immediate postnatal period, it can be assumed that the rate of synthesis of the protein by the *fetus* at the time of birth is equal to or greater than, respectively, the rate of degradation. In addition, the neonatal serum level of the protein under these conditions divided by the normal adult level is an approximation of the amount of protein synthesized per unit weight by the neonate relative to that in the adult. For example, the serum concentration of transferrin during the neonatal period is maintained at a fairly constant level of about 50 to 90% of the adult level (Gitlin and Biasucci, 1969a); the amount of transferrin synthesized per day per kilogram of body weight in the newborn, therefore, is approximately 50 to 90% of that in the adult. On the other hand, if the neonatal serum concentration falls during the immediate postnatal period, the rate of protein synthesis by the neonate is probably less than the rate of degradation, although an increase in the rate of degradation as the cause of this decline cannot be ruled out without additional evidence. Should the rate of decline in the serum concentration of the protein be longer than the half-life of the protein, then it is likely that some neonatal synthesis is taking place. If the rate of decline equals the half-life of the protein, as is the case for IgG, then there is little or no synthesis of the protein by the neonate; a declining neonatal serum concentration equal to the half-life of the protein, of course, does not rule out synthesis by the fetus *prior* to delivery. By studying postnatal changes in serum protein concentrations in the newborn, Hitzig (1961) was able to show that the fetus at term can synthesize albumin, α_1-acid glycoprotein, α_2-macroglobulin, and transferrin, among others.

The phenotype of a protein has proved to be a useful indicator of fetal synthesis for some proteins. It has been demonstrated, for example, that the phenotype of either Gc globulin, transferrin, haptoglobin, or even IgG in the serum of the conceptus can be different from that of the mother (Hirschfeld and Lunell, 1962; Mårtensson and Fudenberg, 1965; Melartin *et al.*, 1966). Obviously, then, the conceptus can synthesize these proteins.

Another method of demonstrating synthesis of a protein by the conceptus is the technique described by Hochwald *et al.* (1961), whereby fetal tissues are cultured or maintained in an appropriate medium containing ^{14}C-labeled amino acids, and the culture fluids are then analyzed by radioimmunoelectrophoresis. Briefly, after the tissues are cultured for 1 to 4 days, the fluids are concentrated, and specific carrier proteins are added. The proteins in the culture fluids are separated and precipitated in agar by means of immunoelectrophoresis, and after drying, the immunoelectrophoretic plates are inverted on sensitive film for radioautography. If suitable controls are employed, the presence of radiolabeled protein in the culture fluid indicates synthesis of the protein by the tissue. Hydrolysis of the labeled protein with specific enzymes followed by high voltage separation of the released peptides, with or without further separation by chromatography, has proved helpful in showing that the radiolabeled amino acids are actually incorporated into the protein

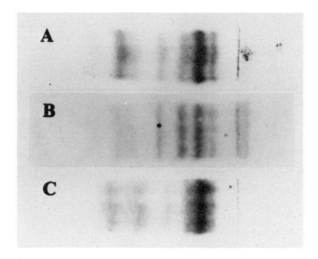

Fig. 8. Chymotryptic hydrolysates separated by high voltage electrophoresis on paper; anode is to the right. A. Purified human growth hormone, developed with ninhydrin. B. Immunochemical precipitate of ^{14}C-labeled growth hormone from a culture of human fetal pituitary, radioautograph. C. Same hydrolysate of labeled growth hormone as in B, but developed with ninhydrin after radioautography. From Gitlin and Biasucci (1969b).

and are not simply bound. For example, in studying the synthesis of growth hormone by cultures of fetal pituitary, the hormone was isolated from the culture fluid by precipitation with antiserum specific for growth hormone. Chymotryptic digests of the precipitated hormone (Fig. 8) contained peptides released from the antibodies in the precipitate as well as from the hormone; the peptide patterns obtained, therefore, when developed with ninhydrin, did *not* resemble the ninhydrin-stained peptide pattern for pure unlabeled growth hormone. However, radioautography revealed a *radiolabeled* peptide pattern for the antibody-precipitated hormone which was similar to the ninhydrin-developed pattern obtained for the pure unlabeled protein (Gitlin and Biasucci, 1969b).

The development of plasma protein synthesis in various organs of the human conceptus has been studied using the radioimmunoelectrophoretic method (Gitlin and Biasucci, 1969a; Gitlin and Perricelli, 1970), and the results obtained are as follows:

A. Plasma Protein Synthesis in the Liver

The embryonic liver at 3 weeks postconception is simply a thickened area of cells forming a small saccule on the ventral side of the entodermal canal between the heart and the yolk sac. The yolk sac at this stage of development is just a pouch with a broad base attached to the midgut. At 4 weeks of gestation, the embryo has grown to 4 or 5 mm in crown–rump length, the liver is a diverticulum of hepatic buds and ducts still without evidence of lobes, and the yolk sac is a distinct vesicle with a relatively narrow yolk stalk. The liver at this early stage of formation can already synthesize prealbumin, albumin, α-fetoprotein, α_1-antitrypsin, C1 esterase inhibitor, α_2-macroglobulin, C3 or β_{1C}, β-lipoprotein, hemopexin, and transferrin. By 4.5 to 5 weeks of gestation the embryo measures 10 to 15 mm in crown–rump length, and hepatic lobes can now be distinguished; at this time, the liver can synthesize α_1-acid glycoprotein and ceruloplasmin as well. In some embryos, the liver at 5.5 weeks of gestation can synthesize fibrinogen, and by 8.5 weeks, hepatic synthesis of fibrinogen is established in all normal embryos. Thus, the liver is capable of synthesizing a number of plasma proteins at a time when hepatic cells are just appearing, and as the liver differentiates morphologically, it develops the capacity to synthesize others as well, biochemical differentiation accompanying morphological differentiation.

At 11 to 12 weeks of gestation, the liver is a source of small amounts of IgG and IgE. Although hepatic synthesis of these immunoglobulins may soon cease thereafter, it has been observed as late as 17.5 weeks of gestation. It should be noted that the liver during embryonic and fetal development is host to a continuously changing hematopoietic cell population. Since lymphoid cells can be found in the mesenteric lymph nodes as early as 8 weeks of gestation, it is probable that hepatic synthesis of IgG and IgE is attributable to lymphopoietic cells in the liver and not the hepatic parenchyma. At 15 to 17 weeks of gestation, the spleen becomes the major organ of synthesis for these and other immunoglobulins.

B. Plasma Protein Synthesis by the Yolk Sac

Although the liver is the principal if not the only organ of synthesis for albumin in adults, this is definitely not so in the embryo. The yolk sac also synthesizes albumin. In fact, by 5.5 weeks of gestation, the yolk sac can synthesize not only albumin, but also prealbumin, α_1-antitrypsin, α-fetoprotein, and transferrin. Whether these proteins are synthesized by the yolk sac earlier than 5.5 weeks is not known, since this was the earliest stage examined. The amount of prealbumin, α_1-antitrypsin, α-fetoprotein, and transferrin produced *in vitro* by the yolk sac appears to be equal to or even greater than that produced *in vitro* by equivalent quantities of liver from the same embryo. On the other hand, the amount of albumin produced by the yolk sac is less than that synthesized by the liver. By 8.5 weeks of gestation, synthesis of each of these proteins by the yolk sac, with the exception of albumin, has decreased noticeably. Yolk sac synthesis of prealbumin and α_1-antitrypsin is below detectable levels at 11.5 weeks of gestation, and at this stage, only relatively small amounts of albumin, α-fetoprotein, and transferrin are produced.

Thus, the human yolk sac during its brief existence as a well-developed structure can synthesize a number of plasma proteins. The human yolk sac becomes atretic toward the end of the first trimester of gestation or the beginning of the second, and a decrease in plasma protein synthesis accompanies this change. In the rat fetus and in the chick embryo, the yolk sac is a prominent membrane which performs biologically important functions throughout antenatal development: in the rat, it is one of the fetal membranes, and during the last quarter of gestation it is the only fetal membrane remaining intact; in the chick, the yolk sac envelopes and absorbs the yolk necessary to nurture the embryo. In both of these species, the yolk sac produces plasma proteins until birth: the rat yolk sac synthesizes α-fetoprotein and transferrin, among others, while the chick yolk sac produces these two proteins and albumin as well.

C. Plasma Protein Synthesis in Other Organs

Embryonic lung apparently can occasionally synthesize trace amounts of transferrin: the lungs from 3 embryos between 8.5 and 12 weeks of gestation proved capable of producing minute amounts of transferrin, but the lungs from 12 other conceptuses between 7.5 and 18 weeks of gestation did not. Cultures of embryonic and fetal lungs also synthesize small amounts of hemopexin and significant amounts of C3 (β_{1C}) beginning as early as 4.5 weeks of gestation or less. The lung can synthesize IgE, and perhaps even IgG, as early as 11 weeks of gestation, but the lung cultures in these studies of necessity also include perihilar lymph nodal tissue.

The gastrointestinal tract also synthesizes plasma proteins. For example, serum α-fetoprotein is synthesized by the gastrointestinal tract beginning as early as 4 weeks of gestation, but the amounts produced are much less than those produced by the liver or by the yolk sac. Cultures of gastrointestinal tract can produce IgG as early as 11 to 12 weeks of gestation; as noted above, lymphoid cells can be identified in the mesenteric lymph nodes by 8 weeks of gestation. The largest amounts of IgG produced by any organ during gestation are produced by the spleen, but splenic synthesis of IgG has not been detected earlier than 15 to 16 weeks of gestation, or about the time that lymphoid cells are first observed in this organ. On the other hand, synthesis of small amounts of IgM does take place in the spleen beginning at about 10.5 weeks of gestation, soon after lymphocytes appear in the peripheral blood. After 17 weeks of gestation, the spleen becomes the principal organ for the synthesis of both IgM and IgG.

Still other organs and tissues may contribute plasma proteins in the conceptus; e.g., trace amounts of serum α-fetoprotein are produced by an occasional kidney or placenta. Cultures of skin and muscle yield β_{1C} and C1 esterase inhibitor at least as early as 4 weeks of gestation. At 10 weeks of gestation, the peripheral blood already contains small numbers of lymphocytes, and by 11.5 weeks, cultures of blood can also produce IgM. Trace amounts of α_1-antitrypsin and β_{1C} and relatively large amounts of both β-lipoprotein and α_2-macroglobulin are also produced by peripheral blood cells as early as 11.5 weeks of gestation. By 17.5 weeks of gestation, peripheral blood cells can synthesize IgG as well.

Throughout this section, a cautious approach has been taken as to when the synthesis of a given protein by a particular organ or tissue actually begins. First, conceptuses earlier than 4 weeks of gestation were not studied, and hence it is not known whether a protein which is synthesized at this stage of development is also produced earlier. Second, the failure to detect synthesis of a protein at any stage does not necessarily mean that the protein is not synthesized, but only that synthesis, if present, is below the limits of detection of the method.

D. Phylogeny versus Fetal Ontogeny

A protein which is synthesized by a given organ or tissue in one animal species may be synthesized by entirely different organs or tissues in other species, or perhaps not even synthesized at all. As noted in Section IV,B, for example, the yolk sacs of both the human embryo and the chick embryo synthesize serum albumin, but the yolk sac of the rat apparently does not (Gitlin and Boesman, 1967a; Gitlin and Kitzes, 1967). Needless to state, there must be some order to this variability among species, the key, of course, as in all differences between species, being evolution. This order is not readily apparent, due to a paucity of data concerning the sites of plasma protein synthesis in embryos and fetuses of different animal classes. However, some information has been obtained concerning at least one protein which exemplifies the orderly changes that have taken place in the sites of plasma protein synthesis during evolution; this protein is serum α-fetoprotein (cf. Section V,E).

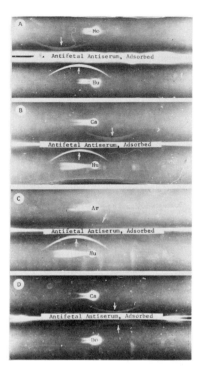

Fig. 9. Detection of α-fetoprotein by immunoelectrophoresis in human fetal serum (Hu) and in fetal serum of the squirrel monkey (Mo), cat (Ca), armadillo (Ar), and dog (Do). Antifetal serum used was prepared in rabbits against human α-fetoprotein and adsorbed with human adult serum to ensure specificity. From Gitlin and Boesman (1967b).

In the human conceptus, α-fetoprotein is synthesized primarily in both the liver and the yolk sac, as was noted above (Section IV,A and B), with lesser amounts being synthesized in the gastrointestinal tract; synthesis of trace amounts by an occasional kidney or placenta has also been observed. All mammals thus far examined, from primates to marsupials (Fig. 9), synthesize α-fetoprotein during the fetal state (Gitlin and Boesman, 1967b; Zizkovsky and Masopust, 1974), and homologs of mammalian α-fetoprotein (Figs. 10 and 11) are produced by avian embryos (Gitlin and Kitzes, 1967) and by shark fetuses (Gitlin *et al.,* 1973). In the shark fetus, serum α-fetoprotein is synthesized principally by the liver and the stomach, with smaller quantities being synthesized by the intestine, yolk sac, and kidney. It has been determined that the α-fetoproteins of different shark species are remarkably similar to each other antigenically, and hence are similar to some extent structurally.

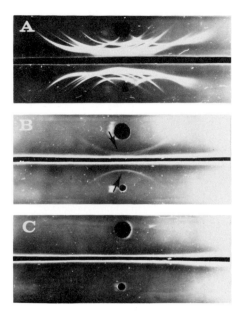

Fig. 10. A. Immunoelectrophoresis of fetal lemon shark serum, *Negaprion brevirostris,* developed with rabbit antiserum prepared against this serum. B. Immunoelectrophoresis of fetal lemon shark serum developed with the same antiserum after adsorption with adult lemon shark serum. C. Immunoelectrophoresis of adult lemon shark serum developed with the adsorbed antiserum used in B: The α-fetoprotein detected in the fetus is absent in an adult shark. Anode to the left in each figure. From Gitlin *et al.* (1973).

Since the shark species studied belong to two different suborders which evolved independently about 180 million years ago, cistrons for α-fetoprotein must have existed before both suborders diverged, or more than 180 million years ago. The data also suggest that α-fetoprotein in sharks has remained structurally quite stable, at least in regard to the antigenic sites detected, since the shark species studied represent 10 separate genera that emerged at different times over a period of at least 60 million years. Synthesis of the avian homolog of human α-fetoprotein occurs chiefly, if not exclusively, in the yolk sac.

The occurrence of α-fetoprotein in so many different species of sharks, mammals, and birds makes it highly improbable that synthesis of this protein appeared as a separate independent event in each class. More likely, an archaic homolog of α-fetoprotein must have existed in an ancestor common to these three classes (Gitlin *et al.,* 1973). The evolutionary stream leading to the development of the elasmobranchs diverged from the stream leading to amphibia, reptiles, and mammals at

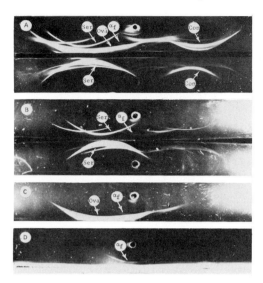

Fig. 11.   Immunoelectrophoresis, anode to the left. A. Chick embryo serum in upper well, hen serum in lower, antiserum in trough between the wells had been prepared in rabbits against chick embryo serum, anti-CE. B. Chick embryo serum in upper well and hen serum in lower; antiserum anti-CE was adsorbed with whites of unfertilized eggs, resulting in the loss of the ovalbumin and conalbumin lines. C. Chick embryo serum; developed with anti-CE adsorbed with hen serum. D. Chick embryo serum; developed with anti-CE adsorbed with yolk from an unfertilized egg. Ser = serum albumin; Ova = ovalbumin; α_f = embryo-specific globulin, or α_f-globulin; Con = conalbumin. From Gitlin and Kitzes (1967).

some time during the Silurian period of the Paleozoic era, or about 400 to 450 million years ago. Mammalian divergence from the reptilian stem probably occurred about 230 to 250 million years ago, and birds began to diverge from the reptiles about 180 million years ago, or 50 million years *after* the emergence of mammals. According to this evolutionary clock, then, the α-fetoproteins present in the animal species of today are in fact descendants of an ancestral α-fetoprotein synthesized by animals which lived and died more than 400 to 450 million years ago. During evolution, there has been a shift caudally among the entoder-mally derived organs in their relative importance for the synthesis of α-fetoprotein. At some time before or during the emergence of the earliest mammals, or more than 230 million years ago, α-fetoprotein synthesis declined in the stomach while it increased in the yolk sac; during this change, the liver remained a principal organ for the synthesis of α-fe-toprotein. At some point in time between the emergence of mammals and the appearance of birds, α-fetoprotein synthesis in the liver *and* the stomach was eliminated, or at least curtailed drastically, and the yolk sac became the most important site for the synthesis in birds.

V. Antenatal and Postnatal Development

A. Prealbumin

Prealbumin is synthesized in the conceptus apparently only by the liver and the yolk sac; it is not produced by fetal lungs, gastrointestinal tract, spleen, kidneys, blood, or placenta. Its synthesis begins very early during development (cf. Section IV), at least as early as 4 weeks post-conception. In one conceptus of 11.5 weeks gestation, the serum concentration of prealbumin was found to be 5 mg per 100 ml, but apparently soon thereafter and for the remainder of gestation the pre-albumin level averages 10 mg per 100 ml (Rossi *et al.,* 1970). The average concentration of prealbumin in the cord serum of full term infants is 13 mg per 100 ml, and in maternal serum at the time of delivery it is 23 mg per 100 ml, the same as in normal adults. During the first year of life, the mean serum prealbumin level is approximately 10 mg per 100 ml. Although the exact development of prealbumin is not yet clear, it is apparent that the maximum rate of prealbumin synthesis in the fetus is only half that of the normal adult, and is still less than in the adult during infancy (Rossi *et al.,* 1970).

B. Albumin

The only organs noted to synthesize albumin in the conceptus are the liver and the yolk sac (cf. Section IV). Synthesis of the protein is already evident at the earliest developmental stages of these organs that were examined, i.e., at 4 weeks and 5.5 weeks of gestation, respectively (Gitlin and Perricelli, 1970). By 6 weeks of gestation (Fig. 12) the al-

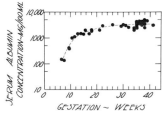

Fig. 12.   Serum concentration of albumin in the human conceptus as a function of gestational age.

bumin concentration in the serum of the conceptus is approximately 0.15 gm per 100 ml (Gitlin and Boesman, 1966). A small fraction of this albumin is of maternal origin, having reached the embryo by transplacental transfer (cf. Section III,B,1). The serum albumin concentration, however, rises rapidly (Fig. 12) to reach a level of 1.0 gm per 100 ml by 12 weeks' gestation and adult levels by 20 to 26 weeks. This rapid increase is attributable entirely to endogenous albumin synthesis by the conceptus, rather than to maternofetal transfer. The amount of albumin produced by the yolk sac decreases relative to the amount produced by the liver after 4 weeks of gestation, due in part to the more rapid increase in liver size and in part to changes in yolk sac development; by 12 weeks, yolk sac albumin synthesis is markedly curtailed. Therefore, the albumin present in the conceptus after 12 weeks is largely of hepatic origin with a relatively small contribution, probably less than 5 to 10% of the total, from the mother. When the fetal serum level is equal to that of the mother, the amount of albumin transferred from the mother to the fetus is balanced by an equal amount transferred from the fetus to the mother. In addition, as indicated by Eq. (5), the rate of albumin synthesis by the fetus then equals the rate at which albumin is degraded by the fetus. As would be expected, the serum albumin concentration normally remains relatively steady at adult levels during the postnatal period unless affected by severe changes in hydration of the infant.

C. α_1-Acid Glycoprotein

Hepatic synthesis of α_1-acid glycoprotein begins at approximately 4.5 weeks of gestation (Gitlin and Biasucci, 1969a) or somewhat later than the onset of albumin synthesis (Section IV,A). Whether tissues other than the liver can produce the protein remains to be investigated; peripheral blood cells do not synthesize it. As noted earlier (cf. Section III,B,1 and Fig. 2), α_1-acid glycoprotein crosses the placenta from mother to fetus by a process which has first-order kinetics (Gitlin et al., 1964a); thus, a small fraction of the protein present in fetal serum is actually of maternal origin. The average serum concentration of α_1-acid glycoprotein in cord blood at term is somewhat less than half of that in the mother (Table II): cord serum levels at term average 32% of the mean adult level, whereas maternal serum at term averages 72% of the mean adult level (Laurell, 1968; Gitlin and Biasucci, 1969a). It has been suggested by Laurell (1968) that the relatively low concentration of α_1-acid glycoprotein in maternal serum at term as compared to levels in nonpregnant adults may represent an estrogen effect induced by increased estrogen levels during pregnancy (Laurell and Skanse, 1963).

TABLE II

**The Relative Concentrations for a Given Protein in the Cord Plasma of the
Infant at Term, Maternal Plasma at Delivery, and in Nonpregnant Adult Plasma**

Protein	Child/mother	Child/adult	Mother/adult
α-Fetoprotein	160	20,000	125
α_2-Macroglobulin	1.5	1.5	1.0
Albumin	1.2	1.0	0.83
IgG	1.0 (0.90–1.2)	1.2	1.2
C1 Esterase inhibitor	0.77	1.1	1.5
α_1-Antitrypsin	0.75	1.5	2.0
Fibrinogen	0.73	1.0	1.4
Transferrin	0.63	0.64	1.0
Prealbumin	0.56	0.56	1.0
Gc Globulin[a]	0.50	0.88	1.8
C3	0.50	0.58	1.2
α_1-Acid glycoprotein[b]	0.44	0.32	0.72
Plasminogen	0.29	0.60	2.1
β-Lipoprotein	0.28	0.24	0.87
Ceruloplasmin	0.18	0.30	1.7
Hemopexin	0.18	0.30	1.6
IgM[a]	0.16	0.13	0.77
Haptoglobin	<0.02	<0.02	0.94
IgA	<0.001	<0.001	1.0

[a] Toivanen *et al.* (1969a).
[b] Laurell (1968).

D. α_1-Antitrypsin

Both the liver and the yolk sac produce α_1-antitrypsin in the conceptus, beginning at or before 4 weeks of gestation (Gitlin and Biasucci, 1969a; Gitlin and Perricelli, 1970). The liver is the principal source of α_1-antitrypsin throughout development; synthesis by the yolk sac decreases significantly by 8.5 weeks of gestation and is undetectable at 11.5 weeks. Whether other fetal organs or tissues produce small amounts of α_1-antitrypsin has not been investigated.

The serum α_1-antitrypsin concentration in the embryo of 6.5 weeks gestation is only 6.5% of the normal adult level, but it rises rapidly to reach an average concentration of about 70% of the adult level between 9.5 and 10.5 weeks of gestation (Fig. 13). The level then rises more slowly to achieve adult levels at about 26 weeks and concentrations from 110 to 175% of the adult level between 27.5 weeks and term; the fetal serum level at term averages about 150% of the adult mean con-

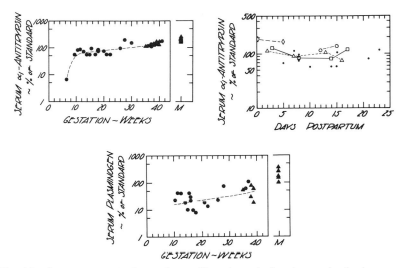

Fig. 13. Serum concentrations of α_1-antitrypsin and plasminogen in the human conceptus as functions of gestational age and of α_1-antitrypsin in the neonate as a function of postpartum age. The following symbols apply to Figures 13 through 18: solid circles and triangles represent individual conceptuses; solid triangles over abscissa marked M are serum concentrations in the mothers of those fetuses indicated by solid triangles to the left; individual neonatal concentrations are indicated by dots and the connected open symbols indicate serial measurements on the same neonate.

centration (Table II). The maternal serum concentration at term averages 200% of that in the normal adult (Ganrot and Bjerre, 1967; Laurell, 1968; Gitlin and Biasucci, 1969a).

During the immediate postnatal period (Fig. 13), the neonatal serum α_1-antitrypsin concentration decreases, and normal adult ranges are reached within 2 weeks. From what has been stated earlier in Section II, it is apparent that this fall could be due to either a decrease in endogenous synthesis or to the catabolism of α_1-antitrypsin transferred from the mother in excess of what can be replaced by neonatal synthesis or both. Although maternofetal transfer of α_1-antitrypsin has not been measured directly, the α_1-antitrypsin phenotypes present in the conceptus are not necessarily those of the mother, suggesting that maternofetal transfer of the protein, like albumin, is relatively small if it does occur (Adinolfi, 1971). Thus, neither the relatively high α_1-antitrypsin levels seen in the fetus at term nor the postnatal decrease in the neonate would seem to be attributable to maternofetal transfer. On the other hand, whatever it is that stimulates *maternal* synthesis of α_1-antitrypsin to levels twice those in the nonpregnant adult, perhaps estrogen, might pass to and operate in the conceptus to stimulate α_1-antitrypsin or vice-versa. If this influence ceases upon delivery, particularly understandable if the stimulus is of maternal origin, *neonatal* synthesis and the neonatal serum level would both decrease.

E. α-Fetoprotein

Serum α-fetoprotein in the human conceptus is principally a product of both the liver and the yolk sac with much smaller amounts being synthesized by the gastrointestinal tract (Gitlin *et al.*, 1972b). The kidneys and the placenta may, on occasion, produce a trace amount of α-fetoprotein in tissue cultures. Synthesis of the protein is evident as early as 29 days of gestation, the earliest stage studied (Gitlin and Biasucci, 1969a). The liver remains the primary site of synthesis throughout intrauterine life, synthesis by the yolk sac decreasing markedly as the organ becomes atretic toward the beginning of the second trimester (Gitlin and Perricilli, 1970).

The serum level of α-fetoprotein in the conceptus (Gitlin and Boesman, 1966) at 6.5 weeks of gestation is only 6.7 mg per 100 ml, but it rises rapidly to reach levels of almost 200 mg per 100 ml by 9.5 weeks gestation and 300 mg per 100 at 10 to 13 weeks (Fig. 14). From about 14 weeks of gestation to approximately 30 to 32 weeks, the serum concentration falls exponentially with a half-life on 32 days. This exponential decline is attributable to the fact that fetal growth during this period increases more rapidly than does the total amount of α-fetoprotein synthesized. The total amount of α-fetoprotein synthesized by the conceptus (Fig. 14) actually increases rapidly after 12 to 14 weeks of gestation to reach maximum levels at about 20 weeks of gestation, and then remains relatively constant until 30 to 32 weeks of gestation, after which it declines rapidly. The rapid decline in α-fetoprotein synthesis after 30 to 32 weeks of gestation is reflected in the precipitous fall seen in the α-fetoprotein serum concentration at this time. The α-fetoprotein concentration at term ranges from 1.3 to 8.6 mg or more per 100 ml; just 1 or 2 weeks earlier, the serum α-fetoprotein range is from 1.4 to 17.8 mg per 100 ml. The wide range of levels encountered at delivery and the differences that 1 or 2 weeks in gestation can make argues for caution in comparing levels in any two different series of infants, whether both series are normal or one of the two groups is believed to be abnormal.

The serum α-fetoprotein level in the newborn normally declines rapidly with an average half-life of 3.5 days during the first weeks of life (Gitlin and Boesman, 1966) and then somewhat more slowly until the normal adult serum level of α-fetoprotein, from 0.1 to 2.0 μg per 100 ml, is reached by 2 years of age (Masseyeff *et al.*, 1974). It is to be noted

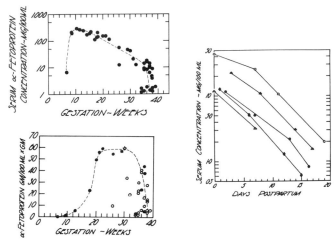

Fig. 14. Development of α-fetoprotein in the human conceptus and neonate. Left upper graph: Serum concentration of α-fetoprotein as a function of gestational age of the conceptus. Left lower graph: Serum concentrations of α-fetoprotein multiplied by the weight of the embryo or fetus as a relative measure of total α-fetoprotein synthesis during gestation. Right graph: Disappearance of α-fetoprotein from plasma of neonates. Adapted from Gitlin and Boesman (1966). See legend to Fig. 13 for explanation of symbols.

that the average serum concentration of α-fetoprotein present at birth is about 20,000 times that found in the normal adult (Table II).

There appears to be some transfer of α-fetoprotein across the placenta, since serum levels up to 50 μg per 100 ml have been reported in normal pregnant women during the third trimester (Seppälä and Ruoslahti, 1972a; Nishi and Hirai, 1973; Ishii, 1973; Massayeff, 1973). Interestingly, the average serum level in the pregnant woman is highest during the third trimester and is usually not elevated above the normal nonpregnant adult level during the first trimester. At 16 weeks of gestation, the maternal serum level averages about 4.5 μg per 100 ml, and at 20 weeks it is about 6.0 μg per 100 ml. The average concentration in the mother then rises exponentially to approximately 45μg per 100 ml at 32 weeks, after which it declines to an average of 25 μg per 100 ml at term. Thus, as the level in the mother is rising from 4.5 μg per 100 ml at 16 weeks to 45 μg per 100 ml at 32 weeks, the fetal concentration is decreasing from approximately 200,000 μg per 100 ml to 20,000 μg per 100 ml (Gitlin and Boesman, 1966). Nevertheless, throughout this period the concentration gradient is from fetus to mother, so that fetomaternal transfer could be responsible for at least part of the elevation of α-fetoprotein in the mother as gestation progresses. Fetomaternal transfer of α-fetoprotein must be quite small, however: at 32 weeks, the maternal level reaches a maximum; at this point, the net transfer of α-fetoprotein between fetus and mother, as noted in Eq. (7), must equal the rate of degradation of α-fetoprotein in the mother less the maternal rate of synthesis (cf. Section II,B). Since the maternal concentration at 32 weeks' gestation averages 45 μg per 100 ml, using Eq. (2) and a half-life of 3.5 days, the rate of α-fetoprotein degradation in a mother weighing 50 kg would be 450 μg per day. Assuming that both the transfer of α-fetoprotein from mother to fetus and the maternal synthesis of α-fetoprotein to be relatively nil, the maximum transfer of the protein from fetus to mother at 32 weeks, when the fetal serum concentration is 20,000 μg per 100 ml, would be 450 μg per day, or a clearance of only about 2.3 ml of fetal serum per day. Yet, this small amount of transfer could account for virtually all of the maternal serum α-fetoprotein and would also explain why the rate of increase of α-fetoprotein in maternal serum is so slow. After 32 weeks, the maternal level declines, in accord with the abrupt decrease that occurs in fetal synthesis at this time. The fact that the decline in the maternal concentration is much slower than in the fetus could also be explained on the basis of fetomaternal transfer: from 32 weeks to term, the fetal concentration is at least 40 to 400 times that found in the mother, and some fetomaternal transfer would continue during this period, despite the rapidity of fall in the fetal level.

Whether some of the increase in the maternal level of α-fetoprotein may be due to an increase in maternal endogenous synthesis is not known. It is also not possible to determine from the data if the placenta becomes increasingly permeable to α-fetoprotein as gestation continues toward term; as noted in Section III,B,2,c, the mouse placenta does become increasingly permeable to albumin as term approaches. That the human placenta can become *abnormally* permeable to α-fetoprotein is indicated by the fact that where there is severe fetal distress or Rh isoimmunization, the maternal level may rise well above 50 μg per 100 ml (Seppälä and Ruoslahti, 1972b,1974; Purves and Purves, 1972; Cohen et al., 1973).

After birth, anomalous serum levels of α-fetoprotein may be found in patients with hepatitis, hepatic cirrhosis, hepatoma, gonadal carcinoma, gastric carcinoma metastatic to the liver, or even in rare instances of gastric carcinoma without hepatic metastases (Masseyeff, 1973; Nishi and Hirai, 1973). Synthesis by gastric carcinoma is in accord with the fetal origin of the protein as is, of course, synthesis in the other conditions mentioned; primitive gonadal carcinomas which synthesize α-fetoprotein are thought to be of yolk sac origin. Synthesis of α-fetoprotein by carcinomas arising from organs or tissues which have the capacity to manufacture the protein during fetal life would seem to represent a depression of the cistron responsible for α-fetoprotein production (Gitlin et al., 1972b).

In some infants born prematurely after the spontaneous onset of labor, the serum α-fetoprotein concentration may be considerably lower than in fetuses of comparable gestation which were delivered by caesarean section in the absence of labor (Gitlin and Boesman, 1966). On the basis of a 3.5 day half-life, it can be calculated from Eq. (2) that α-fetoprotein synthesis in these spontaneously delivered infants decreased abruptly at least 1 to 2 weeks before labor began. It has recently been suggested that α-fetoprotein inhibits cellular immunity. It is fascinating to speculate that the abrupt curtailment of α-fetoprotein synthesis might result in an immunological rejection of the placenta, initiating either spontaneous premature labor or even spontaneous labor at term.

F. Gc Globulin

By comparing the phenotypes of Gc globulin present in fetal and maternal sera, Melartin and her associates (1966) found that the fetus synthesizes this protein as early as 10 weeks of gestation. In accord with this, tissue culture has indicated that Gc globulin is synthesized even as early as 4 weeks of gestation (D. Gitlin and A. Biasucci, unpublished).

The serum concentration of Gc globulin in the conceptus rises steadily from a concentration of approximately 7 mg per 100 ml at 12 to 13 weeks to a mean of 23 mg per 100 ml at term; the maternal level at term is 46 mg per 100 ml, or twice that in the full-term fetus (Toivanen et al., 1969a). Postnatally the concentration continues to increase and by 6 months of age, the mean Gc globulin level is even higher than that in adults, 32 mg per 100 ml in the infant as compared to 26 mg per 100 ml in adults (Table II).

G. Ceruloplasmin

Ceruloplasmin is synthesized exclusively by the liver, beginning in most cases at approximately 4.5 weeks of gestation (Gitlin and Biasucci, 1969a). In one instance, cultures of an 11.5 weeks liver failed to produce the protein. Just as the early synthesis of ceruloplasmin may be variable, so may the serum ceruloplasmin concentration during early gestation vary quite widely. In the 6.5-week embryo, the serum level is about 0.4 mg per 100 ml, but between 9.5 and 26 weeks of gestation, levels from less than 0.2 mg per 100 ml to as much as 3.5 mg per 100 ml are encountered (Fig. 15). During the period of 27 weeks gestation to term, the serum ceruloplasmin concentration ranges from 4.6 to 15.5 mg

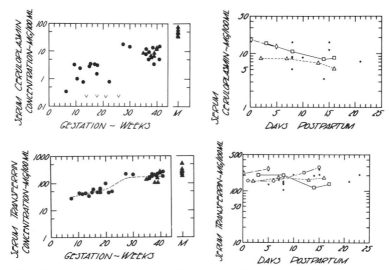

Fig. 15.   Serum concentrations of ceruloplasmin and transferrin in the human conceptus and neonate. From Gitlin and Biasucci (1969a). See Fig. 13 for explanation of symbols.

per 100 ml. Interestingly, the level in the neonate falls during the immediate postnatal period, in some infants with an initial half-life of about 10 days (Fig. 15). Since the half-life of ceruloplasmin in normal adults is 5 to 7 days, it is apparent that both the fetus at term and the neonate must synthesize some ceruloplasmin. In fact, the decline in the neonatal level is presumably due to the termination of maternofetal estrogen transfer at birth. Since estrogen stimulates the synthesis of ceruloplasmin, the decrease in estrogen during the neonatal period may account for the fall in ceruloplasmin concentration.

After its initial decline during the first month of postnatal life (Gitlin and Biasucci, 1969a), the ceruloplasmin serum level slowly rises to reach the normal nonpregnant adult range usually before a year of age (Hitzig, 1961). There are considerable ethnic differences in the normal adult level of ceruloplasmin, the mean ranging from a low of 21 mg per 100 ml in Orientals to 29 mg per 100 ml in Caucasians and 38 mg per 100 ml in American Indian groups (Shokeir, 1970). In pregnant women at term, the mean ceruloplasmin level ranges from 50 mg per 100 ml in some series (Gitlin and Biasucci, 1969a; Shokeir, 1971) to approximately 90 mg per 100 ml in others (Hitzig, 1961; Laurell, 1968).

H. α_2-Macroglobulin

All human fetal tissues produce radiolabeled α_2-macroglobulin when cultured in ^{14}C-labeled amino acids. However, since the labeled protein

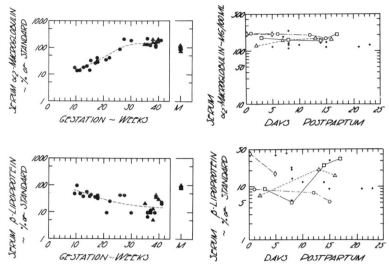

Fig. 16.   Serum concentrations of α_2-macroglobulin and β-lipoprotein in the human conceptus and neonate. From Gitlin and Biasucci (1969a). See legend to Fig. 13 for explanation of symbols.

is also synthesized in cultures of peripheral blood, it cannot be determined whether the labeled protein is synthesized by the tissue or by the blood in that tissue (Gitlin and Biasucci, 1969a). It has been suggested that α_2-macroglobulin becomes radiolabeled in such cultures only through the binding of other labeled products rather than because of endogenous α_2-macroglobulin synthesis (Adinolfi, 1971). However, enzymatic hydrolysis of labeled α_2-macroglobulin produced in fetal liver cultures yields radioactive peptides which correspond in electrophoretic mobility to peptides obtained from purified unlabeled α_2-macroglobulin (Gitlin and Biasucci, 1969a). The evidence suggests that fetal liver, or the blood contained in the liver at the very least, actually synthesizes α_2-macroglobulin.

The serum concentration of α_2-macroglobulin in the conceptus between 9 and 13 weeks of gestation is from 14 to 17% of adult levels (Fig. 16). It then rises exponentially reaching a mean concentration of 150% of that in the adult by 28 to 30 weeks of gestation and is then maintained at that level until term. The serum α_2-macroglobulin concentration present at birth is either sustained at that level or decreases slightly during the neonatal period (Fig. 16). The concentration at 1 year of life may be higher than during the neonatal period (Hitzig, 1961), and it appears (Ganrot and Bjerre, 1967) that in adolescence the mean level is about 175% of the older adult. In the pregnant woman at term, the mean serum level of α_2-macroglobulin is from 103 to 110% of that in the nonpregnant adult of comparable age (Hitzig, 1961; Ganrot and Bjerre, 1967; Gitlin and Biasucci, 1969a).

I. β-Lipoprotein

As with α_2-macroglobulin, all fetal tissues including blood seem capable of producing labeled β-lipoprotein in culture. It is not clear at this time whether the source of the protein is the tissue or only the blood in that tissue, or whether the labeling of the β-lipoprotein is attributable not to synthesis of the protein but rather to synthesis of other proteins which may interact with β-lipoprotein. A comparison of the radiolabeled peptides released by tryptic hydrolysis with unlabeled peptides obtained from purified serum β-lipoprotein indicates that, in hepatic cultures at least, the labeled amino acids are incorporated into protein and are not simply bound (Gitlin and Biasucci, 1969a).

As pregnancy proceeds toward term, the serum β-lipoprotein concentration in the conceptus after 9.5 weeks of gestation actually decreases (Fig. 16): from values of 49 to 95% of adult levels at the end of the first trimester, the serum concentration decreases to values which are only 5 to 42% of the mean adult level. The phenotypes of β-lipoprotein found in cord serum at term may be discordant with those of the mother (Morganti and Beolchini, 1968), in accord with fetal synthesis of the protein. During the neonatal period (Fig. 16), the serum concentration may be somewhat erratic, but overall the levels present at birth are sustained, as might be expected (Gitlin and Biasucci, 1969a). Serum levels then increase, and may even exceed normal adult levels by 9 months of age (Hitzig, 1961).

J. Haptoglobin

The serum concentration of haptoglobin in the conceptus is quite low: of 21 sera from conceptuses ranging from 7.5 weeks to 41 weeks of gestation (Gitlin and Biasucci, 1969a), the concentrations in 12 were below the limit of detection which was 1% of the mean adult level (Fig. 17). The concentrations in the remainder were from 1 to 2.7% of that in the adult. Postnatally, the haptoglobin levels seem unpredictable, rising rapidly and dramatically in some neonates and falling just as rapidly and dramatically in others (Fig. 17).

It is possible that the low haptoglobin levels present *in utero* may be due in part to increased hemolysis in the conceptus, but this speculation has not been proved. Yet, the rapidity with which haptoglobin levels can rise during the immediate postnatal period suggests that the fetus at term

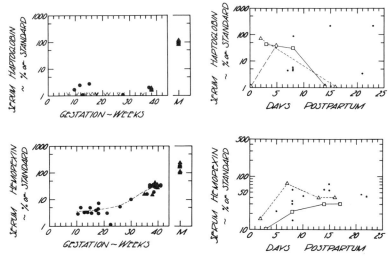

Fig. 17.   Serum concentrations of haptoglobin and hemopexin in the human conceptus and neonate. From Gitlin and Biasucci (1969a). See legend to Figure 13 for explanation of symbols.

has the capacity to synthesize much larger amounts of haptoglobin than may be evident from the levels present before birth. That the fetus can synthesize haptoglobin is substantiated by the observation that the haptoglobin phenotype in fetuses as early as 21 weeks of gestation may differ from those of the mother (Hirschfeld and Lunell, 1962).

K. Hemopexin

Hemopexin in the conceptus is synthesized by the liver and, to a lesser degree, by the lungs (Gitlin and Biasucci, 1969a). The serum concentration of hemopexin between 10.5 and 26 weeks of gestation ranges from 1.0 to 7.2% of the mean concentration in adults, after which it increases to reach an average of 30% of the mean adult level at term (Fig. 17) or only 18% of the maternal level; the maternal level averages more than 1.5 times that in nonpregnant adults (Table II). During the immediate postnatal period, the hemopexin level continues to rise (Fig. 17).

L. Transferrin

In the human conceptus, transferrin is synthesized by the liver and by the yolk sac (cf. Section IV). In an occasional embryo, the lungs also seem to have the capacity to produce small amounts of the protein (Gitlin and Biasucci, 1969a). It has been known for some time that the fetus can synthesize transferrin, since transferrin phenotypes in conceptuses as early as 9 weeks of gestation may differ from the maternal phenotype (Rausen *et al.,* 1961; Melartin *et al.,* 1966). Interestingly, at least some of the transferrin synthesized by the fetus may not be fully "mature": a small fraction of the transferrin present in cord serum at term may be deficient in sialic acid; this partial deficiency is corrected within 3 months postnatally (Parker *et al.,* 1963).

The serum transferrin level in the conceptus rises during gestation from a level of about 28 mg per 100 ml at 7.5 weeks to a mean of approximately 190 mg per 100 ml at term (Fig. 15); the maternal level at term averages 305 mg per 100 ml (Gitlin and Biasucci, 1969a). Postnatally, the serum levels are well sustained (Fig. 15), providing further proof of fetal synthesis, and then increase to reach the normal adult range by 9 months of age (Hitzig, 1961). A similar pattern of transferrin development has been reported by Toivanen and his colleagues (1969a) although their absolute levels for transferrin are somewhat lower overall than those just described.

M. Fibrinogen and Plasminogen

1. Fibrinogen

Fibrinogen synthesis in most human embryos starts at about 5.5 weeks of gestation, but for some, synthesis does not begin until as late as 8.5 weeks of gestation (Gitlin and Biasucci, 1969a). The site of synthesis is the liver. Although there appears to be some maternofetal transfer of fibrinogen (Fig. 2), the rate is relatively slow and the amount transferred is correspondingly small. At term, the cord plasma fibrinogen level averages about 70% of the level in the mother (Table II).

2. Plasminogen

The organs or tissues which synthesize plasminogen in the human conceptus are not known. Plasminogen can be detected in serum at 10.5 weeks of gestation, the earliest stage in which it has been measured (Gitlin and Biasucci, 1969a). The serum plasminogen concentration range during the first half of gestation (Fig. 13) is from 8 to 43% of the adult mean level and from 14% to as much as 110% during the second. There is a distinct trend toward an increasing plasminogen concentration as gestation progresses, the mean level in cord serum at term being 60%

of the normal nonpregnant adult (Table II). The average maternal concentration at term is twice that of the nonpregnant adult.

N. The Immunoglobulins

1. IgM

Synthesis of IgM in the human conceptus begins as early as 10.5 weeks of gestation, the site at this time being the spleen (Gitlin and Biasucci, 1969a). By 11.5 weeks some IgM is manufactured by peripheral blood cells as well as the spleen. The amount of IgM produced by the spleen increases gradually until at 15 to 18 weeks of gestation there is an abrupt increase in splenic IgM synthesis. At about 17.5 weeks of gestation, the thymus can also produce small amounts of IgM.

IgM has been detected in the serum of the conceptus as early as 13 weeks of gestation, the lower limit of sensitivity for the method used being 0.05 mg per 100 ml (Toivanen *et al.,* 1969b). However, the serum IgM level in most conceptuses between 10.5 and 15 weeks in this series was undetectable. In accord with the increase in IgM synthesis by the spleen at 15 to 18 weeks of gestation, more than half of the fetuses between 15 and 20 weeks have detectable serum IgM concentrations, some as high as 4 mg per 100 ml (Fig. 18). The level of IgM then increases steadily, and at term the mean concentration is about 13 to 15 mg per 100 ml; the standard deviation at term, however, is as great as the mean concentration (Toivanen *et al.,* 1969b). The serum IgM continues to increase postnatally, and reaches normal adult levels in about a year (Johansson and Berg, 1967).

Since there is little maternofetal transfer of IgM (cf. Section III,B,1), the concentration of bactericidal antibodies against gram-negative bacilli in the newborn is normally quite low (Kochwa *et al.,* 1961; Gitlin *et al.,* 1963). As the concentration of IgM increases during the first year of life, bactericidins and isohemagglutinins rise concomitantly.

2. IgA

Synthesis of IgA by the conceptus has not been clearly established. Although cultures of embryonic and fetal tissues in ^{14}C-labeled amino acids have failed to yield radiolabeled IgA, the negative results do not preclude synthesis which was less than could be detected by the methods used (van Furth *et al.,* 1965; Gitlin and Biasucci, 1969a). In instances of intrauterine infection, cord serum IgA levels may be higher than normal, suggesting either that the fetus at or near term may have the capacity to synthesize the protein, or that the placenta becomes abnormally permeable to the protein (Stiehm *et al.*, 1966; McFarlane and Udeozo, 1968).

Although it is generally held that IgA does not traverse the placenta, in fact it does, albeit exceedingly slowly; maternofetal transfer of IgA may be greater during the first trimester than during the remainder of gestation (Gitlin and Biasucci, 1969a). Concentrations of 10 mg or less per 100 ml between 6.5 and 17 weeks of gestation (Fig. 18) have been reported with levels of less than 1 mg per ml being found in fetuses during the last trimester (Gitlin and Biasucci, 1969a; Toivanen *et al.*, 1969b). In many instances, however, the serum IgA level is below detectable levels, or less than 0.2 mg per 100 ml. It should be noted that the mean serum concentration at term in the mother is approximately 210 mg per 100 ml. Following birth, the neonatal IgA level remains low

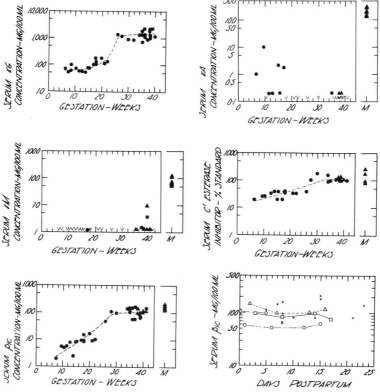

Fig. 18. Serum concentrations of IgG, IgA, IgM, C3 (β_{1C}), and C1 esterase inhibitor in the conceptus or neonate as a function of age. From Gitlin and Biasucci (1969a). See legend to Figure 13 for explanation of symbols.

until the third week of life and then increases slowly. Adult levels may not be achieved until the child is 4 years of age or even older (Johansson and Berg, 1967).

3. IgD

The human conceptus apparently can synthesize IgD in tissue culture beginning at about 11 weeks of gestation (D. L. Miller and D. Gitlin, unpublished). From 5 to 8% of normal infants have cord serum levels of IgD above 2 mg per 100 ml, IgD in the remainder being below this, the limit of detection of the methods used (Evans *et al.,* 1971; Leslie and Swate, 1972). The percentage of infants with detectable levels of IgD increases to 20% by 8 months of age and to 60% by 5 years of age. Only 80% of adults have serum levels of IgD above 1 mg per 100 ml.

4. IgE

Synthesis of IgE by the conceptus begins as early as 11 weeks of gestation, primarily in the lung and the liver (Miller *et al.,* 1973a). By 21 weeks the spleen participates in IgE production. Interestingly, IgE synthesis in adults occurs primarily in plasma cells in the lungs and gastrointestinal tract according to Tada and Ishizaka (1970), with lesser amounts produced by cells in the spleen and peripheral lymph nodes.

The serum levels of IgE in cord blood at term are approximately 1% of those of the mother at delivery (Berg and Johansson, 1969; Bazaral *et al.,* 1971); the mean maternal level is approximately 20 to 25 μg per 100 ml, depending upon the series. Because the low cord serum concentrations do not correlate well with the maternal levels, it has been postulated that IgE is synthesized by the fetus (Johansson, 1968) and does not cross the placenta (Bazaral *et al.,* 1971). However, not only is IgE synthesized by the fetus as noted above, but it also slowly crosses the primate placenta (Miller *et al.,* 1973b) in first-order fashion (cf. Section III,B,1). The apparent lack of correlation between infant and maternal levels at birth is not surprising, in view of the fact that the low cord serum levels are dependent in part upon fetal synthesis and in lesser part upon maternofetal transfer. At 6 weeks of age, the mean serum IgE level is 2.5 times that at birth, and at 6 months, the level has risen 10-fold over that at 6 weeks, or to about 25% of the mean adult level. As might be expected, since IgE synthesis appears sensitive to genetic factors as well as to environmental stimulation, the IgE levels at 6 months of age vary widely from individual to individual, the range extending from that of the newborn to that of adults (Bazaral *et al.,* 1971).

5. IgG

As is the case with IgM and IgE, synthesis of IgG in the human conceptus begins at about 11 weeks of gestation; synthesis at this time occurs in the liver and gastrointestinal tract (Gitlin and Biasucci, 1969a). As noted in Section IV,B, lymphoid cells are present in the mesenteric lymph nodes by 8 weeks of gestation and in peripheral blood by 10 weeks. Since the liver is an active hematopoietic organ from 2 to 7 months of gestation, it is not too surprising that the early liver is capable of producing IgG and other immunoglobulins, although it does not normally do so later. At about 15 to 16 weeks of gestation, the spleen begins to synthesize IgG and is the principal site of IgG synthesis by 17 to 18 weeks of gestation.

The changes that occur in the serum concentration of IgG during normal antenatal and postnatal development are as complex as has been found for any protein. IgG is present in the serum of the human embryo as early as 4.5 weeks of gestation, and the level from this point until 15 weeks of gestation is only 5 to 8% of the mean adult level (Fig. 18). The IgG present in the conceptus during this period is largely of maternal origin transferred to the conceptus across the placenta by a first-order process, possibly diffusion (cf. Section III, B,1); the IgG contributed by endogenous fetal synthesis is nil before 11 weeks and relatively insignificant between 11 and 15 weeks. After 15 weeks of gestation, the serum IgG concentration rises, and between 17 and 20 weeks of gestation the level ranges from 10 to 20% of the average adult level. This increase correlates in time with the increase in IgG synthesis that takes place in the fetal spleen. After 22 weeks of gestation, serum IgG increases rapidly to approximately maternal levels by 26 weeks of gestation. This rapid increase is attributable to the maturation or release of the active transport systems which carry IgG across the placenta (cf. Section III,B,2). From 26 weeks until term, the fetal serum level is similar to that of the mother. Because of the nature of the maternofetal IgG transfer process, i.e., an active but IgG inhibitable system operating most efficiently at relatively low maternal IgG concentrations superimposed on a first-order transfer mechanism, the serum IgG level in the infant tends to be higher than that of the mother when the maternal concentration is less than 1.6 gm per 100 ml and lower than that of the mother when the maternal level exceeds 1.6 gm per 100 ml (Edozien, 1965).

The serum concentration of IgG in the neonate begins to fall immediately after delivery with a half-life of about 30 days. This decline is due to the failure of endogenous synthesis to compensate for the amount of

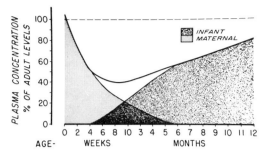

Fig. 19. Serum concentration of IgG in the human neonate as a function of the balance between the degradation of IgG obtained from the mother and the synthesis of IgG by the neonate.

IgG which must be degraded at the serum levels present (cf. Section II,A); as the decline continues, the lowered serum levels result in decreased rates of degradation, and when the rate of degradation equals the rate of synthesis, the decline ceases (Fig. 19). Since IgG synthesis takes a significant upturn at 2 weeks to 2 months of postnatal age, the falling rate of degradation meets a rising rate of synthesis, the two becoming equal by 1 to 3 months of age. The serum IgG level at this low point is usually 300 to 600 mg per 100 ml. As the rate of synthesis increases, the serum IgG level rises. Should the upturn in synthesis be delayed beyond 3 months, however, the serum IgG concentration may fall below 150 mg per 100 ml, and the infant is then highly susceptible to bacterial infection (cf. Chapter 7 on transient hypogammaglobulinemia of infancy). The normal child reaches adult IgG concentrations from 9 months to 5 years of age.

Based on structural differences in the heavy chain, IgG can be separated into 4 subclasses (cf. Chapter 1, Volume III). All traverse the placenta equally well, but each differs in the time and rate at which the postnatal increase in synthesis occurs (Morrel *et al.*, 1972). For example, serum levels of IgG3 at 1 to 2 months of age are about 30 mg per 100 ml, or approximately half of those in adults, but by 3 months of age, they recover to at least 75% of the adult level. The serum concentration of IgG1 also rises relatively rapidly after a low at 2 to 3 months, reaching adult levels at 8 months of age. On the other hand, the postnatal increase in the rates of synthesis for IgG2 and IgG4 are so slow that these subclasses are only half of the adult concentrations at 2 years of age. The postnatal serum changes described above for the total IgG class are, of course, a composite of the changes that occur in the subclasses. The subclass IgG1 constitutes approximately 61% of the total IgG in the adult, and IgG2 accounts for about 30% of the total IgG; the remaining 9% is divided between IgG3 and IgG4.

O. Some Complement Components and C1 Esterase Inhibitor

1. C3 or β_{1C}/β_{1A}

The third component of complement, C3, apparently can be synthesized by many different tissues in the human conceptus beginning at least as early as 29 days of gestation. The largest amounts of C3 are produced by the lung, liver, skin, and subcutaneous tissue and even in blood (Gitlin and Biasucci, 1969a; Adinolfi *et al.*, 1968). Since the macrophage, fibroblast, and lymphoid cell seem to be sites of synthesis for C3, it is not surprising to find C3 production to be a function of many different tissues (Asofsky and Thorbecke, 1961; Stecher and Thorbecke, 1967; Glad and Chessin, 1968). However, Alper and his associates (1969) have reported a conversion of C3 phenotype in a patient who had received an orthotopic liver transplant, the conversion being from the phenotype of the recipient to the phenotype of the donor. Thus, in the adult at least, the liver seems to be the principal site of C3 synthesis *in vivo;* the finding that large amounts of C3 are produced in tissue cultures may be related to the fact that fibroblasts grow much more readily in culture than other types of cells.

The serum concentration of C3 in the conceptus rises almost exponentially from a low of 1.9 mg per 100 ml at 5.5 weeks of gestation to a range of 52 to 167 mg per 100 ml between 28 and 41 weeks of gestation (Fig. 18); the mean level in cord serum at term is approximately 90 mg per 100 ml (Propp and Alper, 1968). The mean level in maternal serum is from 161 to 175 mg per 100 ml, depending on the series; thus the cord serum concentration at term is approximately half of the maternal level (Table II). Propp and Alper (1968) have demonstrated discordance in serum C3 phenotypes between mother and infant at birth; the data are in accord with the observation that C3 is synthesized *in utero,* and suggest that, if C3 does cross from mother to fetus, the maximum amount in fetal serum that could be of maternal origin must be *less* than 5% of the total fetal level, the limit of sensitivity of the phenotyping method used. The maternal serum concentration of C3 at term is slightly higher than in nonpregnant adults (Propp and Alper, 1968). It is interesting, therefore, that, although the levels are half those in the mother, the concentration in the neonate falls slightly after birth (Fig. 18) and recovers before the infant is 3 weeks of age. By 6 months of age, C3 concentrations are at adult levels.

2. C4

Synthesis of C4 by lung and liver, as well as by cells obtained from peritoneal washes, has been reported in conceptuses of 14 weeks of age or older (Adinolfi *et al.,* 1968). Sera from fetuses of 18 weeks or older contain detectable levels of C4, the concentration increasing steadily during development to reach levels about half those in maternal serum at term (Fireman *et al.,* 1969).

3. Complement Activity

The complement activity of fetal sera in terms of the ability to hemolyze sensitized erythrocytes seems to parallel the development of C3, C4, and C5, at least, each of which increases in like manner during gestation. At term the hemolytic activity of cord serum is approximately half that of maternal serum and adult levels are reached at 3 to 6 months of age (Fishel and Pearlman, 1961; Fireman *et al.,* 1969).

4. C1 Esterase Inhibitor

Interestingly, C1 esterase inhibitor is synthesized in culture by all tissues which synthesize C3 except blood. At 6.5 weeks of gestation, the serum concentration of the inhibitor is only 20% of the normal adult level; it rises steadily to reach adult levels by 28 weeks of gestation (Fig. 18). It may be noted that C1 esterase inhibitor levels in the fetus relative to those in the adult are higher than the relative levels of C1; e.g., the serum C1 concentration in the infant at birth is only half that of nonpregnant adults, while C1 esterase inhibitor at term is at adult levels. The average maternal serum concentration of C1 esterase inhibitor at term is slightly higher than the mean level in nonpregnant adults.

VI. Epilogue

In this chapter, we have tried to emphasize the obvious, i.e., that the concentration of a plasma protein, whether in fetal plasma or in maternal plasma, in interstitial fluid or amniotic fluid, is the result of a balance between opposing dynamic metabolic and physiological processes which proceed simultaneously. The plasma proteins present in amniotic fluid, for example, are largely of maternal origin, yet a fraction of each of them, and virtually all of one of them, is a product of the conceptus. The relative amounts of a given amniotic fluid protein that are derived from mother and conceptus will depend in part upon the development of the plasma protein in the conceptus; since most proteins in the conceptus are lower in concentration earlier in gestation, with the notable exception of α-fetoprotein, the contribution of plasma protein to amniotic fluid by the conceptus early in development will be correspondingly less than at or near term. Proteins leave amniotic fluid partly by diffusion but principally through fetal swallowing; little of the protein swallowed by the fetus reaches the fetal circulation, most of it being hydrolyzed in the fetal gastrointestinal tract. Yet some, however small the amount, does enter the fetal circulation, and some, including that of fetal origin, even reaches the maternal plasma. There is, of course, a much greater maternofetal exchange of plasma proteins via the placenta. As has been explained, different proteins traverse the placenta in different ways: some do not cross the placenta at all, but most, including even a molecule the size of fibrinogen, do so by a simple first-order mechanism. Still others cross the placenta by methods which are quite complex, involving cell membrane receptors and intracellular transport systems. Obviously then, the overall contribution of the mother to the fetal plasma concentration of a protein will differ from one protein to the next. Most of the IgG present in the conceptus, for example, even after fetal synthesis of IgG is at maximum, is of maternal origin. Yet IgG *is* synthesized by the fetus, and the transplacental transfer of fetal IgG from fetus to mother can induce maternal synthesis of antibodies against discordant IgG Gm allotypes synthesized by the fetus. For most proteins, however, the rate at which a protein is transferred from mother to fetus at or near term by whatever route is quite small compared to the rate at which the protein is synthesized by the fetus. In these instances, if the techniques used to differentiate the maternal contribution from protein synthesized by the fetus are insufficiently sensitive, as in some phenotyping methods, it may appear as if all of the protein in fetal plasma were of fetal origin. Similarly, the greater contribution by the mother to the plasma protein content of amniotic fluid may easily, but erroneously, lead to the conclusion that all of a given amniotic fluid protein is of maternal origin.

The maintenance of a plasma protein concentration in any of the body fluids of either mother or conceptus, then, is anything but static. With development, both antenatal and postnatal, an additional dimension is added: change. The relative impact on each of the factors which contribute to a plasma protein concentration shifts continuously during development, and not always in the same direction. As stated at the onset of this chapter, there is some apparent order to this chaos. But as chaotic as it may still appear, even a simple tabulation of normal change is essential, for without a knowledge of the normal there can be no diagnosis or understanding of the abnormal.

REFERENCES

Adinolfi, M. (1971). *In* "The Biochemistry of Development" (P. F. Benson, ed.), pp. 224–247. Heinemann, London.

Adinolfi, M., Gardner, B., and Wood, C. B. S. (1968). *Nature (London)* **219**, 189–191.

Allan, L. D., Ferguson-Smith, M. A., Donald, I., Sweet, E. M., and Gibson, A. A. M. (1973). *Lancet* **2**, 522–525.

Alper, C. A., Johnson, A. M., Birtch, A. G., and Moore, F. D. (1969). *Science* **163**, 286–288.

Asofsky, R., and Thorbecke, G. J. (1961). *J. Exp. Med.* **114**, 471–483.

Bazaral, M., Orgel, H. A., and Hamburger, R. N. (1971). *J. Immunol.* **107**, 794–801.

Berg, I., and Johansson, S. G. O. (1969). *Acta Paediat. Scand.* **58**, 513–524.

Brambell, F. W. R. (1966). *Lancet* **2**, 1087–1093.

Brambell, F. W. R., Hemmings, W. A., Oakley, C. L., and Porter, R. R. (1960). *Proc. Roy. Soc., Ser. B* **151**, 478–482.

Brock, D. J. H., and Sutcliffe, R. G. (1972). *Lancet* **2**, 197–199.

Buse, G. B., Roberts, W. J., and Buse, J. (1962). *J. Clin. Invest.* **41**, 29–41.

Chez, R. A., Smith, R. G., and Hutchinson, D. L. (1964). *Amer. J. Obstet. Gynecol.* **90**, 128–135.

Cohen, H., Graham, H., and Lau, H. O. (1973). *Amer. J. Obstet. Gynecol.* **115**, 881–883.

Dancis, J., Lind, J., Oratz, M., Smolens, J., and Vara, P. (1961). *Amer. J. Obstet. Gynecol.* **82**, 167–171.

Derrington, M. M., and Soothill, J. F. (1961). *J. Obstet. Gynaecol. Brit. Commonw.* **68**, 755–761.

Donato, L., Matthews, M. E., Nosslin, B., Segré, G., Vitek, F., Andersen, S. B., Mc-Farlane, A. S., Pavoni, P., and Yalow, R. S. (1966). *In* "Labelled Proteins in Tracer Studies" (L. Donato, G. Milhaud, and J. Sirchis, eds.), p. 375. European Atomic Energy Community, Brussels.

Edozien, J. S. (1965). *In* "Radioisotope Techniques in the Study of Protein Metabolism," Tech. Rep. Ser., No. 45, pp. 202–203. IAEA, Vienna.

Evans, H. E., Akpata, S. O., and Glass, L. (1971). *Amer. J. Clin. Pathol.* **56**, 416–418.

Fireman, P., Zuchowski, D. A., and Taylor, P. M. (1969). *J. Immunol.* **103**, 25–31.

Fishel, C. W., and Pearlman, D. S. (1961). *Proc. Soc. Exp. Biol. Med.* **107**, 695–699.

Freeman, T. (1965). *Ser. Haematol.* **4**, 76–86.

Ganrot, P. O., and Bjerre, B. (1967). *Acta Obstet. Gynecol. Scand.* **46**, 126–137.

Gitlin, D. (1974). *In* "The Placenta, Biological and Clinical Aspects" (K. S. Moghissi, ed.), p. 151, Thomas, Springfield, Illinois.

Gitlin, D., and Biasucci, A. (1969a). *J. Clin. Invest.* **48**, 1433–1446.

Gitlin, D., and Biasucci, A. (1969b). *J. Clin. Endocrinol. Metab.* **29**, 926–935.

Gitlin, D., and Boesman, M. (1966). *J. Clin. Invest.* **45**, 1826–1838.

Gitlin, D., and Boesman, M. (1967a). *J. Clin. Invest.* **46**, 1010–1016.

Gitlin, D., and Boesman, M. (1967b). *Comp. Biochem. Physiol.* **21**, 327–336.

Gitlin, D., and Kitzes, J. (1967). *Biochim. Biophys. Acta* **147**, 334–340.

Gitlin, D., and Koch, C. (1968). *J. Clin. Invest.* **47**, 1204–1209.

Gitlin, D., and Morphis, L. G. (1969). *Nature (London)* **223**, 195–196.

Gitlin, D., and Perricelli, A. (1970). *Nature (London)* **228**, 995–997.

Gitlin, D., Janeway, C. A., and Farr, L. E. (1956). *J. Clin. Invest.* **35**, 44–56.

Gitlin, D., Rosen, F. S., and Michael, J. G. (1963). *Pediatrics* **31**, 197–208.

Gitlin, D., Kumate, J., Urrusti, J., and Morales, C. (1964a). *J. Clin. Invest.* **43**, 1938–1951.

Gitlin, D., Kumate, J., Urrusti, J., and Morales, C. (1964b). *Nature (London)* **203**, 86–87.

Gitlin, D., Kumate, J., and Morales, C. (1965). *J. Clin. Endocrinol. Metab.* **25**, 1599–1608.

Gitlin, D., Kumate, J., Morales, C., Noriega, L., and Arévalo, N. (1972a). *Amer. J. Obstet. Gynecol.* **113,** 632–645.

Gitlin, D., Perricelli, A., and Gitlin, G. M. (1972b). *Cancer Res.* **32,** 979–982.

Gitlin, D., Perricelli, A., and Gitlin, J. D. (1973). *Comp. Biochem. Physiol. B* **46,** 207–215.

Gitlin, J. D., and Gitlin, D. (1973). *Pediat. Res.* **7,** 290.

Glade, P. R., and Chessin, L. N. (1968). *Int. Arch. Allergy Appl. Immunol.* **34,** 181–187.

Hirschfeld, J., and Lunell, N.-O. (1962). *Nature (London)* **196,** 1220.

Hitzig, W. H. (1961). *Helv. Paediat. Acta* **16,** 46–81.

Hochwald, G. M., Thorbecke, G. J., and Asofsky, R. (1961). *J. Exp. Med.* **114,** 459–470.

Ishii, M. (1973). *In* "GANN Monograph on Cancer Research" (H. Hirai and I. Miyaji, eds.), No. 14, pp. 89–98. Univ. Park Press, Tokyo.

Johansson, S. G. O. (1968). *Int. Arch. Allergy Appl. Immunol.* **34,** 1–8.

Johansson, S. G. O., and Berg, T. (1967). *Acta Paediat. Scand.* **56,** 572–579.

Jones, E. A., and Waldmann, T. A. (1972). *J. Clin. Invest.* **51,** 2916–2927.

Kochwa, S., Rosenfield, R. E., Tallal, L., and Wasserman, L. R. (1961). *J. Clin. Invest.* **40,** 874–883.

Laurell, C.-B. (1968). *Scand. J. Clin. Lab. Invest.* **21,** 136–138.

Laurell, C.-B., and Skanse, B. (1963). *J. Clin. Endocrinol. Metab.* **23,** 214–215.

Leslie, G. A., and Swate, T. E. (1972). *J. Immunol.* **109,** 47–50.

McFarlane, H., and Udeozo, I. O. K. (1968). *Arch. Dis. Childhood* **43,** 42–46.

Mårtensson, L., and Fudenberg, H. H. (1965). *J. Immunol.* **94,** 514–520.

Masseyeff, R. (1973). *In* "GANN Monograph on Cancer Research" (H. Hirai and T. Miyaji, eds.), No. 14, pp. 3–18. Univ. Park Press, Tokyo.

Masseyeff, R., Gilli, G., Krebs, B., Bonet, C., and Zrihen, H. (1974). *Proc. Int. Conf. Alpha-Feto-Protein, 1974* pp. 313–322.

Melartin, L., Hirvonen, T., Kaarsalo, E., and Toivanen, P. (1966). *Scand. J. Haematol.* **3,** 117–122.

Miller, D. L., Hirvonen, T., and Gitlin, D. (1973a). *J. Allergy Clin. Immunol.* **52,** 182–188.

Miller, D. L., Zapata, R., Hutchinson, D. L., and Gitlin, D. (1973b). *Fed. Proc., Fed. Amer. Soc. Exp. Biol.* **32,** 1013.

Morell, A., Skavril, G., Hitzig, W. H., and Barandun, S. (1972). *J. Pediat.* **80,** 960–964.

Morganti, G., and Beolchini, P. E. (1968). *Humangenetik* **5,** 98–106.

Morphis, L. G., and Gitlin, D. (1970). *Nature (London)* **228,** 573.

Nencioni, T., Brambati, B., and Crosignani, P. G. (1970). *Gynecol. Obstet.* **69,** 219–226.

Nishi, S., and Hirai, H. (1973). *In* "GANN Monograph on Cancer Research" (H. Hirai and T. Miyaji, eds.), No. 14, pp. 79–87. Univ. Park Press, Tokyo.

Parker, W. C., Hagstrom, I. W., and Bearn, A. G. (1963). *J. Exp. Med.* **118,** 975–989.

Pritchard, J. A. (1965). *Obstet. Gynecol.* **25,** 289–297.

Propp, R. P., and Alper, C. A. (1968). *Science* **162,** 672–673.

Purves, L. R., and Purves, M. (1972). *S. Afr. Med. J.* **46,** 1290–1297.

Rausen, A. R., Gerald, P. S., and Diamond, L. K. (1961). *Nature (London)* **192,** 182.

Rogentine, G. N., Rowe, D. S., Bradley, J., Waldmann, T. A., and Fahey, J. L. (1966). *J. Clin. Invest.* **45,** 1467–1478.

Rossi, T., Hirvonen, T., and Toivanen, P. (1970). *Scand. J. Clin. Lab. Invest.* **26,** 35–36.

Ruoslahti, E., Tallberg, T., and Seppälä, M. (1966). *Nature (London)* **212,** 841.

Seppälä, M., and Ruoslahti, E. (1972a). *Amer. J. Obstet. Gynecol.* **112,** 208–212.

Seppala, M., and Ruoslahti, E. (1972b). *Lancet* **2,** 278–279.

Seppälä, M., and Ruoslahti, E. (1974). *Proc. Int. Conf. Alpha-Feto-Protein, 1974* pp. 387–391.

Seppälä, M., and Ruoslahti, E., and Tallberg, T. (1966). *Ann. Med. Exp. Biol. Fenn.* **44,** 6–7.

Shokeir, M. H. K. (1970). *Clin. Genet.* **1,** 166–170.
Shokeir, M. H. K. (1971). *Clin. Genet.* **2,** 223–227.
Solomon, A., Waldmann, T. A., and Fahey, J. L. (1963). *J. Lab. Clin. Med.* **62,** 1–17.
Stecher, V. J., and Thorbecke, G. J. (1967). *J. Immunol.* **99,** 643–652.
Stiehm, E. R., Ammann, A. J., and Cherry, J. D. (1966). *N. Engl. J. Med.* **275,** 971–977.
Tada, T., and Ishizaka, K. (1970). *J. Immunol.* **104,** 377–387.
Takeda, Y. (1966). *J. Clin. Invest.* **45,** 103–111.
Toivanen, P., Rossi, T., and Hirvonen, T. (1969a). *Scand. J. Haematol.* **6,** 113–118.
Toivanen, P., Rossi, T., and Hirvonen, T. (1969b). *Experientia* **25,** 527–528.
van Furth, R., Schuit, H. R. E., and Hijmans, W. (1965). *J. Exp. Med.* **122,** 1173–1187.
Wladimiroff, J. W., and Campbell, S. (1974). *Lancet* **1,** 151–154.
Zizkovsky, V., and Masopust, J. (1974). *Proc. Int. Conf. Alpha-Feto-Protein, 1974* pp. 125–128.

7 / Genetic Alterations in the Plasma Proteins of Man

David Gitlin and Jonathan D. Gitlin

I. Introduction

The performance of a protein under any given set of conditions, whether *in vivo* or *in vitro,* is fundamentally dependent upon only 2 factors: the structure of the protein and the amount of the protein present, or stated more succinctly, quality and quantity. Both of these factors are, of course, subject to genetic modification, and to paraphrase a fundamental biological law, if change is possible it will.

A. Structural Variants

A detailed consideration of molecular genetics is beyond the purview of this discussion. It will be helpful, however, to remember that alterations in protein structure may result either from a deletion, a change, or an addition in a single base within the gene, or from more substantial changes such as occurs in unequal gene crossovers. Where there is a change in a single base of a given codon, a substitution of one amino acid for another in the protein may result, unless the base change results in a degenerate code for the same amino acid as before. If there is a deletion or an addition of a base in the gene, a shift in the "reading frame" occurs, and there may be an alteration in the structure of the resulting protein beyond this point; the alteration may be a change in amino acid sequence or a shortening of the chain or both. Where the change in base results in a nonsense codon either at that point or further along the gene short of its coding for the entire polypeptide, the polypeptide chain will be terminated at that codon. Unequal crossovers between genes can result in polypeptides much longer or much shorter than the accustomed variety, if the crossover is unequal and operative; the amino acid sequence in the longer chain would contain a segment duplicating part of the amino acid sequence, and both longer and shorter polypeptides may contain a new amino acid as a result of a new codon at the juncture of the crossing genes. Internal crossovers with deletion of portions of the gene can result in polypeptide variants that are shorter than the normal due to a loss of part of the amino acid sequence.

It is almost unnecessary to state that the detection of genetic modifications in protein structure is dependent upon the performance of the protein in the detecting system. Electrophoresis, for example, may readily detect protein variants in which a charged amino acid is substituted for one of opposite charge, but the same method may be virtually useless in discovering differences between proteins in which one uncharged straight chain amino acid is substituted for a similar uncharged amino acid. Ultracentrifugation may be useful in discerning protein products of unequal gene crossovers, but may be of little value in differentiating between proteins which differ by only a single amino acid. Assays of a protein's function may or may not be helpful in detecting variants, although the function of a protein depends upon its primary structure; a single amino acid substitution may either drastically alter a protein's function, may not change it at all, or anything in between.

B. Quantitative Variants

Modification of the amount of a given protein present in the cell or in the body fluids is genetically controlled either through synthesis or through degradation or both (cf. Chapter 6). Genetic control over the rate of degradation is expressed in part through protein structure, and a change in protein structure may be accompanied by a change in the rate at which the protein is degraded. On the other hand, genetic control over the rate of elimination of a given protein may also be expressed more indirectly; e.g., the rate of conversion of very low density β-lipoproteins to low density β-lipoproteins is dependent upon several factors including lipoprotein lipase, and a genetic deficit of lipoprotein lipase results in increased serum levels of the very low density β-lipoproteins.

Synthesis of a protein is also controlled genetically, both directly and indirectly. For example, the complete deletion of a gene or even the formation of a nonsense codon at the beginning of the polypeptide coding sequence will result in the *complete* absence of synthesis of the protein for which the gene is responsible. However, there are comparatively few examples indeed in which the synthesis of a plasma protein is *totally* inhibited genetically; in most inherited plasma protein deficiencies, at least trace amounts of the normal protein are actually synthesized. In these instances, it is not likely that the structural genes are actually deleted, but instead that synthesis of normal mRNA is deficient. A decrease in the amount of normal specific mRNA produced may result in a decrease in the rate of synthesis of the protein for which it codes. The deletion of a gene, the effective inhibition of a gene, or a decrease in the synthesis of normal mRNA are more or less direct genetic modifications of protein synthesis. On the other hand, inhibition of protein synthesis may be controlled genetically more indirectly. For example, immunoglobulins are synthesized primarily, but not exclusively, by plasma cells; genetic defects which interfere with the development of plasma cells, as in certain immunoglobulin deficiencies, will result secondarily in a decreased synthesis of specific immunoglobulins.

C. Genetic Variation and Polymorphism

The frequency with which a given protein variant appears in a population depends upon a number of factors. These include, of course, the rate at which the mutation appears in the population and the rate at which it is lost in the population. A protein mutation, or variant, is either beneficial, neutral, or deleterious in its effects on the host's survival and reproducibility. If deleterious, it is apparent that the mutant allele will be selected against in the population and that recurrent mutations will maintain the variant in the population only at relatively low frequencies. If the variant has a beneficial effect, and thus there is selection for it in the population, the population frequency of the variant allele will increase. When the gene frequency for the variant reaches a level in the population greater than can be accounted for on the basis of recurrent mutation alone, the gene is said to be polymorphic; i.e., polymorphism is the occurrence of two or more alleles in such proportions that the rarest of them is more frequent than could be maintained by recurrent mutation (Ford, 1940, 1945). Generally, the frequency of the least common allele is at least 0.01, or present in at least 1% of the population, before it is held to be polymorphic. When selection for a given variant is unopposed by adverse forces, the variant may eventually replace the normal allele, and the polymorphism is then "transient." The gene frequencies for the polymorphic forms become stable or "balanced" when the selective forces affecting them become balanced. Obviously, the gene frequencies for a given variant may differ from one population to another, since the selective forces, often obscure or unknown, may differ in different populations. Some populations may become so circumscribed by environmental conditions or cultural customs that a variant normally rare elsewhere may reach polymorphic levels within that population, dependent as always, of course, upon local selection conditions. On the other side of the coin, when a variant is so rare as to be restricted to only a few families, its relative uniqueness is sometimes noted by being referred to as a "private" variant.

II. The Albumins

Both structural and quantitative albumin variants are known. The structural variants can be divided into two major categories: one of these is the class of albumins which has been called variously paralbuminemia, bisalbuminemia, alloalbuminemia, or simply double albuminemia, and the other is a group of albumins which appear to be unusually prone to dimerization. The quantitative albumin variant is characterized by a marked deficiency in albumin synthesis and has been termed analbuminemia.

A. The Paralbumins: Structural Variants

1. Monomeric Variants

In 1957, it was found that human serum may contain more than just one class of albumins; Knedel (1958) and Nennstiel and Becht (1957) reported observing two electrophoretically distinct albumin bands in a single serum. Knedel called the disorder "double-albuminemia," and designated the two albumins as A_1 and A_2. Earle and his colleagues (1958) independently reported a similar albumin anomaly in 25 individuals of a pedigree of 56 living persons, and unaware of Knedel's study, termed the two albumins A and B (Fig. 1). It was evident even from these early studies that: (a) B was a genetic variant of A, and that A was probably normal serum albumin; (b) the presence of both albumin B (or A_2) and albumin A (or A_1) in the same serum represented the het-

PAPER ELECTROPHORESIS OF URINE AND SERUM PROTEINS

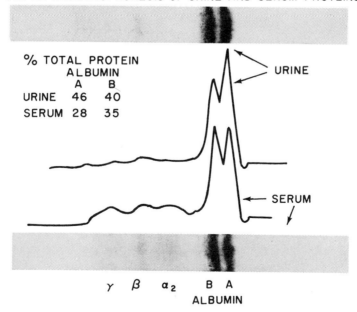

```
% TOTAL PROTEIN
     ALBUMIN
       A    B
URINE  46   40
SERUM  28   35
```

Fig. 1. Electrophoretic patterns of serum and urinary proteins of a patient heterozygous for a monomeric paralbumin, albumin B. From Earle *et al.* (1959).

erozygous state; (c) the total albumin concentration in sera containing both albumins was normal, the concentration of each of the two albumins being half of the total and equal to the other; (d) synthesis of albumin B probably represented a point mutation in gene A^A, an amino acid which was positively charged between pH 4.5 and 10 in albumin B being substituted for an amino acid with a free carboxyl residue in albumin A; and (e) albumins A and B differed in their relative ability to bind certain dyes, although the two albumins were indistinguishable immunochemically with the antisera used (Earle *et al.,* 1959). The anomalous albumin was not associated with detectable disease, and the equal expression of gene A^B indicated that genes A^A and A^B exercised equal influence over the rate of albumin synthesis. Although the two genes are said to be codominant, the use of this and similar terms for the expression of genes related to protein synthesis may be somewhat semantic in view of molecular genetic mechanisms involved. Certainly in the case of the double-albumin variation, A^B is neither dominant nor recessive to A^A.

Since these early reports, at least 20 genetic variants of albumin have been described in which the heterozygous state is characterized by the presence of 2 separate and distinct albumin bands on serum electrophoresis. To distinguish this form of structural variation from that typified by excessive dimerization, the term "monomeric variant" has been suggested (Weitkamp *et al.,* 1973). Unfortunately, however, only a fraction of the dimeric variant is actually in the dimer form, as will be noted below, the remainder being monomeric. In addition, the distinction between monomeric and dimeric variants is probably artificial, since both may be variations of point mutations, all being the products of alleles at a single albumin locus. Tertiary structure is dependent, of course, upon the primary structure or amino acid sequence, and the "dimeric" variant may still be the result of but a single amino acid substitution. Nevertheless, for the present it is at least convenient to separate the albumin variants into monomeric and dimeric forms, if only to distinguish the structural consequences of the mutations.

As general terms for the condition in which an individual possesses a genetic albumin variant, neither bisalbuminemia nor double-albuminemia are adequate. While eminently descriptive of the heterozygous state, the reader is reminded that only one albumin is found in the homozygous state and not two albumins. Paralbuminemia or even the later term alloalbuminemia would seem to be more acceptable general designations for the state in which an albumin variant is present, and the term paralbumin has been used to designate the albumin variant.

It is necessary to emphasize, however, that "normal" serum albumin is *not* necessarily a single species in different individuals or even in the same individual (Earle *et al.,* 1959). Albumin considered to be "normal" could, in fact, be polymorphic. A single amino acid substitution in the proper place in the polypeptide chain need not change the measurable gross properties of the albumin, especially if the substitution involves only uncharged amino acids. A suggestion of this possibility lies in the results of Sarcione and Aungst (1962), who reported that the albumin A found in their patient with paralbuminemia did not bind thyroxine normally. Other instances of anomalous binding behavior of the "normal" albumin in patients with paralbuminemia have been reported (Tárnoky and Lestas, 1964). Yet, if the "normal" albumin in these patients is, in fact, a polymorphic form of albumin, it would have to occur with relatively high frequency in the population, if one is to find it in association with a relatively rare albumin variant.

A collaborative group study of most of the genetic albumin variants thus far reported revealed at least 20 different monomers (Weitkamp *et al.,* 1973). The investigation was done using vertical starch gel electrophoresis at pH 5.0, pH 6.0, and pH 6.9; in this system, 14 of the variants migrated more slowly and six migrated more rapidly than the normal albumin component. The variants were distinguished from each other on the basis of their relative electrophoretic mobilities in the three buffer systems. Clearly, there will be others.

The most frequent albumin variant among Europeans and their lineage is albumin B; of the 29 European albumin variants reported, 18 seem to be the same albumin, albumin B (Weitkamp *et al.,* 1973). Tryptic digestion of albumin B yields two peptides and chymotryptic digestion yields one peptide not found in albumin A (Gitlin *et al.,* 1961). These data, coupled with measurements of the electrophoretic mobilities of albumins A and B from pH 2.5 to pH 12.1, indicated that a lysine residue in albumin B replaced a glutamic or aspartic acid residue in albumin A (Gitlin *et al.,* 1961). Support for this conclusion came from the data of Winter and his associates (1972): using trypsin and chymotrypsin to hydrolyze albumin Ann Arbor and albumin Oliphant, both slow migrating albumin variants, amino acid sequencing of anomalous peptides revealed that: (a) both albumins are the result of a point mutation whereby lysine is substituted for glutamic acid in normal albumin, and (b) both variants are the same, and are probably identical to albumin B.

The complete amino acid sequence of human serum albumin provided by J. R. Brown in advance of publication (J. R. Brown, personal communication, 1974) permits identification of the point of substitution and confirms the earlier studies. Winter *et al.* (1972) reported that the variant sequence is present in a chymotryptic peptide with the sequence Ala-LYS-Glu-Gly-Lys-Lys-Leu whereas the corresponding chymotryptic peptide from normal albumin had the sequence Ala-GLU-Glu-Gly-Lys-

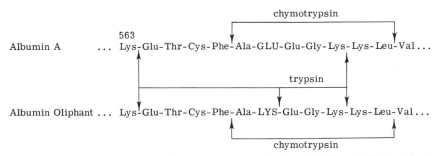

Fig. 2. Amino acid sequence of human serum albumin A and of albumin Oliphant in the region where the substitution of lysine for glutamic acid occurs. The arrows indicate the different peptides obtained by trypsin and chymotrypsin cleavage as shown by Gitlin *et al.* (1961) and Winter *et al.* (1972). The sequence of albumin A is shown beginning with Lys-563 in the complete structure kindly made available in advance of publication by J. R. Brown (personal communication, 1974).

Lys-Leu. Substitution of glutamic acid in the normal by lysine in albumin Oliphant gave a new point of tryptic cleavage yielding the variant peptide Glu-Gly-Lys. This is shown in Fig. 2 which gives the sequence of normal albumin beginning at position 563 in the provisional numbering system of J. R. Brown (personal communication, 1974). In accord with the early report of Gitlin *et al.* (1961) for albumin B tryptic digestion of the variant albumin yields two peptides and chymotryptic digestion yields one peptide not found in albumin A.

Reference to the complete sequence of human albumin given in Fig. 4 of Chapter 3, Volume I by Peters shows that the amino acid substitution occurs in the C-terminus of the albumin molecule, just beyond the last disulfide bridge. This small tail is apparently not essential to the compact disulfide-locked domain structure of albumin and hence is in an area more susceptible to mutation.

Monomeric paralbumins in European populations or in populations of European origin are relatively rare, the gene frequencies for the variants ranging from less than 10^{-4} among the English (Cooke *et al.*, 1961) to somewhat less than 10^{-3} among the French and Italians (Bonazzi, 1968; Fine, 1970). On the other hand, some albumin variants are so frequent among certain populations that the albumins are polymorphic. The gene frequency of albumin Naskapi, a fast moving albumin variant found in North American Indians (Melartin and Blumberg, 1966), is 0.138 among the Naskapi, 0.090 among the Montagnais, 0.07 among the Sioux, and approximately 0.01 among North American Eskimos. Albumin Naskapi has not as yet been reported in Caucasians, Negroes, or South American Indians. What selective advantage albumin Naskapi has that would result in this polymorphism is not clear, although Blumberg and his associates (1968) point to the selective binding properties of albumins in general as one possible factor: as noted earlier, different albumin variants may have different binding abilities for small molecules. At the other end of the scale, albumin variants have been found which seem to be unique to certain families in some South American tribes. Based on a study of such "private" variants involving 15 different serum and erythrocyte proteins, Neel (1973) suggests that the mutation rate among these Indians may be as high as 8×10^{-5} per locus per generation or about 8 times that assumed for other populations; he points to the high rate of chromosomal breakage among these tribes, and to mercury, infection, and hallucinogens as possible factors.

2. Dimeric Variants

In 1959, Fraser, Harris, and Robson described a genetic albumin variant identifiable by a retardation of somewhat less than 10% of the total serum albumin on starch gel electrophoresis. The individuals who possessed the variant were thought to be heterozygous for a gene necessary for its synthesis. In 1966, Laurell and Niléhn reported a similar variant characterized by a slight decrease in charge and solubility of approximately a fourth of the total serum albumin. On agarose electrophoresis, sera containing the variant showed an albumin band that spread cathodally more than normal. On vertical starch gel electrophoresis, the albumin band was not broader than normal, but there was a band in the postalbumin region which was shown to be albumin immunochemically; the band contained somewhat less than 10% of the total albumin. Normal serum produces a band of similar mobility under the same electrophoretic conditions, but in these instances, the amount of albumin in the band is only 1% of the total. After mild treatment with 0.1 M mercaptoethanol, the slow albumin band in both normal and variant sera disappeared. Laurell and Niléhn cautiously concluded that either the sera contained an albumin variant that was abnormally sensitive to dimerization or there was an increased amount of a positively charged substance which was bound to albumin, sensitizing the mercaptalbumin to oxidation. In 1969, Jamieson and Ganguly reported a similar dimeric variant: no differences could be found between normal albumin and the variant in the number or reactivity of the free sulfhydryls, but treatment with mercaptoethanol reduced only half of the dimer unless 8 M urea was also used. These authors concluded that the dimerization in this case was attributable at least in part to noncovalent bonds.

Weitkamp and his associates (1972) state that they could not detect any differences in mobility in either the monomeric or dimeric albumin zones among the albumin variants described by Fraser et al. (1959), Laurell and Niléhn (1966), and Jamieson and Ganguly (1969), implying that the three variants were the same. Wietkamp et al. (1972) also reported finding two additional dimeric albumins in South American Indian tribes, albumin Makiritare and albumin Yanomama. In the starch gel system used by these investigators, there were differences observed between these variants in the cathodal elongation of the monomeric albumin band as well as in the mobility of the dimeric albumin band. The cathodal elongation of the monomeric band and the cathodal mobility of the dimeric band was greatest for albumin Makiritare, less for albumin Yanomama, still less for the other three variants and least for normal albumin. There was a correlation between the relative cathodal spread of the monomeric band and the relative migration of the dimeric band. Therefore, Weitkamp and his associates (1972) concluded that the dimeric variants were probably monomeric variants with increased tendency to dimerize. In this regard, it may be noted that other monomeric variants may have structural instability: albumin Paris, which is a monomeric variant apparently identical to albumin Gomback, seems to be easily denatured on prolonged storage (Lie-Injo et al., 1971).

None of the paralbumins appear to be associated with specific disease, and as noted earlier, all appear to be products of alleles acting at a single structural locus. There is some evidence that this locus may be loosely linked to the locus for Gc globulin; the map distance between them is estimated to be 1.5% (Weitkamp et al., 1966).

B. A Quantitative Variant: Analbuminemia

In 1953, a 31-year-old woman was referred to Bennhold and his colleagues (1954) because she was found to have an elevated erythrocyte sedimentation rate. The patient was a field worker and appeared to be quite healthy. Electrophoretic analysis of her serum, however, failed to reveal any serum albumin. A study of sera from the patient, her brother, her parents, and 220 relatives disclosed (Bennhold et al., 1954; Ott, 1957; Bennhold and Kallee, 1959) that: (a) her total serum protein level and that of her brother was 4.8 and 5.4 gm per 100 ml, respectively, but both the patient and her brother lacked detectable serum albumin; (b) the total serum protein concentrations in the patient's father and mother were 6.3 and 6.4 gm per 100 ml, respectively, the albumin level being 3.3 and 3.1 gm per 100 ml, respectively; (c) no other instance of the serum albumin deficiency was found in the family. The disorder was called analbuminemia, and only 10 additional persons with analbuminemia have since been reported as of this writing. All but three of the individuals were adults at the time the condition was first discovered, and no definite disease or disorder other than a relatively mild edema seems directly linked to the analbuminemic state (Keller *et al.,* 1972). The three patients described by Irunberry *et al.* (1971) were 10 to 15 years of age when they were found to have analbuminemia.

1. Nature of the Defect

From what little data are available, it appears that analbuminemia is probably the homozygous expression of an autosomal allele. It is to be emphasized that albumin is not entirely lacking in at least some of these individuals: using an immunochemical method, Ott (1957) found only 1.6 mg of albumin per 100 ml of serum in the analbuminemic brother of Bennhold's patient. Although this concentration is but 0.005 times the normal, the presence of even this small amount of albumin is highly significant. In other patients, from 5 to 37 mg of albumin per 100 ml of serum have been detected immunochemically (Irunberry *et al.,* 1971; Keller *et al.,* 1972). If there is, in fact, only one structural locus for albumin, then the defect in analbuminemia cannot be a homozygous deletion of that locus. Since the analbuminemic individual can actually synthesize *some* albumin, the defect must be instead in the mechanisms which regulate the rate of albumin synthesis.

The reader need hardly be reminded that the genetic defect in one analbuminemic pedigree may not necessarily be the same as that in others. Higher serum albumin levels, from 0.15 to 0.29 gm per 100 ml, have been reported in other patients with analbuminemia before any albumin infusions were given, but these determinations were made using either salt fractionation or serum electrophoresis. Both of the latter methods are notoriously unreliable at low albumin concentrations. In this regard, Ott (1957) noted that although his patient had only 1.6 mg of albumin per 100 ml of serum when measured immunochemically, electrophoresis of the same serum revealed the presence of approximately 0.27 gm of protein per 100 ml of serum with the mobility of serum albumin at pH 8.6. The protein had a sedimentation constant of 3.39 S and was not related immunochemically, and hence structurally, to albumin.

That the lack of albumin in analbuminemia is attributable to a deficiency in albumin synthesis rather than to an excess in albumin degradation is indicated by the fact that the half-life of the protein in this condition is actually longer than normal (cf. Chapter 6, Section II,A). The half-life of albumin in normal individuals is approximately 15 days: in analbuminemia, the albumin half-life is about 50 to 115 days (Bennhold and Kallee, 1959; Waldmann et al., 1964; Keller et al., 1972). After the albumin level is raised to 2 gm or more per 100 ml by intravenous infusions of albumin, the albumin half-life ranges from 50 to 110 days in some patients (Bennhold and Kallee, 1959; Waldmann et al., 1964) or approximately the same as during the analbuminemic state. In other patients, the albumin half-life after the albumin level is raised is normal or 15 to 17 days (Keller et al., 1972). In either event, the paucity of serum albumin in analbuminemia cannot be ascribed to excessive degradation.

The similarity of the half-life of albumin at high and low serum albumin concentrations in some of these patients is in accord with other evidence (Gitlin and Janeway, 1960b) that the degradation of albumin may be a first-order process (cf. Chapter 6); i.e., the fractional rate of degradation, and hence the half-life, is independent of the serum concentration of the protein. Under these circumstances, since the half-life of albumin in analbuminemia is actually 3 to 7 times *longer* than normal, there would appear to be a defect in some patients in the rate at which albumin is degraded as well as in the rate at which it is synthesized (Waldmann et al., 1964). As to what this defect might possibly be, it is important to note that Brambell (1966) has suggested that both the degradation of plasma proteins and the transport of proteins across tissue barriers may have a common underlying basis (cf. Chapter 6, Section III,B). He proposed that plasma proteins are selectively bound by specific receptors on the cell membrane, and that, during pinocytosis, free plasma proteins together with receptor-bound proteins would be invaginated intracellularly. The unbound proteins would be degraded, but the bound proteins would resist hydrolysis and be released from the cell intact, or in effect, be transported. Applied to albumin metabolism, the hypothesis suggests that the fractional rate of degradation would be inversely related to the number and avidity of those cell receptors which bind albumin. Investigation has revealed that there are cell membrane receptors that selectively bind specific plasma proteins (Jones and Waldmann, 1972; Gitlin and Gitlin, 1973). The binding of a protein by cell receptors does seem to be a necessary initial step in the transport of the protein across a tissue barrier, but actual transport involves other mechanisms as well: a protein can be bound and not transported, but a protein is not transported unless it is first bound (Gitlin and Gitlin, 1973). If degradation of a plasma protein is inversely related to binding by specific cell receptors, the relationship is by no means absolute, and specific factors other than or in addition to cell membrane receptors determine the rate at which a protein is degraded.

It was mentioned earlier that analbuminemia is the expression of a pair of autosomal alleles. That the anomalous allele, which we shall term A^{ANA}, is possibly "recessive" is based on the accepted but unproved presumption that the normal serum albumin concentrations in the parents of analbuminemic patients reflect normal states of albumin metabolism. The rates of albumin synthesis and degradation, however, have not been measured in these parents. The serum concentration of a protein is a balance between the rate of synthesis of the protein and the fractional rate of degradation, or half-life; a rate of albumin synthesis which is only half of normal will result in a normal serum concentration if the half-life of the protein is twice normal (cf. Chapter 6, Section II). In the homozygous expression of A^{ANA}, synthesis of albumin is markedly deficient, and there is a 3- to 7-fold decrease in the fractional rate of albumin degradation. If the A^{ANA} allele had *equal* expression in the heterozygote and the other allele were normal, then the serum albumin concentrations in the parents of analbuminemic individuals *should* be normal. In other words, A^{ANA} may actually be equal in expression to the normal albumin allele and not "recessive" at all.

2. Clinical and Physiological Implications

Although a number of clinical conditions have occurred in patients with analbuminemia, none seems directly related to the analbuminemic state except persistent mild edema, hypotension, and an elevation of serum globulins including the lipoproteins. The rates of degradation of plasma proteins other than albumin are entirely normal, and their distribution between the plasma and extravascular compartments (cf. Chapter 6, Section II) is also normal (Waldmann *et al.,* 1964). Thus, the elevation in serum globulins is attributable to increased synthesis. When the serum albumin level is raised in these patients by intravenous infusions of albumin, the serum globulin levels decrease in relation to the increase in albumin concentration. Although part of the reduction in serum globulin concentration after albumin infusion is attributable to an expansion of plasma volume, half of the decrease is due to other factors.

The total serum globulin concentration in these patients ranges from 4.4 to 5.7 gm per 100 ml. The colloid osmotic pressure of analbuminemic serum is approximately half of normal (Ott, 1957) despite the paucity of serum albumin, evidently due to the elevation of serum globulins. Although patients with analbuminemia do exhibit some edema, the amount of edema appears relatively mild clinically, a surprising finding in view of the marked reduction in colloid osmotic pressure. Bennhold (1956) has suggested that the relatively low blood pressure which accompanies this disorder may decrease edema formation by decreasing the mean capillary hydrostatic pressure, but the latter has not been measured. Ott (1957) has suggested that the extravascular colloid osmotic pressure might be low in analbuminemia, and this would contribute to reducing edema formation. Although the distribution of globulins between extravascular and intravascular compartments is normal (Waldmann *et al.*, 1964), the volume of the extravascular compartment is expanded in this disorder and hence the concentrations of serum globulin in interstitial fluids must be less than normal, as indicated by Ott (1957). In view of the copious diuresis that occurs upon administration of diuretics to analbuminemic patients, intravascular to extravascular protein concentrations could easily be 10 or more to 1 instead of the normal 4 or 5 to 1 (Gitlin, 1957).

In view of the extreme ease with which analbuminemia can be diagnosed by means of serum electrophoresis and the widespread use of serum electrophoresis in hospitals and clinics in many countries of the world, it is surprising that so few patients with analbuminemia have thus far been reported. Since heterozygous advantage is the most important single factor leading to polymorphism, Cohen (1965) has pointed to analbuminemia as a probable reason for the apparent lack of albumin polymorphism; i.e., albumin may not be essential to life.

III. The α_1-Antitrypsins

Well over 20 different variants of α_1-antitrypsin have been recognized, and undoubtedly more are still to come (Fagerhol and Laurell, 1970; Kueppers, 1973). Collectively, they are known as the Pi system for the obvious reason that α_1-antitrypsin accounts for approximately 90% of the protease inhibitor activity of normal plasma (cf. Chapter 5, Volume I).

A. Structural and Quantitative Variants

Using acid starch gel electrophoresis in one dimension followed by electrophoresis at 90° into agarose containing specific antibodies, i.e., the crossed antigen–antibody electrophoresis method of Laurell (1965), α_1-antitrypsin can be separated into 8 different peaks or zones, the amount of protein in each peak being characteristic of the phenotype (Fagerhol, 1969). All alleles presently known appear to act at a single locus, and each apparently has equal expression. The eight peaks or zones are due to the microheterogeneity of α_1-antitrypsin.

The most frequent gene has been termed Pi^M, and of course, its product is type M α_1-antitrypsin. Variants are named in accordance with their relative electrophoretic mobility (Fagerhol and Laurell, 1970). At present, Pi^B represents the gene for the fastest variant and Pi^Z the slowest. Since the product of each allele behaves differently on electrophoresis, it has been assumed that the differences between variants are structural, presumably the result of point mutations. Among Europeans and North Americans, α_1-antitrypsin is polymorphic (Fagerhol and Laurell, 1970): the gene frequency of Pi^M ranges from 0.86 to 0.99, that of Pi^S ranges from 0.02 to 0.14, and the frequency of Pi^Z is from 0.01 to 0.024. The selective forces for this polymorphism can only be guessed at. Among Finns and Laplanders, Pi^S and Pi^Z are far less frequent.

In addition to being structural variants, type Z and type S α_1-antitrypsins are also quantitative variants: the concentrations of these variants in serum are much lower than for other Pi types. In individuals of phenotype ZZ, the α_1-antitrypsin level is only 10 to 15% of that in individuals of phenotype MM, the most prevalent phenotype (Ganrot *et al.*, 1967); i.e., the concentration of α_1-antitrypsin is approximately 25 mg per 100 ml in ZZ individuals as compared to 180 to 250 mg per 100 ml in MM individuals (Kueppers, 1972). It has been suggested, therefore, that each Pi^Z gene yields about 10 to 15% of the amount produced by each Pi^M gene, i.e., an amount equal to 7% of the total α_1-antitrypsin found in normal plasma (Ganrot *et al.*, 1967). Similarly, each Pi^S gene seems to yield about 60% of the α_1-antitrypsin produced by each Pi^M gene, i.e., an amount equal to about 30% of the total α_1-antitrypsin found in normal plasma. The average serum concentrations of phenotypes MZ and MS are, in fact, close to the predicted, about 60 and 80%, respectively, of that in type MM plasma (Fagerhol, 1969). There are data to suggest that the genes Pi^P and Pi^W may also yield lower α_1-antitrypsin levels than does Pi^M (Fagerhol and Hauge, 1968; Fagerhol and Hauge, 1969). In addition to these, there is one allele, Pi^-, which may represent a gene deletion: in the homozygous state no serum α_1-antitrypsin could be detected by any of the techniques used, including electroimmunoassay capable of detecting as little as 70 μg of α_1-antitrypsin per 100 ml of serum (Talamo *et al.*, 1973). As would be expected, type M$-$ individuals have lower α_1-antitrypsin levels than are present in individuals of type MM, but the phenotype in M$-$ individuals, of course, would appear to be type MM. In the absence of the homozygous state, Pi^- would be difficult to detect with certainty. In any event, it is highly desirable to confirm the absence of α_1-antitrypsin in patients of type $--$: in the complete absence of α_1-antitrypsin, Pi^- could represent a relatively uncommon example among plasma protein variants, a deletion of an allele.

Theoretically, the low serum concentrations of α_1-antitrypsin associated with Pi^Z and Pi^S could be due to decreased synthesis secondary to alteration of regulator genes. However, studies in patients with α_1-antitrypsin who developed hepatic disease have revealed intracellular hepatic accumulations of α_1-antitrypsin (Sharp, 1971; Sharp and Freier, 1972; Gordon et al., 1972; DeLellis et al., 1972). It has been suggested, therefore, that the α_1-antitrypsin deficiency in these patients may be due to a block in the release of α_1-antitrypsin from the endoplasmic reticulum of the cell (Sharp, 1971). Support for this concept comes from the fact that serum α_1-antitrypsin levels in type ZZ individuals increase only slightly in response to estrogen stimulation compared to the increases obtained in type MM individuals (Lieberman and Mittman, 1973); type MZ persons show an intermediate increase. Similarly, SS and SZ individuals show less of a response to estrogen than is seen with type MM. That the low serum levels of α_1-antitrypsin in individuals of either phenotype ZZ or — — are not due to increased degradation is suggested, but not proved, by the observation that the half-life of M type α_1-antitrypsin in such individuals is 5 to 6 days (Talamo et al., 1973), similar to that in normal individuals (Kueppers and Fallat, 1969).

B. Variants and Human Pathology

Individuals with primary α_1-antitrypsin deficiency are unusually prone to specific forms of either hepatic disease or pulmonary disease or both.

1. Hepatic Disorders

In 1968, Sharp et al. suggested an association between severe deficiency of serum α_1-antitrypsin and a familial form of hepatic cirrhosis which begins in infancy. Since then, at least two score such patients have been reported (Sharp et al., 1969; Johnson and Alper, 1970; Aagenaes et al., 1972; Porter et al., 1972), and many more have remained unreported. It has been estimated that as many as 20 to 25% of infants with hepatic disease may have α_1-antitrypsin deficiency underlying the disorder (C. A. Alper, personal communication). Of the reported patients, almost all had hepatic cirrhosis demonstrable in infancy or early childhood. Clinical manifestations typically begin during the first year of life with hepatomegaly or hepatosplenomegaly. Jaundice is often present and serum levels of hepatic enzymes are elevated. A few patients present as "neonatal hepatitis." Jaundice, when present, tends to disappear, but in almost all patients, the cirrhosis is progressive and may result in portal hypertension with all the complications thereof. In a

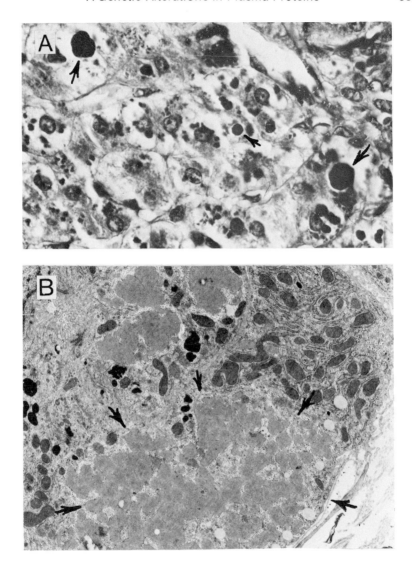

Fig. 3. Liver of a child who succumbed to infantile hepatic cirrhosis associated with α_1-antitrypsin deficiency. A. Light photomicrograph; arrows indicate intracellular hyaline masses of α_1-antitrypsin. B. Electron micrograph of a portion of an hepatocyte with α_1-antitrypsin mass at bottom outlined by arrows; endoplasmic reticulum at upper right; $\times 6200$. These photographs were made available through the generosity of Drs. E. Yunis and F. Sherman of the Children's Hospital of Pittsburgh.

rare patient with neonatal hepatitis due to α_1-antitrypsin deficiency, only a few residua may result. The disease is, of course, familial, and it appears in individuals who have very low α_1-antitrypsin levels; of those individuals with the disease who have been typed, the phenotype was ZZ. The hepatic disease appears as an autosomal "recessive" characteristic, although, of course, the Pi^Z allele has a penetrance equal to that of the other Pi alleles. As noted above, the liver in children with this disorder contains intracellular granules or masses of α_1-antitrypsin (Fig. 3), suggesting either a defect in the intracellular transport of the protein or a defect in the release of the protein from the ribosome (Sharp, 1971). Less than 20 to 30% of infants homozygous for Z type α_1-antitrypsin develop hepatic disease, and it has been suggested, therefore, that additional factors may enter into the α_1-antitrypsin deficient state to determine whether a given individual develops hepatic disease or not (Gans, 1972).

Hepatic cirrhosis associated with α_1-antitrypsin deficiency has been described in adults, and at least 3 such patients have developed hepatomas (Ganrot *et al.*, 1967; Berg and Eriksson, 1972; DeLellis *et al.*, 1972).

2. Familial Emphysema

Endowment with a ZZ phenotype is like being forced to voyage for a lifetime on a ship that must navigate a course between Scylla and Charybdis. And one should remember that at least one European or North American in approximately 1500 is phenotypically ZZ. If such an individual escapes the scourge of familial infantile hepatic cirrhosis, other potential dangers lie ahead.

Called by whatever name, chronic obstructive pulmonary disease or early onset familial emphysema, a rose may be a rose, but the disease can be disastrous. Soon after Laurell and Eriksson (1963) found α_1-antitrypsin deficiency, the association between the deficiency and emphysema in adults was made (Eriksson, 1965). The emphysema is manifest relatively early clinically, as early as adolescence in a few patients, but most often it appears in patients between 30 and 40 years of age. The disease is characterized by a loss of pulmonary perfusion, vascularity, and tissue at the bases (Guenter *et al.*, 1968; Levine *et al.*, 1970). This is most easily demonstrated using [133]xenon for pulmonary perfusion (Fallat *et al.*, 1973) and angiography for pulmonary blood flow (Welch *et al.*, 1969).

It has been estimated that approximately 1% of all emphysema is associated with α_1-antitrypsin deficiency. Although data are conflicting, it is generally felt that other α_1-antitrypsin phenotypes may also result in emphysema. There seems to be little argument that adults with phenotypes SS and SZ are prone to the disorder (Fagerhol and Hauge, 1969), but opinion regarding the susceptibility of MZ or even MS individuals is divided. It has been reported that [133]xenon ventilation can distinguish among ZZ, MZ, MS, and MM individuals, in accord with the concept that MZ and MS adults are more predisposed to emphysema than MM adults (Kanner *et al.*, 1973). Certainly individuals of phenotype —— must be prone to emphysema; in fact, this phenotype was discovered in a 24-year-old patient with advanced pulmonary emphysema (Talamo *et al.*, 1973).

Conversely, not all adults of phenotype ZZ develop pulmonary disease. Exactly how many such persons do escape is not clear, since onset of the disease may occur relatively late, but certainly many pass 60 without overt signs of pulmonary difficulty (Fagerhol and Laurell, 1970). Why some ZZ individuals develop emphysema and some do not is unknown, just as it is not clear why some develop familial infantile hepatic cirrhosis and some do not. Since it is generally thought that α_1-antitrypsin inhibits proteases derived from leukocytes and macrophages, alterations in the levels of these proteases or in factors which release them may be additional components in the development of the disease, or lack of it (cf. Chapter 5, Volume I). Although it had originally been thought that patients with emphysema due to α_1-antitrypsin deficiency do not develop hepatic disease, a combination of the two disorders has been reported (Glasgow *et al.*, 1973).

Respiratory distress syndrome, otherwise known as hyaline membrane disease of the newborn, has been thought to be associated with primary α_1-antitrypsin deficiency (Evans *et al.*, 1970). However, other studies have not been able to corroborate an α_1-antitrypsin deficiency in this disorder (Hyvarinen *et al.*, 1970). In any event, it has been shown that any α_1-antitrypsin deficiency in this syndrome, if it occurs, is temporary, and hence secondary (Evans *et al.*, 1972).

IV. The Ceruloplasmins

The color of ceruloplasmin is so startling and so strikingly beautiful, it is noteworthy that there are few experienced investigators indeed who have begun a discussion of the protein without mentioning it. The color, of course, as the name implies, is sky blue (Holmberg and Laurell, 1948) and is attributable to the presence of 8 atoms of copper per molecule of protein. The protein is an α_2-globulin (cf. Chapter 2), and its serum concentration in normal adults averages approximately 21 mg per 100 ml in

Orientals, 29 mg per 100 ml in Caucasians and Negroes, and 38 mg per 100 ml in American Indians (Shokeir, 1970). The changes that occur in serum ceruloplasmin concentration during human development are described in Chapter 6. There are at least 6 genetically determined structural variants of ceruloplasmin recognized as of the time of this writing, and one genetically related clinical entity in which the rate of ceruloplasmin synthesis is altered. The latter disorder is hepatolenticular degeneration or Wilson's disease (Wilson, 1912).

A. Hepatolenticular Degeneration (Wilson's Disease)

1. Clinical Considerations

Hepatolenticular degeneration is aptly named. In adults, it is characterized by a gradual deterioration of the cerebral lenticular nuclei and progressive cirrhosis of the liver. The neurological symptoms usually predominate in adults, and there is often only minimal clinical evidence of the hepatic disorder. In children, the hepatic aspects of the disease are paramount. Thus, the disease may present with neurological manifestations alone or with signs of hepatic dysfunction alone, or both together. The disorder is attributable to a genetic defect in copper metabolism: the tissues, particularly the liver and brain, have elevated concentrations of copper, and even the pathognomonic sign of Wilson's disease, the Kayser-Fleischer ring, is due to copper deposition in Descemet's membrane at the junction of cornea and sclera. Since 95 to 98% of the total plasma copper is normally in the form of ceruloplasmin (Holmberg and Laurell, 1948), Scheinberg investigated the level of ceruloplasmin in Wilson's disease and found it to be much lower than normal (Scheinberg and Gitlin, 1952).

2. Copper Metabolism, the Ceruloplasmin Deficiency, and the Genetic Defect

The amount of copper present in the tissues, and hence in the total body, is a balance between the amount of copper absorbed via the gastrointestinal tract and the amount of copper excreted. The primary route of copper excretion in man is normally via the liver into the gastrointestinal tract, with comparatively small amounts being lost from the plasma into the urine. When tracer doses of copper are administered orally to patients with hepatolenticular degeneration, the fraction of the dose recovered in the feces over a period of several days is less than in normal individuals (Zimdahl *et al.*, 1953; Earl *et al.*, 1954; Matthews, 1954; Bearn and Kunkel, 1955; Bush *et al.*, 1955; Jensen and Kamin,

1957). On the basis of these data, it has been suggested that the basic metabolic defect in this disease is excessive copper absorption.

When normal copper metabolism was studied in mice, it was found (Gitlin *et al.,* 1960) that copper given orally is absorbed by two different mechanisms: one of these is nonsaturable and first-order, the amount of copper absorbed by this process being directly proportional to the amount of copper presented to the gastrointestinal tract; the other is an enzymatic or carrier-mediated process which is saturable at lower doses of copper. Thus, whatever the oral intake of copper, the fraction absorbed depends upon the amount of copper ingested: as the amount of oral copper increases, the fraction absorbed decreases. When mice are given different amounts of copper intravenously, most of the copper accumulates in the liver within minutes, just as in man, and is then excreted into the gastrointestinal tract more slowly via the bile. The rate of biliary excretion is approximately proportional to the intravenous copper dose, and hence, is also proportional to the hepatic copper pool.

In view of the data obtained on the normal metabolism of copper in mice, it is interesting to note that the concentration of copper in bile in Wilson's disease is in the *normal* range, despite the increased hepatic copper pool that is found in this disorder (Denny-Brown and Porter, 1951; Bush *et al.,* 1955). Since the concentration of copper in bile is normally approximately proportional to the size of the hepatic copper pool, the presence of normal biliary copper levels in Wilson's disease in the face of an increased hepatic copper pool clearly denotes a defect in hepatic *excretion.* As noted earlier, the fraction of an oral tracer dose of copper recoverable in the feces of Wilson's disease patients is less than normal, and this has been interpreted as indicating excessive copper absorption. However, over the period of time that the feces are collected, a given fraction of the oral dose is not only absorbed, but part of the absorbed copper is actually excreted back into the gastrointestinal tract. The hepatic defect in copper excretion in Wilson's disease would prevent some of the tracer dose which had been absorbed from getting back into the gastrointestinal tract during the period of fecal collection, and less of the tracer dose would be found in the feces than normally even in the absence of *any* increase in absorption. The accumulation of copper in Wilson's disease, therefore, appears to be due entirely to the hepatic defect in copper excretion rather than to excessive copper absorption. The fact that the biliary concentration of copper in adults with this disorder is relatively normal is simply a reflection of the balance achieved between copper absorption and copper excretion. With a defect in excretion, the amount of copper in the liver will increase until the amount of copper excreted via the bile per unit time is equal to the amount of copper absorbed per unit time. The copper intake being normal, in the steady state the biliary copper concentration must also be normal, even in Wilson's disease.

Part of the hepatic copper normally reappears in the plasma as a component of ceruloplasmin, and about 95% of the total plasma copper is in this form. Approximately 5% of the plasma copper is relatively loosely bound to albumin. In approximately 95% of patients with Wilson's disease, however, the serum ceruloplasmin concentration is less than two-thirds of the average normal level, well below the normal range: in symptomatic patients, the average ceruloplasmin concentration is about 6 mg per 100 ml and in asymptomatic patients it is even lower (Sternlieb and Scheinberg, 1968). The *total* plasma copper level in Wilson's disease is also usually low, but this is attributable to the low levels of ceruloplasmin in these patients; nonceruloplasmin plasma copper levels in Wilson's disease are actually above normal. Approximately 5% of the patients with Wilson's disease have normal serum levels of ceruloplasmin, but it has been noted that these patients all seem to have severe liver disease at the time (Scheinberg and Sternlieb, 1963). Since ceruloplasmin levels are increased above normal in patients with hepatic cirrhosis due to causes other than Wilson's disease, it is presumed that in some of the Wilson's disease patients with severe hepatic disease who have ceruloplasmin levels in the normal range, the synthesis of ceruloplasmin is stimulated above the "basic" level. In favor of this view is the fact that when the serum ceruloplasmin concentration is only moderately depressed, it can be raised to the normal range by pregnancy or estrogen administration, both of which can increase ceruloplasmin levels in the normal individual as well (Cartwright *et al.,* 1960); Sternleib and Scheinberg, 1961; German and Bearn, 1961).

The deficiency of ceruloplasmin in Wilson's disease is due to a defect in the rate of ceruloplasmin synthesis, despite the fact that both nonceruloplasmin copper and hepatic copper are elevated. The half-life of unlabeled purified ceruloplasmin in patients with Wilson's disease is 5.6 to 7.2 days (Scheinberg and Sternlieb, 1960); when labeled with ^{67}Cu, the half-life of ceruloplasmin in two patients was 4.4 and 5.2 days, respectively (Sternlieb *et al.,* 1961). In individuals with chronic illnesses unrelated to Wilson's disease, radioiodinated ceruloplasmin was shown to have a half-life of 5 to 7 days (Gitlin and Janeway, 1958) and in one normal person, ^{67}Cu-labeled ceruloplasmin had a half-life of 5.4 days (Sternlieb *et al.,* 1961). Thus, there would not appear to be any increase in ceruloplasmin degradation in Wilson's disease, and the low serum ceruloplasmin levels encountered in this disease must be attributed to deficient synthesis.

It appears most likely at this time that the deficiency in ceruloplasmin synthesis is a secondary consequence of a more basic metabolic defect. It had been suggested (Scheinberg and Morell, 1957) that the absorption of copper from the gastrointestinal tract might be controlled by a dissociation of ceruloplasmin copper in the intestinal plasma: a low ceruloplasmin level would presumably result in increased intestinal absorption. However, the exchange of copper in ceruloplasmin *in vivo* is far too small for ceruloplasmin to function either as a regulator of copper absorption or as a transport vehicle for the transfer to copper from the intestines (Gitlin and Janeway, 1960a; Sternlieb *et al.,* 1961). That the copper in ceruloplasmin *may* exchange *in vivo,* albeit very slowly, is suggested by the slight difference in turnover rates between ceruloplasmin copper and the polypeptide moiety (Gitlin and Janeway, 1960a); ceruloplasmin labeled with radioactive copper does seem to have a slightly faster turnover in mice than does ceruloplasmin labeled in the polypeptide moiety with radioiodine. Although Sternlieb *et al.* (1961) state that ceruloplasmin copper does not exchange *in vivo* in man; a study of their data indicates that copper-labeled ceruloplasmin may indeed have a slightly faster half-life than polypeptide-labeled ceruloplasmin. Marceau *et al.* (1970) and Shokeir and Shreffler (1970) have proposed that ceruloplasmin functions to transfer copper to copper-containing enzymes such as cytochrome oxidase. Whether ceruloplasmin does serve in this capacity or has a slight function as a plasma oxidase, or both, must await more precise data on the turnover of ceruloplasmin, ceruloplasmin copper, and intracellular copper-containing enzymes.

It is clear that ceruloplasmin is synthesized in the liver (cf. Chapter 6). Although the presence of apoceruloplasmin, or ceruloplasmin less its copper, has been reported in normal plasma (Carrico *et al.,* 1969), copper apparently becomes an integral part of ceruloplasmin prior to release of the protein from the hepatocyte. Since an increase in the hepatic copper pool increases serum ceruloplasmin levels (Gitlin *et al.,* 1960), it would appear that the amount of copper in the hepatic pool shares in regulating the rate of ceruloplasmin synthesis. We would like to suggest, therefore, that the decreased synthesis of ceruloplasmin in Wilson's disease *and* the decrease in the hepatic excretion of copper in this disorder have the same underlying etiology: an enzymatic defect which prevents or inhibits the normal intracellular transfer of copper, either *from* a given copper pool to both bile and ceruloplasmin or, alternatively, *into* that pool.

About 20% of individuals who are heterozygous for the allele responsible for the metabolic defect in Wilson's disease have serum ceruloplasmin concentrations less than 20 mg per 100 ml (Sternlieb and Scheinberg, 1968). Interestingly, hepatic copper levels in heterozygous individuals average more than 3 times the normal (Sternlieb and Schein-berg, 1968). The data, at least superficially, are in accord with the expression of an anomalous allele which produces an error in the transfer of copper from or into the common intracellular pool as suggested above.

Clearly, the liver is not the only organ specifically involved in Wilson's disease. The brain also accumulates high levels of copper, a phenomenon not duplicated in normal animals given either a high copper diet or repeated injections of sublethal doses of copper. If the same defect postulated for the hepatocyte, i.e., an error in the intracellular transfer of copper, were present in such sites as well, it would account for the unusual tissue distribution of copper in this disease and the gen-eralized nature of the disorder. Even the leukocyte cytochrome oxidase deficiency observed in Wilson's disease (Shokeir and Shreffler, 1969) might best be explained on this basis.

Wilson's disease is inherited as an autosomal recessive characteristic; neither the parents nor the children of patients with Wilson's disease show any clinical symptoms of the disorder, although chemical signs of the anomalous allele are usually present as noted above. By restricting copper intake and by increasing the excretion of copper via the urine with such agents as D-penicillamine, the tissue copper pool in patients with Wilson's disease can be reduced. Such therapy can ameliorate symptomatology in affected patients or prevent symptoms in patients still asymptomatic (Sternlieb and Scheinberg, 1968).

B. Structural Variants

Ceruloplasmin B, or CpB, is the predominating form of this protein in all races. Although variants of ceruloplasmin seem to be rare among Caucasians, at least four structural variants of CpB have been found among Negroes and a fifth, CpTh, has been observed in Thailand (Sho-keir and Shreffler, 1970; Shokeir, 1971). In order of their decreasing electrophoretic mobility in starch gel at pH 9, the ceruloplasmin variants are CpA, CpBpt (for Bridgeport), CpNH (for New Haven), and CpC. Ceruloplasmin B migrates between CpBpt and CpNH under these con-ditions, and CpTh is said to have a mobility similar to that of CpA. Ceruloplasmins B, A, and NH are polymorphic among Negroes; the other ceruloplasmins have gene frequencies of less than 0.3%. The alleles appear to have equal expression in the heterozygous state. Each of the ceruloplasmins seem to have the same molecular size, although each displays a small degree of polymerization (Shokeir, 1971); under the best of testing conditions, the amount of ceruloplasmin which is found in the polymerized state is not more than 2 to 3% of the total (Poulik and Bearn, 1962). The structural differences between ceruloplasmins, therefore, are presumed to be amino acid substitutions arising as a consequence of point mutations.

V. The Transferrins

More than a score of transferrin variants have thus far been reported, each of the alleles acting at a single locus and each having equal expression (cf. Chapter 6, Volume I). All but one of these appear to be structural variants; one, at least, is a quantitative variant resulting in congenital atransferrinemia.

A. Structural Variants

The universal transferrin, i.e., the transferrin present in all population groups in highest frequency by far, is called transferrin C or TfC. At least 20 variants are now recognized which differ from TfC in electrophoretic mobility in starch gels. Those transferrins which migrate faster than TfC under standard conditions are termed Type B transferrins, TfB, and those which migrate more slowly are designated as Type D transferrins, TfD. To unify the classification of these variants and to provide sufficient flexibility of the classification to include new ones when recognized, the transferrins are designated first as to type and then identified by subscripts which reflect their relative electrophoretic mobilities or their origin. Thus, variant TfB_{0-1} has an electrophoretic mobility slower than TfB_0 and faster than TfB_1; similarly, TfD_{0-1} is slower than TfD_0 which in turn is slower than TfC. The subscript system becomes less than ideal when transferrin types are designated by subscripts of origin rather than relative mobility; the relative mobilities of such transferrins as D_{Wigan}, $D_{Finland}$, and $D_{Adelaide}$ may be somewhat difficult to remember. Most transferrin variants are relatively rare, but a few are polymorphic in some populations (Parker and Bearn, 1961): the gene frequency for TfD_1 among Negroes, for example, is 0.06, while that for TfB_{0-1} among certain North American Indians is 0.04 and the frequency of TfD_{Chi} among Chinese is 0.03.

The differences between these electrophoretic variants seem to be structural, probably due to point mutation, since transferrin is a single polypeptide chain. Single amino acid substitutions have been described for several variants (Wang *et al.,* 1966, 1967a,b). As noted above, each of the alleles seems to act at a single locus, and each has equal expression.

B. Congenital Atransferrinemia: A Quantitative Variant

At least four patients with hereditary deficiency of transferrin have been reported to date (Heilmeyer *et al.,* 1961; Cáp *et al.,* 1968; Sakata, 1969; Goya *et al.,* 1972). In only one of these patients was serum transferrin not detected; immunochemical assays indicated the presence of less than 3 mg to as much as 39 mg per 100 ml of serum in the remaining 3. The amounts of transferrin found were not due to preceding transfusions, and hence, in these children, the deficiency would seem to represent a defect in the regulation of transferrin synthesis rather than a structural gene deletion. Each of the patients had marked hypochromic anemia beginning in early infancy and required repeated blood transfusions. In accord with the marked deficiency in serum transferrin, total iron binding capacity of the serum was from 10 to 20% of normal, and serum iron was less than a third of normal. The half-life of radioiodinated transferrin in one patient was found to be 7 days as compared to a range of 6.9 to 8.0 days in five other members of the family (Goya *et al.,* 1972); the half-life of transferrin in normal individuals is 6.7 to 8.4 days (Katz, 1961). Thus, the transferrin defect in this patient was one of synthesis. The half-time of plasma iron clearance was 25 min as compared to the normal of 80 to 120 min, indicating a more rapid turnover of iron in the transferrin present (Goya *et al.,* 1972).

The parents of these children had low serum transferrin concentrations, about half of normal, suggesting that each of the two alleles, the normal and the anomalous, have equal expression. Two of the patient's siblings in one family, a brother and a sister, had serum transferrin levels of 12 to 14 mg per 100 ml (Goya *et al.,* 1972); a third sibling, a brother, had a transferrin level of 135 mg per 100 ml. The normal serum transferrin level is from 200 to 300 mg per 100 ml. Thus, congenital atransferrinemia seems to represent the homozygous expression of an autosomal allele.

Transferrin, of course, is responsible for the transport of iron in plasma, and the protein has a special affinity for immature red cells. The administration of transferrin in one patient resulted in a modest increase in reticulocytes followed by an increase in hemoglobin (Goya *et al.,* 1972). The infusion of transferrin in this patient at intervals of 3 to 6 months resulted in a similar response each time which was sustained for several months. The data are in accord with the role of transferrin in the transfer of iron for hemopoiesis. Interestingly, Goya *et al.* (1972) observed an increase in gastrointestinal iron absorption after an oral dose, indicating to these investigators that transferrin may not be essential for iron absorption.

It is a bit disturbing to note that the siblings of Goya's patient had serum transferrin levels of only 12 to 14 mg per 100 ml, but did not have anemia (Goya *et al.,* 1972). Admittedly, the patient had increased hemoglobin synthesis and reticulocyte formation when sufficient transferrin had been infused to raise the serum transferrin level from less than 3 mg per 100 ml before infusion to 15 mg per 100 ml after the infusion. However, at transferrin levels of 12 to 14 mg per 100 ml, the siblings were probably homozygous for the anomalous allele, yet they did *not* have anemia even at 6 and 9 years of age, respectively. It would seem then that severe hypochromic anemia may not be an inevitable consequence of congenital atransferrinemia, depending upon other factors as well.

VI. The Immunoglobulins

In 1952, three children who had had repeated serious infections since infancy were reported to have an absence of "γ-globulin" in their sera on moving boundary electrophoresis (Bruton *et al.,* 1952); the disorder was called agammaglobulinemia (Bruton, 1952). Soon thereafter it was observed that patients with agammaglobulinemia lacked not only "γ-globulin" but also two additional proteins that were found to be present in normal serum; the presence of the two proteins in normal serum was noted only as a consequence of their apparent absence in agammaglobulinemic serum (Gitlin *et al.,* 1956). The two proteins were easily distinguished from "γ-globulin" and from each other with appropriate antisera, and their absence in agammaglobulinemia assured them a firm role as "immune globulins." After a progression of names, the two proteins became known as γM or IgM and γA or IgA; of course, what was then identified simply as "γ-globulin" became γG or IgG. Since then, two additional immunoglobulin classes have been identified, γD or IgD and γE or IgE.

A committee of World Health Organization (WHO) has since recommended that the symbol γ not be used to identify the immunoglobulins (World Health Organization, 1972) because γ is also used to identify the heavy chain of IgG (cf. Chapter 1, Volume III). Thus, the five classes of human immunoglobulins are to be designated IgG, IgA, IgM, IgD, and IgE. This rule will be followed in the present discussion.

Before entering the morass known colloquially as "the immunoglobulin deficiencies," a brief review of normal immunoglobulin metabolism is definitely in order.

A. Normal Immunoglobulin Metabolism

1. The Assay of Immunoglobulins

Structurally, the immunoglobulins are almost bewilderingly heterogeneous even within a given immunoglobulin class. This heterogeneity is entirely genetically determined, and is only in part related to the varied functions of the immunoglobulins as specific antibodies (cf. Chapters 1 and 2, Volume III). The IgG class of immunoglobulins, for example, is presently divided into four subclasses based on antigenic, and hence structural, differences in the γ chain, and each of the four subclasses can be divided further into allotypes based on antigenically different Gm groups. In fact, every specific antibody differs structurally from all other antibodies, even of the same immunoglobulin class or subclass, which have different specificities. Even two immunoglobulin molecules which react specifically with the same hapten or antigen may not have the same primary structure.

Immunoglobulin concentrations in body fluids are most accurately determined at present by immunochemical techniques: an antiserum is prepared against a specific class or subclass of immunoglobulins, and the antiserum is then used to assay the immunoglobulin by a variety of methods, including precipitation in liquids or gels, with and without the adjunct use of radioisotopic labeling of either the antigen or the antibody. It is a rather widespread delusion, however, that the techniques currently employed, regardless of the degree of sophistication of either the method or the investigator, provide more than just an acceptable approximation of the immunoglobulin concentration. As noted above, the immunoglobulins being assayed are remarkably heterogeneous in structure, and hence equally heterogeneous in the sites which may react with the antiserum; in addition, the antibodies in the antiserum are likewise heterogeneous in both structure and specificity, since these, too, are immunoglobulins. Thus, unless the immunoglobulin used as a standard or reference for the assay method is structurally identical to the immunoglobulin being assessed, a condition rarely fulfilled, the relative estimations of immunoglobulin can be only approximate. Unless two different antisera are identical in every way in terms of hapten specificity, quantity, and class of every antibody in those antisera, a condition also rarely fulfilled, comparison of immunoglobulin values obtained with the two antisera must also be approximate. The WHO has recommended and implemented the use of specific sera to be employed as international immunoglobulin reference standards for assaying serum immunoglobulin concentrations in an attempt to obviate some of these difficulties. Unfortunately, the use of an international reference standard does not help in estimating absolute immunoglobulin levels. Also, it can accomplish little more, and perhaps less, in standardizing immunoglobulin levels estimated in different laboratories than if each laboratory used its own large, local normal serum pool as a reference standard. A universal "standard" cannot solve the critical problem of differences in immunoglobulins from one serum to the next nor the differences in antibodies from one antiserum to the next. Now that these caveats have been offered the reader, serum immunoglobulin determinations obtained by immunochemical methods *can* be very useful clinically, because normal biological variation in immunoglobulin metabolism is broader than the degree of uncertainty in the determinations.

2. Sites of Synthesis

The normal development of immunoglobulin metabolism, both antenatally and postnatally, is given in Chapter 6; the serum concentration of each immunoglobulin class or subclass is age dependent.

Synthesis of the plasma immunoglobulins occurs in lymphoid cells, primarily in plasma cells but also in some lymphocytes. A given cell produces only one class of immunoglobulins and may produce only a given subgroup of a given class of immunoglobulins (Mellors and Korngold, 1963; Solomon *et al.*, 1963b; Bernier and Cebra, 1964; Lundberg *et al.*, 1965). Light chains and heavy chains for a given specific immunoglobulin are synthesized in the same cell (Bernier and Cebra, 1964). In fact, most cells which produce antibodies will synthesize antibodies which will react with only one antigen, although some cells will produce two antibodies and perhaps more (Attardi *et al.*, 1964). Thus, the cells which synthesize immunoglobulins produce immunoglobulin molecules of only one specific structure or at most a limited number of structures within the same immunoglobulin subgroup. Cells which synthesize IgM can be distinguished morphologically in certain abnormal conditions such as dysgammaglobulinemia or Waldenström's macroglobulinemia, and these cells are lymphocytoid, i.e., neither mature plasma cells nor lymphocytes and resembling most closely the transitional phases of the plasma cells which synthesize IgG (Dutcher and Fahey, 1959; Kritzman *et al.*, 1961; Cruchaud *et al.*, 1962). Only a small fraction of tissue lymphoid cells are engaged in significant immunoglobulin synthesis, at least at the same time (Gitlin and Sasaki, 1969). Immunoglobulins also seem to be produced in some cells of the germinal follicles of lymphoid organs (Gitlin et al., 1953; Craig et al., 1954; Coons et al., 1955). Although IgG is consistently found in the Hassall's corpuscles of the thymus, its significance at this site is not clear (Gitlin et al., 1953).

Approximately 20% of the peripheral blood lymphocytes carry immunoglobulins on the surface of their cell membranes detectable by means of fluorescent antibodies against μ, γ, and α chains (Pernis et al., 1970; Papamichail et al., 1971). From 25% to more than 90% of the cells which carry surface-bound immunoglobulins seem to carry IgM; less than half of the cells carry IgG and less than 10% carry IgA. This is in sharp contrast to the numbers of tissue lymphoid cells with ribosomal-bound immunoglobulin: in the tonsil, for example, only one in approximately 7000 cells contains detectable IgG, one in 67,000 cells contains IgA and but one in 190,000 contains IgM (Gitlin and Sasaki, 1969). In those tonsillar lymphoid cells which contain ribosomal-bound immunoglobulin, the average amount of IgA per cell is 5.6 times the amount of IgG per cell, and the amount of IgM per cell is 3.7 times the amount of IgG per cell. Multiplying the average cell content of specific immunoglobulin by the number of cells producing that protein, the tonsillar content of ribosomal-bound IgG is almost twice that of IgA and almost 8 times that of IgM; the normal rate of synthesis of IgG in the total body, interestingly enough, is twice that of IgA and 5 times that of IgM. Whatever the nature of the immunoglobulins bound to peripheral blood lymphocytes, it would seem unlikely that the immunoglobulins are products of most of the cells which carry them. Despite the plethora of theories regarding "T" and "B" cells and the relationship of the immunoglobulin-bearing lymphocytes to "B" cells, little is really known about the function or origin of these cells. Perhaps the most persuasive suggestion is that the surface-bound immunoglobulin provides the lymphocyte with a mechanism for the identification of a specific antigen with consequent stimulation, multiplication, transformation when appropriate, and antibody synthesis.

B. Primary Deficiencies in Immunoglobulin Synthesis: Quantitative Variants

The synthesis of each of the immunoglobulin classes in man is a genetically determined characteristic which is independent of the synthesis of the others (Gitlin, 1967). Thus, a genetic insufficiency in the synthesis of one may occur either alone or in combination with an insufficiency in the synthesis of any or all of the others. For example, deficient synthesis of

TABLE I

Synthesis of IgG, IgA, and IgM: Clinical Combinations Thus Far Reported

Clinical state	*IgG*	*IgA*	*IgM*
A. With normal numbers of small lymphocytes			
Normal individual	+[a]	+	+
Agammaglobulinemia	−	−	−
IgG, IgA deficiency	−	−	+
(dysgammaglobulinemia type 1)			
IgG, IgM deficiency	−	+	−
IgA, IgM deficiency	+	−	−
(dysgammaglobulinemia type 2)			
IgG deficiency	−	+	+
(dysgammaglobulinemia type 3)			
IgM deficiency	+	+	−
(dysgammaglobulinemia type 4)			
IgA deficiency	+	−	+
B. With thymic alymphoplasia			
Normal or elevated immunoglobulins	+	+	+
Agammaglobulinemia	−	−	−
IgG, IgA deficiency	−	−	+
IgG deficiency	−	+	+
IgM deficiency	+	+	−

[a] + indicates normal or increased; − indicates markedly deficient.

the three major immunoglobulins IgG, IgM, and IgA, alone or in combination, could result in seven different deficiency states as indicated in Table I. Clinical instances of each of these seven possible variations have now been reported, and all but two of these have been shown to be inheritable; whether the latter two deficiency states, i.e., IgA, IgM deficiency and IgM deficiency alone, are also inheritable remains to be proved. Agammaglobulinemia, as noted above, is characterized by deficient synthesis of each of the three major immunoglobulin classes: the serum concentration of IgG is less than 100 mg per 100 ml, and both serum IgM and IgA are either undetectable or almost entirely absent. The dysgammaglobulinemias are characterized by a deficiency in the synthesis of one or more immunoglobulin classes in the presence of normal or increased synthesis of at least one immunoglobulin class.

1. The Agammaglobulinemias

a. CLINICAL VARIANTS. There are *at least* three different major genetic variants of agammaglobulinemia: two of these are "congenital" and the third occurs in adolescents and adults. A fourth form of agammaglobulinemia is a transient state appearing in infants (Gitlin, 1955).

i. Congenital agammaglobulinemia. There are two genetically different forms of congenital agammaglobulinemia; the more common variant of the two is inherited as an X-linked recessive characteristic appearing in males; the other, even more rare, is an autosomal recessive trait manifested in both males and females. Each of these two forms of agammaglobulinemia is probably genetically heterogeneous, since each seems to include two or more variants.

Interestingly, in the majority of children with congenital agammaglobulinemia the severe recurrent bacterial infections that typify this disorder usually do *not* begin until the child is between 9 months and 2 years of life, although it may start earlier in some. The reason for a relatively late onset of infections in some children when the disorder is presumed to be congenital is not clear; certainly virtually all IgG of maternal origin has been degraded by the infant before 9 months of age (cf. Chapter 6, Section V,N). It is of note, therefore, that one child with indisputable X-linked congenital agammaglobulinemia, who had his first serious infection at age $2\frac{1}{2}$ years when his serum IgG level was only 20 mg per 100 ml, was known to have a serum IgG level of 500 mg per 100 ml at 5 months of age (Gitlin, 1966). A serum IgG concentration of 500 mg per 100 ml is far too high for a child of 5 months who supposedly was unable to synthesize IgG from birth (cf. Chapter 6). Thus, this child was able to synthesize a significant amount of IgG during infancy. It would seem, therefore, that "congenital" X-linked agammaglobulinemia may occur in some children as an hereditary abiotrophy; i.e., attributable to a gene of decreased penetrance with expression manifested during the first 3 years of life.

ii. Adult agammaglobulinemia. The majority of the patients with this form of agammaglobulinemia are between 17 and 54 years of age at the time of onset of their recurrent infections, although one patient was as young as 7 years and another as old as 71 years. In a few patients, adult agammaglobulinemia is clearly inherited as an autosomal recessive characteristic. However, in most patients, an hereditary basis to the disorder cannot be demonstrated. Of all reported patients with adult agammaglobulinemia, approximately a third are females. The relationship between this disorder and the form of congenital agammaglobulinemia which is attributable to an autosomal recessive allele is not clear; delayed expression of the latter would yield "adult" agammaglobulinemia.

iii. Transient hypogammaglobulinemia of infancy. The serum IgG concentration present in the infant at birth is approximately equal to that of the mother, and almost all of that IgG is of maternal origin transferred to the child *in utero* across the placenta (cf. Chapter 6, Section III). The normal infant does not synthesize significant amounts of IgG during the first 4 weeks of life, and as a consequence, the serum IgG level falls after birth with a half-life of about 1 month, due to degradation of the IgG by the infant (cf. Chapter 6, Fig. 19). At some point between 4 and 12 weeks of age, the amount of IgG synthesized by the infant equals the amount of IgG being degraded, and the decline in serum IgG ceases. Endogeneous IgG synthesis normally then increases, and as it exceeds the amount of IgG being degraded, the serum IgG concentration rises. This decrease and subsequent increase in serum IgG concentration occurs in all normal infants, and hence is a genetically determined sequence of events. In some infants, however, the normal increase in IgG synthesis is delayed beyond 3 months; as a result, the serum IgG level may fall below 100 to 150 mg per 100 ml. Should this occur, the infant becomes "agammaglobulinemic"; comparatively little IgM or IgA is actually transferred from mother to child antenatally, and the rate of synthesis of these immunoglobulins during early infancy is but a fraction of that in the older child or adult (cf. Chapter 6). In contrast to the congenital and adult forms of agammaglobulinemia which are permanent states, this form of hypogammaglobulinemia is temporary, lasting as short as 1 month in some infants and as long as a year in others. The duration, of course, depends upon when the child starts to synthesize increased amounts of immunoglobulin, particularly IgG. The disorder is seen in both males and females, and may not easily be distinguished from congenital agammaglobulinemia except in retrospect when immunoglobulin levels return toward normal. In some infants, the IgM and IgA levels are not as low as are seen in congenital agammaglobulinemia, and this may offer a clue in anterospectively differentiating the two conditions. Whether the delay in immunoglobulin synthesis seen in this disorder is genetic in origin or acquired is not yet known.

b. Clinical implications. The serum IgG level in untreated patients with congenital or adult agammaglobulinemia is less than 100 mg per 100 ml. In congenital agammaglobulinemia, it is usually less than 25 mg per 100 ml, and in the adult form, it is most frequently between 25 and 75 mg per 100 ml. As noted above, IgM and IgA synthesis is usually negligible. When patients with congenital agammaglobulinemia are treated with injections of concentrated IgG obtained from the pooled plasma of normal adults, their resistance to bacterial infection is not usually improved unless the serum concentration of *administered* IgG is maintained above 100 to 150 mg per 100 ml (Gitlin *et al.,* 1962). For this reason, a serum IgG level of 100 to 150 mg per 100 ml is considered to be the upper limit for the diagnosis of transient hypogammaglobulinemia of infancy.

Clearly, the effectiveness of an immunoglobulin in protecting an individual against infection depends upon the nature and quantity of specific antibodies and not upon the concentration of the immunoglobulin as a class of proteins. However, the serum immunoglobulin concentration is a partial reflection of the individual's ability to synthesize specific antibodies. Despite the low levels of IgG found in patients with congenital or adult agammaglobulinemia, sufficient antibodies against the measles virus and a number of other viruses can often be synthesized as to provide immunity against reinfection with those viruses, but the amounts of antibacterial antibodies produced, when produced at all, are far too small to provide adequate protection against bacterial invasion. Thus, patients with agammaglobulinemia are highly susceptible to infection with certain bacteria, particularly those of the pyogenic group, and fungi such as *Monilia*. The clinical course of these patients varies widely, but the lungs are involved most often in almost all patients (Gitlin *et al.*, 1962).

Patients with agammaglobulinemia have normal numbers of peripheral blood lymphocytes, and they have relatively normal numbers of lymphocytes in their tissues. In accord with these observations, these patients can and do develop the delayed type of hypersensitivity (Porter, 1955), and this explains why these children can become immune to such organisms as vaccinia virus and varicella virus; immunity to these viruses is dependent more upon cellular immunity than humoral immunity. It also may explain why there is an extraordinarily high incidence of collagen disease in these patients (Janeway *et al.*, 1956) and why skin homografts are rejected (Schubert *et al.*, 1960).

c. THE METABOLIC DEFECT AND ITS GENETIC IMPLICATIONS. The deficiency in immunoglobulins in agammaglobulinemia is attributable to deficient synthesis and is not due to increased degradation; the half-life of IgG in this disorder is longer than in the normal individual (Gitlin, 1957; Solomon *et al.*, 1963a). The plasma deficit in immunoglobulins in agammaglobulinemia is secondary to a cellular deficit: the tissues are virtually devoid of plasma cells, and plasma cells as well as transitional cells fail to appear in response to antigenic stimulation (Craig *et al.*, 1954). Primary follicles in lymph nodes are poorly defined when present, and secondary germinal centers are absent (Fig. 4). Peripheral blood lymphocytes are normal in numbers, but when the lymphocytes are examined by immunofluorescence for surface-bound immunoglobulins, patients with congenital X-linked agammaglobulinemia can be divided into two groups: most of the patients are deficient in lymphocytes with receptors for both immunoglobulins and the third component of complement; a small number of patients have low normal numbers of lympho-

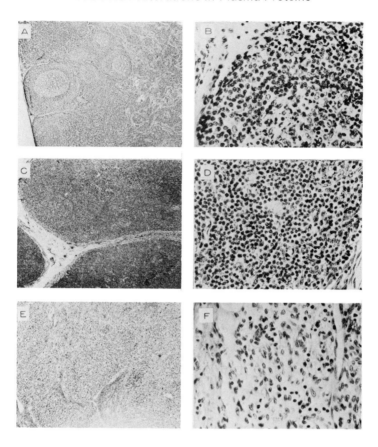

Fig. 4. Photomicrographs of lymph nodes in normal, agammaglobulinemic, and thymic alymphoplastic children. A. Normal infant 8 days after antigenic stimulation; primary follicles are large with prominent secondary reaction centers. B. Higher power of A, showing numerous lymphocytes in primary follicle; part of a reaction center is seen in lower right of figure. C. Lymph node from a child with X-linked congenital agammaglobulinemia; there are normal numbers of lymphocytes, but no secondary follicles. D. Higher power of A. E. Lymph node from a child with X-linked thymic alymphoplasia and agammaglobulinemia, showing lymphocytic hypoplasia and absence of secondary follicles. F. Higher power of E showing marked paucity of lymphocytes. Adapted from Gitlin and Craig (1963).

cytes with surface-bound immunoglobulins (Geha *et al.*, 1973). Whether patients with autosomal recessive agammaglobulinemia can also be divided into two such groups remains to be seen, but this is obviously a distinct possibility (Siegal *et al.*, 1971). It has been suggested that in those patients with X-linked agammaglobulinemia who have lymphocytes which bind immunoglobulins, the paucity of plasma cells may be due to a failure in differentiation, i.e., a failure in the cells to respond to antigenic stimulation (Cooper *et al.,* 1971a; Geha *et al.,* 1973). This presumes, of course, that immunoglobulin-bearing lymphocytes are those which differentiate into plasma cells or at least mediate that differentiation. The suggestion is appealing, but then it is not clear why most normal lymphocytes bear IgM rather than IgG, when the numbers of plasma cells synthesizing IgM are normally only a third those producing IgG. In any event, it is to be expected that each of the 3 major types of agammaglobulinemia will prove to be heterogeneous in etiology, since a failure in the development of plasma cells may result from a genetic defect in any one of undoubtedly many substances required for the development and differentiation of these cells. A paucity in plasma cells results in deficient immunoglobulin synthesis.

It may be apparent to the reader, if he has survived this far, that we have carefully refrained from a discussion of the so-called "B" cells. This omission is deliberate in the hopes of not revealing our bias concerning "B" cells as presently conceived. For a discussion of such cells with another point of view, the reader is referred to Fudenberg *et al.* (1971). We wish to state only that we believe that a man is not a chicken, despite the claims of Good to the contrary (Good, 1971). In the chicken, the data clearly indicate that the bursa of Fabricius is a site where precursor cells may be induced during early development to differentiate along plasma cell lines (Glick *et al.,* 1956). An equivalent of the chicken's bursa has not yet been found in man, although early claims have pointed, in turn, to the tonsils, the appendix, and Peyer's patches (Cooper *et al.,* 1971b). The mammalian bone marrow has been shown to contain cells which can differentiate into immunoglobulin producing cells (Tyan and Herzenberg, 1968; Mitchell and Miller, 1968); this does not mean, of course, that the bone marrow is the mammalian equivalent of the chicken's bursa of Fabricius. All this is semantics, perhaps, since obviously there *must* be precursor cells, wherever they are, which when properly induced will differentiate into plasma cells (Fig. 5). But the use of the term "B" cells presumes that man has a "bursa-equivalent," and, like the Emperor's new clothes (Andersen, 1846), this presumption may not only be misleading, but it may also be untrue. Hence, our caution in the use of the term "B" cells as it is now applied to man.

As of this writing, we prefer to classify the primary agammaglobulinemias (Gitlin *et al.,* 1962) as follows:

    1. Congenital agammaglobulinemia
      A. X-linked recessive
        (a). Absence or paucity of plasma cell precursors
        (b). Failure in differentiation of plasma cell precursors

B. Autosomal recessive
2. Adult agammaglobulinemia
   A. Autosomal recessive
   B. Sporadic, etiology unknown
3. Transient hypogammaglobulinemia of infancy

The problem of distinguishing between a lack of plasma cell precursors and a suppression of the differentiation of such precursors is exemplified by the observation that one child, who clearly had agammaglobulinemia for the first 9 years of his life, suddenly developed the ability to synthesize large amounts of IgM (Rosen *et al.*, 1961).

In many if not most patients with agammaglobulinemia, lack of famil-

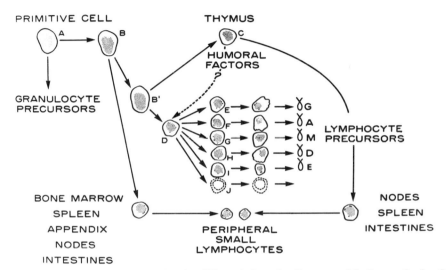

Fig. 5. A proposed scheme for the differentiation of cells responsible for synthesis of the specific immune factors. The differentiation sequence from primitive cell A to cell C takes place before 8 to 10 weeks of gestation. The differentiation of cell D to cells E, G, H, and I takes place at about 10 weeks of gestation (cf. Chapter 6). It will be noted that a failure of differentiation of primitive cell A would result in thymic alymphoplasia and agranulocytosis as seen in reticular dysgenesis; whether or not agammaglobulinemia is also a part of the picture of reticular dysgenesis, as predicted by this scheme, is not known. Failure of cell B to develop would result in thymic alymphoplasia and agammaglobulinemia with alymphocytosis, whereas failure at the level of cell B′ would result in thymic alymphoplasia and agammaglobulinemia without alymphocytosis. Failure of cell C to differentiate would result in thymic alymphoplasia with relatively normal immunoglobulin synthesis rates, whereas failure in cell D would result in agammaglobulinemia without thymic alymphoplasia. For simplicity, the differentiation of only the individual immunoglobulin classes based on the synthesis of different heavy chains is depicted, but it is recognized that the cells of each class differentiate to the point where only one to three different antibodies are synthesized per cell. Failure of one or more, but less than all, of the cells synthesizing individual γ-globulin classes would result in dysgammaglobulinemia. From Gitlin (1967).

ial data precludes intelligent judgment regarding the inheritability of the condition; usually, the patient is the only one with agammaglobulinemia in the sibship and adequate details of the kindred are not obtainable. The heterozygote, as yet, cannot be identified with any degree of certainty. For this reason, it is not known whether agammaglobulinemia in most adult patients is inheritable or acquired, although it is evidently inherited as an autosomal recessive characteristic in some.

2. The Dysgammaglobulinemias

a. CLASSIFICATION. Although the primary dysgammaglobulinemias have been classified sequentially as type 1, type 2, etc., in the past (Gitlin *et al.*, 1962). the number of different forms of dysgammaglobulinemia has increased to the point where this classification is now cumbersome and unrevealing. It seems more logical simply to classify the dysgammaglobulinemias according to the immunoglobulin deficiency present (Gitlin, 1968). As noted above, on the basis of deficient synthesis of one or more of the three major immunoglobulins, six different forms of dysgammaglobulinemia are possible, and patients with each of these possibilities have been found. Obviously, since there are four subclasses of IgG as well as two additional immunoglobulin classes, IgD and IgE, other forms of dysgammaglobulinemia will be found, and some of these, in fact, have been reported.

b. CLINICAL MANIFESTATIONS. When there is deficient synthesis of IgG, regardless of the status of the other immunoglobulin classes, the patient will have an increased susceptibility to serious bacterial infection. In addition to agammaglobulinemia, deficient IgG synthesis occurs in three different forms of dysgammaglobulinemia (Table I): IgG deficiency in association with either a normal synthesis of both IgA and IgM or a deficient synthesis of either IgA or IgM. If the dysgammaglobulinemia is characterized by normal IgG synthesis but deficient synthesis of both IgA and IgM, such patients also have an increased susceptibility to bacterial infection. Patients with dysgammaglobulinemias marked by deficient synthesis of either IgM alone or IgA alone may or may not have recurrent infections, depending upon a number of additional factors. Deficient synthesis of IgM alone, for example, has been found in some patients with congenital spherocytosis (P. Fireman and D. Gitlin, unpublished data), and IgA deficiency as an isolated finding has been seen in otherwise normal persons (Rockey *et al.*, 1964). On the other hand, IgA deficiency in patients with ataxia telangiectasia is associated with an increased incidence of bacterial invasion, particularly of the lungs (Peterson *et al.,* 1964; Fireman *et al.,* 1964; Young *et al.,* 1964). In other patients, it may be associated with coeliac disease or chronic malabsorption (Crabbé and Heremans, 1967; Tomkin *et al.,* 1971).

In accordance with the definition of dysgammaglobulinemia, synthesis of the immunoglobulin which is *not* deficient may be either normal or increased. It is not surprising that patients who are deficient in IgG and IgA and have repeated bacterial infections, for example, may have elevated serum IgM levels. But there is at least one category of dysgammaglobulinemia in which increased synthesis of an immunoglobulin may cause considerable confusion, and that is dysgammaglobulinemia characterized by deficient synthesis of an immunoglobulin subclass. It has long been known that some patients with clinical courses typical of agammaglobulinemia may have serum IgG levels which are below normal but yet well above 250 mg per 100 ml. Since the IgG levels in these patients are not typical of agammaglobulinemia, it has been difficult to classify the disorder. It has been found, however, that at least some of these patients have marked deficits of IgG1 and/or IgG2. Since approximately 60% of serum IgG is of the subclass IgG1 and 30% is of subclass IgG2, deficient synthesis of these subclasses is likely to be accompanied by decreased resistance to bacterial infection. The synthesis of IgG3 in these patients is greatly increased, so that the serum level of IgG as a class is above the IgG range usually found in patients with agammaglobulinemia. In these instances, then, the dysgammaglobulinemia is due to deficient synthesis of major immunoglobulin subclasses. The nature of the antibodies in IgG3, however, is inadequate to compensate the individual for the absence of those antibodies normally associated with IgG1 and IgG2, and hence these patients are predisposed to infection.

c. THE DEFECT.   As in agammaglobulinemia, deficient synthesis of an immunoglobulin appears to be due to a lack of those cells which synthesize the protein: examination of lymphoid tissues from patients with these disorders is certainly compatible with this concept. Conversely, where there is increased synthesis of a given immunoglobulin class, increased numbers of characteristic cells which produce the protein may be found (Rosen *et al.,* 1961).

Again, the lack of data does not permit even tentative conclusions about the inheritability of some forms of dysgammaglobulinemia. Deficient synthesis of IgG and IgA in the presence of normal or increased synthesis of IgM can be inherited in some families as an X-linked recessive trait (Jamieson and Kerr, 1962) and possibly as an autosomal recessive in others (Barth *et al.,* 1965). Selective deficiency of IgA can be inherited as an autosomal dominant trait (Stocker *et al.,* 1968; Tomkin *et al.,* 1971).

3. Specific Humoral Antibody Deficiencies

The Wiskott-Aldrich syndrome is inherited as an X-linked recessive trait and is manifested by thrombocytopenia, eczema, and recurrent infections. Synthesis of IgG and IgA are usually normal and that of IgM is often increased in this disorder. Although not apparently related to the clinical pathology of the disease, there is said to be a deficiency in the synthesis of isohemagglutinins and other antibodies against polysaccharides in these patients.

Although specific antibody deficiencies have been reported in patients with progressive vaccinia and in patients with fatal giant cell pneumonia caused by measles, these deficiencies do not appear to be inherited.

4. Cellular Antibody Deficiencies

An antibody, by definition, is any substance synthesized by the body in response to antigenic stimulation which will react specifically or almost exclusively with that antigen. After synthesis, antibodies either remain as an integral part of the cells which synthesize them or they are released into the body fluids as free molecules. The latter, of course, are the immunoglobulins. Synthesis of the cell-associated or cellular antibodies involves primarily the small lymphocyte. There is an inheritable anomaly of thymic development called either thymic alymphoplasia or hereditary thymic dysplasia, which is associated with a marked deficiency of lymphocytes in all lymphoid tissues (Hitzig and Willi, 1961; Gitlin and Craig, 1963) and a marked deficiency in the synthesis of cell-associated antibodies (Rosen *et al.,* 1962; Gitlin *et al.,* 1964). Whether the thymic defect and the lymphocytic hypoplasia of the lymphoid tissues are related as cause and effect or whether both are the result of a single genetic defect is not known. In both the rat and in the mouse, thymectomy at birth results in generalized lymphocytic hypoplasia and depression of cell-mediated immune responses (Miller, 1961; Waksman *et al.,* 1962), although Good and his colleagues had previously concluded that the thymus in the young rabbit does not participate in the control of the immune response (McLean *et al.,* 1957).

The thymic anomaly in thymic alymphoplasia (Fig. 6) appears to be due to a defect in cellular differentiation occurring at or before 8 to 10 weeks of gestation; the thymus in this disorder is characterized by a

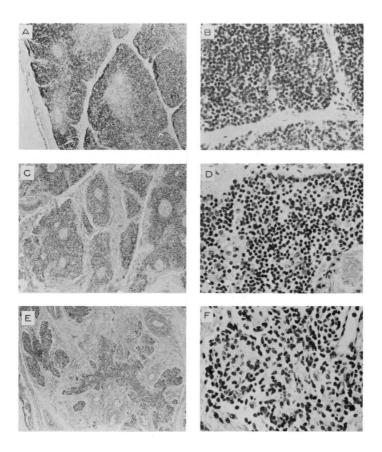

Fig. 6. Photomicrographs of the thymus in normal, agammaglobulinemic, and thymic alymphoplastic children. A. Normal thymus showing lobular structure, well-differentiated outer cortex and central medulla in each lobule, with Hassall's corpuscles in medulla. B. Higher power of A, showing lymphocytes. C. Child with X-linked agammaglobulinemia, with well-developed lobules and prominent Hassall's corpuscles. D. Higher power of C, showing normal numbers of lymphocytes; part of a Hassall's corpuscle is at lower right of figure. E. Thymus from a child with X-linked thymic alymphoplasia combined with agammaglobulinemia, showing poorly developed lobules, no differentiation into cortex and medulla, absence of lymphocytes and absence of Hassall's corpuscles. F. Higher power of E; there are very few if any lymphocytes, the cells present being almost entirely reticular cells. Adapted from Gitlin and Craig (1963).

rudimentary lobular structure, the virtual absence of small lymphocytes and the absence of Hassall's corpuscles (Gitlin and Craig, 1963). Since immunity in man to such diverse organisms as vaccinia, chicken pox, and tuberculosis is due to cell-associated antibodies, the deficiency in the synthesis of these antibodies in these patients results in an extraordinary susceptibility to grave infections. Vaccination with vaccinia or with BCG vaccine can be fatal. The deficiency is due to the failure in the development of those cells which produce these antibodies, a population of small lymphocytes. While not a plasma protein defect, the disorder is mentioned here because of its disastrous effect on patients with primary immunoglobulin deficiencies: the disorder may occur alone or in combination with the immunoglobulin deficiencies (Table I). The most frequent combination is with congenital agammaglobulinemia, when it is sometimes referred to, somewhat incorrectly perhaps, as combined immunodeficiency disease or Swiss-type agammaglobulinemia (Fudenberg *et al.*, 1971). In some families, this combination appears in both males and females and is inherited as an autosomal recessive trait (Hitzig and Willi, 1961); in other families, the combination is inherited as an X-linked recessive trait (Gitlin and Craig, 1963). This form of combined immunodeficiency disease appears to be due to a failure of development or differentiation of a cell which is precursor to both plasma cells and that population of lymphocytes responsible for delayed hypersensitivity (Gitlin, 1967) as noted in Fig. 5. Thymic alymphoplasia has also been seen in conjunction with several forms of dysgammaglobulinemia, particularly IgG, IgA deficiency (Fireman *et al.*, 1966); patients seen with the latter combination thus far have been males. Thymic alymphoplasia in the absence of any primary immunoglobulin deficiency is known as Nezelof's syndrome (Nezelof *et al.*, 1964). Other combinations have been reported and these, too, are listed in Table I.

Agenesis of the thymus also results in lymphocytic hypoplasia. Since the thymus arises from the epithelium of the third branchial pouch during embryonic development and the parathyroids arise from the third and fourth pouches, thymic agenesis is associated with hypoparathyroidism. This disorder is known either as the "third and fourth branchial pouch syndrome" or simply DiGeorge's syndrome. The plasma cell system is not involved directly, and such patients, like those with Nezelof's syndrome, are not deficient in serum immunoglobulins.

A particularly virulent combination of immune deficits is thymic alymphoplasia in association with congenital aleukocytosis, a syndrome known as reticular dysgenesis (DeVaal and Seynhaeve, 1959; Gitlin *et al.*, 1964). In this disorder, all lymphocytes and granulocytes are absent, and no patient has yet survived beyond 2 weeks of age.

5. Normal Differentiation of Immune Cells

Based in large part upon the defects in cellular development observed in patients with immune deficiencies, a scheme (Fig. 5) for the normal differentiation of immune cells has been proposed (Gitlin, 1967).

Although simplistic, it will serve the reader in sorting out the numerous genetic combinations and permutations that are possible which result in specific immune deficits.

VII. The Complement System

The nine components of complement, together with the inhibitors and inactivators that impinge upon their activity, are discussed both individually and collectively in Chapter 8, Volume I. At this point, we wish only to review briefly some of the genetic alterations in the complement system that have been recognized thus far.

A. The First Component

An hereditary deficiency of C1r and 2 hereditary disorders of C1 esterase inhibitor have been reported.

1. C1r Deficiency

A deficiency of C1r, one of the subcomponents of C1, has been reported in a brother and sister of a family in which three siblings had died in infancy (Day *et al.*, 1972). The deficiency is said to be associated with disseminated lupus erythematosis, arthralgia, and recurrent rhinobronchitis (Day *et al.*, 1972). Although the authors state that C1r was undetectable immunochemically in the two patients studied, the method used was qualitative and the lower limit of sensitivity was not given.

2. C1 Esterase Inhibitor

There are 2 genetic variants of C1 esterase inhibitor (Donaldson and Rosen, 1966): one is a quantitative variant manifested by a deficiency of this inhibitor in serum (Donaldson and Evans, 1963), and the other is a structural variant which is inactive (Rosen *et al.*, 1965). Both variants result in the same clinical picture: hereditary angioedema. When C1 esterase is injected into the skin together with C4 and C2, edema is the result (Granerus *et al.*, 1967); this reaction is normally suppressed by C1 esterase inhibitor. In patients with hereditary angioedema, activation of C1 results in the appearance of subcutaneous edema which persists for several days and then subsides. In some patients, edema of the gastrointestinal tract occurs, accompanied by cramps or severe abdominal pain. Unfortunately, acute laryngeal edema may suddenly appear in the course of an attack and may result in the patient's demise. The angioedema occurs in attacks which last for several days to a week or more, and the interval between attacks may be as short as days or as long as years. What precipitates the sudden activation of C1 in this disorder is not known. The serum levels of C4 and C2 are usually below normal in patients with hereditary angioedema, even in the absence of clinical symptoms, due to increased utilization of these components; during an attack of angioedema, the levels of C4 and C2 decrease even further.

The deficiency of C1 esterase which is seen in most families with hereditary angioedema is attributable to deficient synthesis; the half-life of the inhibitor in these patients is normal and the inhibitor present has normal activity. Since small amounts of C1 esterase inhibitor are always present, the deficiency is not due to a structural gene deletion. Interestingly, the frequency of attacks of angioedema in some patients tends to decrease after adolescence, although the serum concentration of inhibitor remains relatively unchanged. The disorder is inherited as an autosomal dominant.

The nonfunctional variant differs from normal C1 esterase inhibitor in electrophoretic mobility, and electrophoretic studies of different kindreds with nonfunctional C1 esterase inhibitor suggest that there may be several nonfunctional variants (F. S. Rosen, unpublished data).

B. The Second Component

An inheritable deficiency of C2 has been reported in at least four families to date (Klemperer *et al.,* 1966; Ruddy *et al.,* 1970). Synthesis of no other complement component, activator, or inhibitor appears to be affected (Klemperer *et al.,* 1966). The variant is a specific deficiency of C2 synthesis, and the heterozygote has serum levels of C2 that are approximately half of normal (Klemperer, 1969). In the homozygotic state, estimation of C2 using a sensitive radioiodinated C3 uptake technique has revealed C2 levels from 0.5 to 4% of normal, although none could be detected by hemolytic methods (Cooper *et al.,* 1968). Using an immunochemical precipitation method, Polley (1968) failed to find C2 in the serum of homozygotes, but the sensitivity of the method used was so low that levels less than 25% of normal could not be detected. The homozygous deficit of C2 is not associated with any clinical disease, despite the fact that C2 is involved in enhancement of phagocytosis. Apparently C2 is present in serum in the homozygotic deficiency state only in very small amounts, but enough so that the individual is not unusually predisposed to infection. Since some C2 can be found, the genetic defect is one of regulation of synthesis, and not due to a structural gene deletion.

C. The Third Component

There are at least two and possibly three different genetically determined defects in the metabolism of C3 thus far reported, and each is associated with an increased susceptibility to infection: of these, one is definitely a primary deficiency in C3 synthesis (Alper *et al.*, 1969, 1972a) and two are manifested by an increase in the rate of C3 degradation (Alper *et al.*, 1970, 1973; Abramson *et al.*, 1971). Of the C3 deficiencies associated with increased catabolism, one is apparently secondary to a deficiency of serum C3 inactivator, and the other is attributed in part to decreased C3 synthesis and in part to a serum enzyme, "C3-ase," which hydrolyzes C3. In addition to these three anomalies in C3 regulation, at least nine structural variants of C3 are known, none of which are associated with clinical disease.

1. Primary Deficiency of C3 Synthesis

In 1969, Alper, Rosen, and their colleagues (Alper *et al.*, 1969) reported a kindred in which 7 of 16 individuals had serum concentrations of C3 that were only half of normal. Of the two allotypes of C3 found in this family, F and S, those individuals with C3 deficiency had only one, F or S, whereas normal siblings were phenotypically FS or SS. The data suggested to the investigators that the C3 deficiency is probably due to a silent allele. Four years later, a patient homozygous for this silent allele was found (Alper *et al.*, 1972a): the patient, a girl 15 years of age, had less than a thousandth of the normal serum concentration of C3; in both father and mother and in each of 5 brothers and sisters, the serum C3 level was only 72 to 84 mg per 100 ml, and in the remaining brother the level was 158 mg per 100 ml. The normal serum concentrations of C3 in this study was from 100 to 200 mg per 100 ml. Thus, both parents and all but one of the six siblings had half the normal serum concentrations of C3. Clearly, the anomalous allele and the normal allele in the heterozygote have equal expression. Since the serum C3 level in the homozygous patient was less than a thousandth of normal, it is possible that in this instance the anomalous allele could represent a gene deletion. Serum concentrations of C2, C4, C5, C6, C1 esterase inhibitor, and C3 inactivator in the patient were all in the normal range.

The patient, obviously homozygous for the anomalous allele and thus phenotypically ——, had had serious recurrent infections since early infancy, including 14 bouts with pneumonia and two attacks of meningococcal meningitis. The clinical course was not unlike that of a patient with congenital agammaglobulinemia. Neither the patient's siblings nor her parents showed any increased predisposition to infection. Interestingly, the patient did not develop leukocytosis in the presence of infection, yet she had a skin rash which was infiltrated with granulocytes. The investigators concluded that C3 or one of its derivatives is required for leukocytosis but not for chemotaxis (Alper *et al.*, 1972a).

2. Enzyme-Associated Deficiencies of C3

To recapitulate the C3 sequence in the complement cascade, C3 convertase fragments C3 into C3a, which is anaphylotoxin, and C3b, which binds to cell surfaces and as such is involved in immune adherence, enhancement of phagocytosis, and activation of the remainder of the complement sequence. C3 inactivator blocks C3b activity and converts C3b to C3c.

a. PRIMARY C3 INACTIVATOR DEFICIENCY.   In 1970, Alper *et al.* reported a patient, 26 years of age, who had had repeated infections since infancy, much as do patients with congenital agammaglobulinemia. The patient was found to have a serum C3 concentration of about 27 mg per 100 ml, or less than a quarter of normal. Radioiodinated C3 turnover studies revealed a markedly shortened half-life of C3, a fifth of normal. The disorder was, therefore, termed "Type I essential hypercatabolism of C3" (Alper *et al.*, 1973). As expected from the low C3 levels, the patient's serum supported complement related activities only poorly, including enhancement of phagocytosis and bactericidal action against gram-negative bacilli. The patient's serum was found to lack C3 inactivator (Abramson *et al.*, 1971), as well as several other components, and the disorder has been ascribed to this deficiency (Alper *et al.*, 1972b). It has been found (Alper *et al.*, 1972b) that C3 inactivator normally inhibits activation of the properdin system and in its absence, the properdin pathway is activated spontaneously with consequent consumption of many complement components. The deficiency in C3 inactivator is inherited, and the patient just described represents the homozygous state. Since production of C3a from C3 is accelerated in this disorder, the patient suffered from recurrent hives and showed increased urinary excretion of histamine.

b. PRIMARY DEFECT IN C3ASE METABOLISM.   Normal plasma apparently contains an enzyme, which, when activated, hydrolyzes C3 to C3c without releasing C3a (Alper *et al.*, 1973). A woman, 30 years of age, was found to have only 8 mg of C3 per 100 ml of serum, and the small amount present was divided equally between C3 and C3c (Alper *et al.,* 1973). The patient had lipodystrophy and had been predisposed to frequent pulmonary and upper respiratory infections for much of her life. The C3 deficiency was attributable at least in part to rapid hydrolysis of C3 by a proteolyic enzyme the investigators called C3ase, and the disorder was termed "Type II essential hypercatabolism of C3." The enzyme is not generated by the coagulation cascade and is not trypsin-like in its activity. Whether this defect is inheritable is not known, since the patient has had four normal children, at least two of whom have normal C3 levels. Since C3a was not released in the hydrolysis of C3 by C3ase, the patient did not manifest urticaria or increased urinary excretion of histamine. Turnover studies in this patient using radioiodinated C3 (Alper *et al.,* 1973) revealed a marked increase in the initial disappearance of the tracer protein from the plasma after intravenous injection; the half-life of the labeled C3 was within the normal range. The data were interpreted as indicating an exchangeable extravascular C3 pool about 5 times normal and a rate of C3 synthesis that was only a fifth to a tenth of normal. Even if the initial disappearance of labeled C3 were due not to an expanded C3 body pool but rather to denaturation of the C3 during labeling, an unlikely event in view of the quality of the investigators, the conclusion that the deficiency must be due in large measure to decreased synthesis remains unaltered, since the method used corrects internally for such denaturation (Gitlin and Janeway, 1960b). Since the four children of the patient had normal serum C3 levels, the deficient synthesis of C3 seen in this patient was not due to a "silent" allele.

3. Structural Variants

The third component of complement is polymorphic among Caucasians, Negroes, and Orientals with respect to two types (Alper and Propp, 1968). Since one type is slower than the other on electrophoresis in agarose gels, one was called S and the other F. The gene frequencies of S and F among Caucasians are 0.75 and 0.25, respectively; among Negroes, the respective frequencies are 0.90 and 0.10, and among Orientals, they are 0.98 and 0.02 (Alper and Propp, 1968). At least a dozen variants of these two types have been reported and they have been designated by subscripts in accordance with their relative electrophoretic mobilities. The fastest variant known at the time that the system of nomenclature was adopted was designated as $F_{1.0}$ and the slowest variant $S_{1.0}$. All fast variants are named in terms of the relative distance between $F_{1.0}$ and F, and all slow variants are named relative to the distance between S and $S_{1.0}$. Thus, the position of $F_{0.6}$ under the conditions of electrophoresis would be at 0.6 times the distance between F and $F_{1.0}$. The variants are presumed to differ structurally, probably as the result of point mutation, and all alleles act at the same locus. Each allele, with one possible exception, has equal expression so that equal amounts of each allele product are present in the heterozygote. In one individual of phenotype FS, the concentration of F was about 60 to 70% of that of S, the total C3 level being normal (Alper and Rosen, 1971); it was concluded that the F allele was a hypomorphic variant in this person, i.e., produced less C3 of type F than normal and was designated C3f. Of seven variants tested, all have similar hemolytic activity (Colten and Alper, 1972).

D. Other Complement Components

Genetic alterations in C4, C5, and C6 have been reported. The C4 variations known thus far appear to be structural modifications, but the mode of allelic action is not yet clear (Rosenfeld *et al.,* 1969).

A familial defect in phagocytosis attributable to a plasma factor has been observed by Miller *et al.* (1968), and the defect in the proband was associated with recurrent infections with gram-negative bacteria. When given plasma, the patient improved clinically and the phagocytosis defect was corrected. It has been suggested that the disorder is attributable to a defect in C5 activity (Miller and Nilsson, 1970).

An inheritable serum deficiency of C6 has been described by Leddy *et al.* (1974). The defect appears to be due to a silent allele, since C6 is not detectable in the serum of the homozygote using an extremely sensitive technique. Heterozygotes have serum C6 levels which are 50 to 70% of normal. Serum from the homozygous individual had a total absence of bactericidal activity against selected gram-negative bacilli, but it did have the capacity to develop chemotactic properties and to mediate immune adherence. No obvious clinical disease was associated with the deficiency at the time of the report.

VIII. The Epilogue: An Apologia

To reach the end of the chapter at this point may seem somewhat premature—much like being abandoned by a guide in the middle of a tour when a great deal evidently remains to be explored. Soon after we accepted the invitation to distill plasma protein genetics into 40 printed pages or less, we realized that we had an unhappy choice to make: either we would write a little about everything or a bit more about less. We opted for the latter, and selected a few plasma proteins to exemplify the types of genetic alterations that have been encountered. Perforce, however reluctantly, we have omitted the α_1-acid glycoproteins, the α- and β-lipoproteins, the Gc globulins, the haptoglobins, the serum cholinesterases, and the blood coagulation proteins. Much of that which was omitted would have been repetitious and would have served primarily to complete the genetic catalog; e.g., structural modifications due to point mutations analogous to those described for albumin have been recognized in each of these groups of proteins; greater heterogeneity due to recurrent mutation, much like that noted for IgG, has been observed among the β-lipoproteins; the accumulation of chylomicra in patients with type I hyperlipoproteinemia is secondary to a deficiency of lipoprotein lipase. Yet, being unable to discuss these proteins for want of space still leaves us with a sense of incompleteness, since the clinical consequences of these alterations are quite different from one protein to the next, depending upon the function of the protein involved.

This chapter, clearly then, is not a review—it cannot even be considered a primer. Judge it instead to be a simple guide for a selected tour.

REFERENCES

Aagenes, O., Mattary, A., Elgjo, K., Munthie, F., and Fagerhol, M. (1972). *Acta Paediat. Scand.* **61,** 632–642.

Abramson, N., Alper, C. A., Lachmann, P. J., Rosen, F. S., and Jandl, J. H. (1971). *J. Immunol.* **107,** 19–27.

Alper, C. A., and Propp, R. P. (1968). *J. Clin. Invest.* **47,** 2181–2191.

Alper, C. A., and Rosen, F. S. (1971). *J. Clin. Invest.* **50,** 324–331.

Alper, C. A., Propp, R. P., Klemperer, M. R., and Rosen, F. S. (1969). *J. Clin. Invest.* **48,** 553–557.

Alper, C. A., Abramson, N., Johnston, R. B., Jr., Jandl, J. H., and Rosen, F. S. (1970). *J. Clin. Invest.* **49,** 1975–1985.

Alper, C. A., Colten, H. R., Rosen, F. S., Rabson, A. R., Macnab, G. M., and Gear, J. S. S. (1972a). *Lancet* **2,** 1179–1181.

Alper, C. A., Rosen, F. S., and Lachmann, P. J. (1972b). *Proc. Nat. Acad. Sci. U.S.* **69,** 2910–2913.

Alper, C. A., Bloch, K. J., and Rosen, F. S. (1973). *N. Engl. J. Med.* **288,** 601–606.

Andersen, H. C. (1846). *In* "Fairy Tales" (S. Larsen, ed.), pp. 171–181. Flensted, Odense, Denmark, 1950.

Attardi, G., Cohn, M., Haribata, K., and Lennox, E. S. (1964). *J. Immunol.* **92,** 347–355.

Barth, W. F., Asofsky, R., Liddy, T. J., Tanaka, Y., Rowe, D. S., and Fahey, J. L. (1965). *Amer. J. Med.* **39,** 319–334.

Bearn, A. G., and Kunkel, H. G. (1955). *J. Lab. Clin. Med.* **45,** 623–631.

Bennhold, H. (1956). *Verh. Deut. Ges. Inn. Med.* **62,** 657–667.

Bennhold, H., and Kallee, E. (1959). *J. Clin. Invest.* **38,** 863–872.

Bennhold, H., Peters, H., and Roth, E. (1954). *Verh. Deut. Ges. Inn. Med.* **60,** 630–634.

Berg, N., and Eriksson, S. (1972). *N. Engl. J. Med.* **287,** 1264–1267.
Bernier, G. M., and Cebra, J. J. (1964). *Science* **144,** 1590–1591.
Blumberg, B. S., Martin, J. R., and Melartin, L. (1968). *J. Amer. Med. Ass.* **203,** 114–119.
Bonazzi, L. (1968). *Clin. Chim. Acta* **20,** 362–363.
Brambell, F. W. R. (1966). *Lancet* **2,** 1087–1093.
Bruton, O. C. (1952). *Pediatrics* **9,** 722–728.
Bruton, O. C., Apt., L., Gitlin, D., and Janeway, C. A. (1952). *Amer. J. Dis. Child.* **84,** 632–636.
Bush, J. A., Mahoney, J. P., Markowitz, H., Gubler, C. J., Cartwright, G. E., and Wintrobe, M. M. (1955). *J. Clin. Invest.* **34,** 1766–1778.
Cáp, J., Lehotská, V., and Mayerová, A. (1968). *Cesk. Pediat.* **23,** 1020–1025.
Carrico, R. J., Deutsch, H. F., Beinert, H., and Orme-Johnson, W. H. (1969). *J. Biol. Chem.* **244,** 4141–4146.
Cartwright, G. E., Markowitz, H., Shields, G. S., and Wintrobe, M. M. (1960). *Amer. J. Med.* **28,** 555–563.
Cohen, B. L. (1965). *Nature (London)* **207,** 1109–1110.
Colten, H. R., and Alper, C. A. (1972). *J. Immunol.* **108,** 1184–1187.
Cooke, K. B., Cleghorn, T. E., and Lockey, E. (1961). *Biochem. J.* **81,** 39P–40P.
Coons, A. H., Leduc, E. H., and Connolly, J. M. (1955). *J. Exp. Med.* **102,** 49–59.
Cooper, M. D., Lawton, A., and Bockman, D. E. (1971a). *Lancet* **2,** 791–795.
Cooper, M. D., Kincade, P. W., and Lawton, A. R. (1971b). *In* "Immunologic Incompetence" (B. M. Kagen and E. R. Stiehm, eds.), pp. 81–101. Yearbook Publ., Chicago, Illinois.
Cooper, N. R., ten Bensel, R., and Kohler, P. F. (1968). *J. Immunol.* **101,** 1176–1182.
Crabbé, P. A., and Heremans, J. F. (1967). *Amer. J. Med.* **42,** 319–326.
Craig, J., Gitlin, D., and Jewett, T. (1954). *Amer. J. Dis. Child.* **88,** 626–629.
Cruchaud, A., Rosen, F. S., Craig, J. M., Janeway, C. A., and Gitlin, D. (1962). *J. Exp. Med.* **115,** 1141–1148.
Day, N. K., Geiger, H., Stroud, R., deBracco, M., Mancada, B., Windhorst, D., and Good, R. A. (1972). *J. Clin. Invest.* **51,** 1102–1108.
DeLellis, R. A., Balogh, K., Merk, F. B., and Chirife, A. M. (1972). *Arch. Pathol.* **94,** 308–316.
Denny-Brown, D., and Porter, H. (1951). *N. Engl. J. Med.* **245,** 917–925.
DeVaal, O. M., and Seynhaeve, V. (1959). *Lancet* **2,** 1123–1125.
Donaldson, V. H., and Evans, R. R. (1963). *Amer. J. Med.* **35,** 37–44.
Donaldson, V. H., and Rosen, F. S. (1966). *Pediatrics* **37,** 1017–1027.
Dutcher, T. F., and Fahey, J. L. (1959). *J. Nat. Cancer Inst.* **22,** 887–917.
Earl, C. J., Moulton, M. J., and Selverstone, B. (1954). *Amer. J. Med.* **17,** 205–213.
Earle, D. P., Hutt, M. P., Schmid, K., and Gitlin, D. (1958). *Trans. Ass. Amer. Physicians* **71,** 69–76.
Earle, D. P., Hutt, M. P., Schmid, K., and Gitlin, D. (1959). *J. Clin. Invest.* **38,** 1412–1420.
Eriksson, S. (1965). *Acta Med. Scand.* **177,** Suppl. 432, 1–85.
Evans, H. E., Levi, M., and Mandl, I. (1970). *Amer. Rev. Resp. Dis.* **101,** 359–363.
Evans, H. E., Keller, S., and Mandl, I. (1972). *J. Pediat.* **81,** 588–592.
Fagerhol, M. K., (1969). *Scand. J. Clin. Lab. Invest.* **23,** 97–103.
Fagerhol, M. K., and Hauge, H. E. (1968). *Vox Sang.* **15,** 396–400.
Fagerhol, M. K., and Hauge, H. E. (1969). *Acta Allergol.* **24,** 107–114.
Fagerhol, M. K., and Laurell, C.-B. (1970). *Progr. Med. Genet.* **7,** 96–111.
Fallat, R. J., Powell, M. R., Kueppers, F., and Lilker, E. (1973). *J. Nucl. Med.* **14,** 5–13.

Fine, J. M. (1970). *Rev. Eur. Etud. Clin. Biol.* **15**, 113–118.

Fireman, P., Boesman, M., and Gitlin, D. (1964). *Lancet* **1**, 1193–1195.

Fireman, P., Johnson, H. A., and Gitlin, D. (1966). *Pediatrics* **37**, 485–492.

Ford, E. B. (1940). *In* "The New Systematics," pp. 493–513. Oxford Univ. Press, London and New York.

Ford, E. B. (1945). *Biol. Rev. Cambridge Phil. Soc.* **20**, 73–88.

Fraser, G. R., Harris, H., and Robson, E. B. (1959). *Lancet* **1**, 1023–1024.

Fudenberg, H. H., Good, R. A., Goodman, H. C., Hitzig, W., Kunkel, H. G., Roitt, I. M., Rosen, F. S., Rowe, D. S., Seligman, M., and Soothill, J. R. (1971). *Pediatrics* **47**, 927–946.

Ganrot, P. O., Laurell, C.-B., and Eriksson, S. (1967). *Scand. J. Clin. Lab. Invest.* **19**, 205–208.

Gans, H. (1972). *In* "Pulmonary Emphysema and Proteolysis" (C. Mittman, ed.), pp. 115–119. Academic Press, New York.

Geha, R. S., Rosen, F. S., and Merler, E. (1973). *J. Clin. Invest.* **52**, 1726–1734.

German, J. L., and Bearn, A. G. (1961). *J. Clin. Invest.* **40**, 445–453.

Gitlin, D. (1955). *Bull. N.Y. Acad. Med.* [2] **31**, 359–365.

Gitlin, D. (1957). *Ann. N.Y. Acad. Sci.* **70**, 122–136.

Gitlin, D. (1966). *Annu. Rev. Med.* **17**, 1–22.

Gitlin, D. (1967). *Acta Paediat. Scand., Suppl.* **172**, 60–74.

Gitlin, D. (1968). *In* "Pediatrics" (H. Barnett, ed.), 14th ed., pp. 500–518, Appleton, New York.

Gitlin, D., and Craig, J. M. (1963). *Pediatrics* **32**, 517–530.

Gitlin, D., and Janeway, C. A. (1958). *Pediatrics* **21**, 1034–1038.

Gitlin, D., and Janeway, C. A. (1960a). *Nature (London)* **185**, 693.

Gitlin, D., and Janeway, C. A. (1960b). *Advan. Biol. Med. Phys.* **7**, 249–293.

Gitlin, D., and Sasaki, T. (1969). *Science* **164**, 1532–1534.

Gitlin, D., Landing, B. H., and Whipple, A. (1953). *J. Exp. Med.* **97**, 163–176.

Gitlin, D., Hitzig, W. H., and Janeway, C. A. (1956). *J. Clin. Invest.* **35**, 1199–1204.

Gitlin, D., Hughes, W. L., and Janeway, C. A. (1960). *Nature (London)* **188**, 150–151.

Gitlin, D., Schmid, K., Earle, D. P., and Givelber, H. (1961). *J. Clin. Invest.* **40**, 820–827.

Gitlin, D., Rosen, F. S., and Janeway, C. A. (1962). *Pediat. Clin. N. Amer.* **9**, 405–423.

Gitlin, D., Vawter, G., and Craig, J. M. (1964). *Pediatrics* **33**, 184–192.

Gitlin, J. D., and Gitlin, D. (1973). *Pediat. Res.* **7**, 290.

Glasgow, J. F. T., Hercz, A., Levison, H., Lynch, M. J., and Sass-Kortsak, A. (1973). *Amer. J. Med.* **54**, 181–194.

Glick, B., Chang, T. S., and Jaap, R. G. (1956). *Poultry Sci.* **35**, 224–225.

Good, R. (1971). *In* "Immunologic Incompetence" (B. M. Kagen and E. R. Stiehm, eds.), pp. 15–16. Yearbook Publ., Chicago, Illinois.

Gordon, H. W., Dixon, J., Rogers, J. C., Mittman, C., and Lieberman, J. (1972). *Hum. Pathol.* **3**, 361–370.

Goya, N., Miyazaki, S., Kodate, S., and Ushio, B. (1972). *Blood* **40**, 239–245.

Granerus, G., Hallberg, L., Laurell, A.-B., and Wetterquist, H. (1967). *Acta Med. Scand.* **182**, 11–22.

Guenter, C. A., Welch, M. H., Russel, T. R., Hyde, R. M., and Hammarsten, J. F. (1968). *Arch. Intern. Med.* **122**, 254–257.

Heilmeyer, L., Keller, W., Vivell, O., Keiderling, W., Betke, K., Wöhler, F., and Schultze, H. E. (1961). *Deut. Med. Wochenschr.* **86**, 1745–1751.

Hitzig, W. H., and Willi, H. (1961). *Schweiz. Med. Wochenschr.* **91**, 1625–1633.

Holmberg, C. G., and Laurell, C.-B. (1948). *Acta Chem. Scand.* **2**, 550–556.

Hyvarinen, M., Graven, S. N., and Stiehm, E. R. (1970). *Pediat. Res.* **4,** 470.

Irunberry, J., Abbadi, M., Khati, B., Benabadji, M., and Racha, E. (1971). *Rev. Eur. Etud. Clin. Biol.* **16,** 372–379.

Jamieson, G. A., and Ganguly, P. (1969). *Biochem. Genet.* **3,** 403–416.

Jamieson, W. M., and Kerr, M. R. (1962). *Arch. Dis. Childhood* **37,** 330–336.

Janeway, C. A., Gitlin, D., Craig, J. M., and Grice, D. S. (1956). *Trans. Ass. Amer. Physicians* **69,** 93–97.

Jensen, W. N., and Kamin, H. (1957). *J. Lab. Clin. Med.* **49,** 200–210.

Johnson, A. M., and Alper, C. A. (1970). *Pediatrics* **46,** 921–925.

Jones, E. A., and Waldmann, T. A. (1972). *J. Clin. Invest.* **51,** 2916–2927.

Kanner, R. E., Klauber, M. R., Watanabe, S., Renzetti, A. D., and Bigler, A. (1973). *Amer. J. Med.* **54,** 706–712.

Katz, J. H. (1961). *J. Clin. Invest.* **40,** 2143–2152.

Keller, H., Morell, A., Noseda, G., and Riva, G. (1972). *Schweiz. Med. Wochenschr.* **102,** 33–41 and 71–78.

Klemperer, M. R. (1969). *J. Immunol.* **102,** 168–171.

Klemperer, M. R., Woodworth, H. C., Rosen, F. S., and Austen, K. F. (1966). *J. Clin. Invest.* **45,** 880–890.

Knedel, M. (1958). *Clin. Chim. Acta* **3,** 72–75.

Kritzman, J., Kunkel, H. G., McCarthy, J., and Mellors, R. C. (1961). *J. Lab. Clin. Med.* **57,** 905–917.

Kueppers, F. (1972). *Humangenetik* **15,** 1–16.

Kueppers, F. (1973). *Amer. J. Hum. Genet.* **25,** 677–686.

Kueppers, F., and Fallat, R. J. (1969). *Clin. Chim. Acta* **24,** 401–403.

Laurell, C.-B. (1965). *Anal. Biochem.* **10,** 358–361.

Laurell, C.-B., and Eriksson, S. (1963). *Scand. J. Clin. Lab. Invest.* **15,** 132–140.

Laurell, C.-B., and Niléhn, J.-E. (1966). *J. Clin. Invest.* **45,** 1935–1945.

Leddy, J. P., Frank, M. M., Gaither, T., Baum, J., and Klemperer, M. R. (1974). *J. Clin. Invest.* **53,** 544–553.

Levine, B. W., Talamo, R. C., and Shannon, D. C. (1970). *Ann. Intern. Med.* **73,** 397–401.

Lieberman, J., and Mittman, C. (1973). *Amer. J. Hum. Genet.* **25,** 610–617.

Lie-Injo, L. E., Weitkamp, L. R., Kosiah, E. N., Bolton, J. M., and Moore, C. L. (1971). *Hum. Hered.* **21,** 376–383.

Lundberg, C., Boesman, M., Fireman, P., and Gitlin, D. (1965). *Fed. Proc., Fed. Amer. Soc. Exp. Biol.* **24,** 502.

McLean, L. D., Zak, S. J., Varco, R. L., and Good, R. A. (1957). *Transplant. Bull.* **4,** 21–22.

Marceau, N., Aspin, N., and Sass-Kortsak, A. (1970). *Can. Fed. Biol. Soc. Abst.* **13,** 127.

Matthews, W. B. (1954). *J. Neurol., Neurosurg. Psychiat.* [N.S.] **17,** 242–246.

Melartin, L., and Blumberg, B. S. (1966). *Science* **153,** 1664–1666.

Mellors, R. C., and Korngold, L. (1963). *J. Exp. Med.* **118,** 387–396.

Miller, J. F. A. P. (1961). *Lancet* **2,** 748–749.

Miller, M. E., and Nilsson, U. R. (1970). *N. Engl. J. Med.* **282,** 354–358.

Miller, M. E., Seals, J., Kaye, R., and Lentsky, L. (1968). *Lancet* **2,** 60–63.

Mitchell, G. F., and Miller, J. F. (1968). *J. Exp. Med.* **128,** 821–837.

Neel, J. V. (1973). *Proc. Nat. Acad. Sci. U.S.* **70,** 3311–3315.

Nennstiel, H.-J., and Becht, T. (1957). *Klin. Wochenschr.* **35,** 689.

Nezelof, C., Jammet, M. L., Lortholary, P., Labrune, B., and Lamy, M. (1964). *Arch. Fr. Pediat.* **21,** 897–920.

Ott, H. (1957). *Z. Gesamte Exp. Med.* **128,** 340–360.

Papamichail, M., Broom, J. C., and Holbrow, E. J. (1971). *Lancet* **2,** 850–852.
Parker, W. C., and Bearn, A. G. (1961). *Ann. Hum. Genet.* **25,** 227–241.
Pernis, B., Forni, L., and Amante, L. (1970). *J. Exp. Med.* **132,** 1001–1018.
Peterson, R. D. A., Kelly, W. D., and Good, R. A. (1964). *Lancet* **1,** 1189–1193.
Polley, M. J. (1968). *Science* **161,** 1149–1150.
Porter, C. A., Mowat, A. P., Cook, P. J. L., Haynes, D. W. G., Shilkin, K. B., and Williams, R. (1972). *Brit. Med. J.* **3,** 435–439.
Porter, H. (1955). *AMA Amer. J. Dis. Child.* **90,** 617–618.
Poulik, M. D., and Bearn, A. G. (1962). *Clin. Chim. Acta* **7,** 374–382.
Rockey, J. H., Hanson, L. A., Heremans, J. F., and Kunkel, H. G. (1964). *J. Lab. Clin. Med.* **63,** 205–212.
Rosen, F. S., Kevy, S. V., Merler, E., Janeway, C. A., and Gitlin, D. (1961). *Pediatrics* **28,** 182–195.
Rosen, F. S., Gitlin, D., and Janeway, C. A. (1962). *Lancet* **2,** 380–381.
Rosen, F. S., Charache, P., Pensky, J., and Donaldson, V. (1965). *Science* **148,** 957–958.
Rosenfeld, S. I., Ruddy, S., and Austen, K. F. (1969). *J. Clin. Invest.* **48,** 2283–2292.
Ruddy, S., Klemperer, M. R., Rosen, F. S., Austen, K. F., and Kumate, J. (1970). *Immunology* **18,** 943–954.
Sakata, T. (1969). *Shonika Shinryo* **32,** 1523.
Sarcione, E. J., and Aungst, C. W. (1962). *Blood* **20,** 156–164.
Scheinberg, I. H., and Gitlin, D. (1952). *Science* **116,** 484–485.
Scheinberg, I. H., and Morell, A. G. (1957). *J. Clin. Invest.* **36,** 1193–1201.
Scheinberg, I. H., and Sternlieb, I. (1960). *Ann. Intern. Med.* **53,** 1151–1161.
Scheinberg, I. H., and Sternlieb, I. (1963). *Lancet* **1,** 1420–1421.
Schubert, W. K., Fowler, R., Jr., Martin, L. W., and West, C. D. (1960). *Transplant. Bull.* **60,** 125–128.
Sharp, H. L. (1971). *Hosp. Pract.* **6,** 83–96.
Sharp, H. L., and Freier, E. F. (1972). *In* "Pulmonary Emphysema and Proteolysis" (C. Mittman, ed.), pp. 101–113. Academic Press, New York.
Sharp, H. L., Freier, E., and Bridges, R. (1968). *Pediat. Res.* **2,** 298.
Sharp, H. L., Bridges, R. A., Krivit, W., and Freier, E. F. (1969). *J. Lab. Clin. Med.* **73,** 934–939.
Shokeir, M. H. K. (1970). *Clin. Genet.* **1,** 166–170.
Shokeir, M. H. K. (1971). *Clin. Genet.* **2,** 41–49.
Shokeir, M. H. K., and Shreffler, D. C. (1969). *Proc. Nat. Acad. Sci. U.S.* **62,** 867–872.
Shokeir, M. H. K., and Shreffler, D. C. (1970). *Biochem. Genet.* **4,** 517–528.
Siegal, F. P., Pernis, B., and Kunkel, H. G. (1971). *Eur. J. Immunol.* **1,** 482–486.
Solomon, A., Waldmann, T. A., and Fahey, J. L. (1963a). *J. Lab. Clin. Med.* **62,** 1–17.
Solomon, A., Fahey, J. L., and Malmgren, R. A. (1963b). *Blood* **21,** 403–423.
Sternlieb, I., and Scheinberg, I. H. (1961). *Ann. N. Y. Acad. Sci.* **94,** 71–76.
Sternlieb, I., and Scheinberg, I. H. (1968). *N. Engl. J. Med.* **278,** 352–359.
Sternlieb, I., Morell, A. G., Tucker, W. D., Greene, M. W., and Scheinberg, I. H. (1961). *J. Clin. Invest.* **40,** 1834–1840.
Stocker, F., Ammann, P., and Rossi, E. (1968). *Arch. Dis. Childhood* **43,** 585–588.
Talamo, R. C., Langley, C. E., Reed, C. E., and Makino, S. (1973). *Science* **181,** 70–71.
Tárnoky, A. L., and Lestas, A. N. (1964). *Clin. Chim. Acta* **9,** 551–558.
Tomkin, G. H., Mawhinney, H., and Nevin, N. C. (1971). *Lancet* **2,** 124–125.
Tyan, M. L., and Herzenberg, L. A. (1968). *J. Immunol.* **101,** 446–450.
Waksman, B. H., Arnason, B. G., and Jankovic, B. D. (1962). *J. Exp. Med.* **116,** 187–205.
Waldmann, T. A., Gordon, R. S., Jr., and Rosse, W. (1964). *Amer. J. Med.* **37,** 960–968.

Wang, A. C., Sutton, H. E., and Riggs, A. (1966). *Amer. J. Hum. Genet.* **18**, 454–458.
Wang, A. C., Sutton, H. E., and Howard, P. N. (1967a). *Biochem. Genet.* **1**, 55–59.
Wang, A. C., Sutton, H. E., and Scott, I. D. (1967b). *Science* **156**, 936–937.
Weitkamp, L. R., Rucknagel, D. L., and Gershowitz, H. (1966). *Amer. J. Hum. Genet.* **18**, 559–571.
Weitkamp, L. R., Arends, T., Gallengo, M. L., Neel, J. V., Schultz, J., and Shreffler, D. C. (1972). *Ann. Hum. Genet.* **35**, 271–279.
Weitkamp, L. R., Salzano, F. M., Neel, J. V., Porta, F., Geerdink, R. A., and Tárnoky, A. L. (1973). *Ann. Hum. Genet.* **36**, 381–392.
Welch, M. H., Richardson, R. H., Whitcomb, W. H., Hammersten, H. F., and Guenter, C. A. (1969). *J. Nucl. Med.* **10**, 687–690.
Wilson, S. A. K. (1912). *Brain* **34**, 295–509.
Winter, W. P., Weitkamp, L. R., and Rucknagel, D. L. (1972). *Biochemistry* **11**, 889–896.
World Health Organization. (1972). *J. Immunol.* **108**, 1733–1734.
Young, R. R., Austen, K. F., and Moser, H. W. (1964). *Medicine (Baltimore)* **43**, 423–433.
Zimdahl, W. T., Hyman, T., and Cook, E. D. (1953). *Neurology* **3**, 569–576.

8 / Automated Immunoprecipitation Analysis of Serum Proteins

Robert F. Ritchie

I. Introduction

Immunology has been late in receiving the benefits of modern technology. As far back as 1939, however, the knowledge existed that a light scattering precipitate produced by mixing antigen and antibody could be used for the practical measurement of the potency of anti-pneumococcal antiserum. No efforts were made to quantitate soluble plasma proteins in liquid media for a considerable time. It is interesting to speculate on what may have prevented the knowledge examined theoretically and experimentally over 55 years ago from developing into the practical system introduced only in 1971. One prominent contender for this dubious distinction must be the general inability to consistently produce high potency and monospecific animal antiserum to human plasma proteins at a reasonable cost. Intimately related has been the general disinterest both in the laboratory and at the bedside, in determining the levels of individual plasma proteins.

The apparent clinical need, or in other words, the practical utilization of a test, has been the driving force that induces the medical industry to respond to a new concept. Despite hundreds of millions of tests being performed in 1972 for the determination of cellular or biochemical blood constituents, less than five million samples were examined for the levels of individual plasma proteins. The automation of immunological testing for specific proteins has therefore occurred at an unusual time. Manual performance of massive numbers of tests for blood elements, enzymes, and metabolites traditionally has preceded the development of semiautomated or fully automated hardware. Laboratory workers, therefore, welcomed with enthusiasm these devices that freed their technologists from tedium, decreased the number of errors, and at least theoretically, increased testing speed and lowered costs. The automated analysis of plasma proteins has been developed at a time when quantitative clinical protein chemistry is in its early infancy and still not weaned from its parents, electrophoresis and radial immunodiffusion (RID).

Increasing interest in plasma protein analysis may perhaps be related to the recognized value of these analyses in the detection of early or subclinical human disease. The majority of laboratory tests have application in urgent situations where biochemical abnormalities occur in close temporal proximity to the time of overt clinical disease. Tests for specific proteins, on the other hand, may have long range or genetic implications such as the analysis of α_1-antitrypsin, ceruloplasmin, low density lipoprotein, and C2. Others are sensitive indices of subclinical disease such as tests for the acute phase reactants and the immunoglobulins.

In view of the fact that over 100 individual plasma proteins have been described, each presumably possessing an antigenic identity and biological function it is reasonable to expect immunological analysis to be successful and justifiable. The recent demand for genetic counseling, early disease detection, and preventive medicine could be significantly aided by this new form of analysis.

II. Historical

The precipitate developed on the addition of soluble antigen to specific antibody is believed to have been first observed by Kraus, who in 1897 noted the reaction on mixing sterile serum from a goat immunized with cholera bacilli with the sterile broth of a culture of the same organism. Further experiments indicated that the reaction with the culture broth was "just as specific as with the agglutination of living or killed bacilli." In 1899, Tchistovich amplified Kraus's observations and showed that the initial opalescence increased with time and with the extent of immunization of the animal whose serum was used. He further noted that animals would produce precipitating antibodies to the serum proteins of other species when appropriately immunized. Bordet, in 1900 confirmed this work and suggested that more than one type of antibody coexisted in the serum of immunized animals. In 1904, Nuttall described in some detail the precipitin reaction and its products and characterized the serum factor responsible for the precipitin reaction as a euglobulin and postulated that "it would appear that precipitation constitutes a reaction with definite chemical groups. . . ." Many workers soon entered the field and within the next three decades carefully studied the nuances of immunochemical reactions as exemplified by the detailed studies of Heidelberger and Kendall (1932).

Instrumentation played a key role in the evolution of accurate immunochemical analysis. Light scattering techniques were used initially in the early 1900's but were replaced by turbidimetry only to revert again in the late 1960's toward nephelometry with the help of greatly improved electronic instruments. The development of optical analysis in immunology vacillated between these two techniques as instruments improved.

The predecessor of an instrument to analyze light scattering dates to 1895 when Richards described a nephelometer for determining the concentration of inorganic salts. The Duboscq colorimeter was modified by Kober (1912–1913, 1917) together with Klett (1921) and by Bloor (1915) to improve on the original instrument which simply measured the amount of unfiltered light that had succeeded in traversing a sample as compared with that of a standard. The new instrument, rather than measuring light having passed directly through the sample, measured light that had been scattered by particulate material suspended in the solution. Bloor, in 1914, used this instrument to measure fat particles in blood and milk in what may have been the first determination of a plasma organic substance by the technique. Kober (1917) used this approach for the first time to measure the concentration of soluble proteins having determined the amount of casein that was precipitated by the addition of sulfosalicylic acid. Nephelometry enjoyed considerable popularity in the early part of the twentieth century until the various problems inherent in the early equipment stimulated investigators to seek a better approach. In 1921, Denis discussed the substitution of turbidimetry for nephelometry. He stated that "the amount of light reflected is not strictly proportional to the weight of the precipitate under observation but seems to be influenced by a variety of factors." Because of the relative insensitivity of the equipment available in 1921, the concentration of light scattering materials had to be great. The criticisms described by Denis (1921) were undoubtedly valid. However, the net result was that during the next 18 years very few publications dealing with nephelometry appeared.

It was not until the work of Libby (1938b) on the reaction of anti-pneumoccal serum and pneumoccal polysaccharides that efforts were directed once again toward the light scattering properties of immune precipitates. The instrument described by Libby (1938a) introduced a collimated light source, the use of a variable resistor to adjust the intensity of the analytical beam, a photoreceptive surface, and an electronic output in the form of a galvanometer. Slightly over a year later, the same author described the use of the photronreflectometer to determine the potency of anti-pneumococcal serums in the first effort at standardization of immune reagents. Recognizing that quantitative analysis performed by the precipitin reaction or by flocculation tests often yielded disparate results, Boyden (1942) carried out an extensive and careful study of comparative serology using a photoelectric technique very similar to that described by Libby. This study of comparative serology marked the beginning of a gradual return in interest in the use of nephelometry as a research tool. Subsequent work by Boyden and Defalco (1943) again carefully analyzed several test systems and suggested that nephelometric analysis had several advantages over the more popular quantitative precipitin data. He described in some detail the difficulties encountered with the photronreflectometer due to improper operation.

In 1947 Chow described a turbidimetric method for determining plasma albumin using rabbit antiserum prepared from electrophoretically pure human albumin. The results paralleled those obtained by analyzing the Kjeldahl nitrogen present in the precipitate, thus emphasizing that the far simpler turbidimetric assay yielded values after 2 hr equivalent to the much longer and more difficult nitrogen assay. Bolton (1947) examined turbidimetry and the ring test with diluted antigen and antibody rather than at the high concentrations used by previous workers and concluded that the latter may actually produce misleading data. Baier (1947) carefully studied the theoretical and applied relationships of turbidimetry and nephelometry emphasizing the importance of using low concentrations of reactants. In the low ranges, the relationship between light scattering and the inverse of the light transmitted in the measurement of an antigen–antibody mixture were parallel. A further study by Boyden and co-workers (1947) approached the important question of whether or not there is a definite relationship between the actual amounts of precipitate and the galvanometric readings obtained in photoelectric instruments such as the photronreflectometer. They concluded that this relationship is quite definite and showed parallelism between nitrogen content of immune precipitates and light scattering. This was shown to be the case with animal as well as plant protein antigens. They further showed that a prozone phenomenon did occur in the situation of antibody excess and that environmental factors such as salt concentration and pH had greatest effect in the range of antigen excess, an observation not put to important use in nephelometry for the next 20 years. Bolton *et al.* (1948) also agreed on the value of photoelectric assay but stressed that moderate changes in particle size distribution in the analyzed precipitates had little effect on nephelometric determinations but did effect turbidimetric results in a predictable manner. Their comparison of several instruments indicated the variability in sensitivity between these instruments which, despite great improvements in electronic circuitry over the years, remains with us and is largely due to the lack of improvement in the optical systems.

Gitlin and Edelhoch (1951) studied light scattering by human serum albumin and specific equine antibody. They found that the angle at which the scattered light was received had a marked effect on the sensitivity of the instrument, particularly in situations of antigen excess.

Light scattering analysis or turbidimetry had, until 1953, relied on unfiltered incandescent light sources. Marrack and Grant (1953) employed a mercury arc lamp and filtered light at 545 nm in their analytical in-

strument. This work and that of Aladjem and Liebermann (1952) illustrated the effect of pH and salt concentration on the light scattering
precipitates. Johnson and Ottewill (1954) used a newer instrument
confirming the work of Pope and Healey (1938) and Gitlin and Edelhoch (1951) and showed that the light scattering ability of a system
could be divided into two phases; the first, a very rapid rise in light scattering that lasted only a few minutes and later a slower increase that
could last for hours. Only recently has additional basic work extended
these observations to the first few seconds of antigen–antibody reaction (Nishi and Kestner, 1974; Savory *et al.*, 1974; Tiffany *et al.*, 1974).

Little new work was presented during the mid-1950's. Despite the excellent basic work laid by previous workers, a comparative evaluation of
quantitative immunochemistry made no reference to optical analysis of
suspended precipitates (McDuffie and Kabat, 1956). Until this point, optical analysis of suspended plasma protein–antibody precipitates had
been limited to studies of albumin and an occasional "globulin mixture."
Several had studied bacterial proteins as well. No worker, however, had
approached the analysis of what had been clearly realized by the late
1950's as the enormously complex and interrelated population of proteins in plasma. In 1959, Schultze and Schwick illustrated that many
human plasma proteins could be accurately and quite easily quantitated
by turbidimetry of antigen–monospecific antibody precipitates. Why this
seemingly valuable technique did not gain acceptance is not clear but
could have been related to the high cost of antibody and the general
unavailability of commercial quantities of the reagents. Nevertheless,
work continued at a low level in many laboratories. Several instruments
were studied at the Rutgers Serological Museum by MacDonald (1960)
who reported that instruments varied in their response to different particle size and at the angle at which the light was received. He indicated
that this variation could be put to good use in evaluating the physical
size of the light scattering particles. Leone (1960) studied the reaction of
a hemocyanin and specific antibody mixture by turbidimetry and emphasized the rapidity with which visual precipitates formed. This information was not put to practical use until workers, approximately 10 years
later, became interested in accelerating the reaction rate for practical
purposes.

Six years later, Stone and Thorp (1966) utilized a newly developed
micronephelometer to estimate the concentration of triglyceride-rich
lipoproteins. Their work led to the development of a new instrument that
used red filtered light at 600 nm. In the same year, Kahan and Sundblad
basing their work on the observations of Heiskell *et al.* (1961)
used — probably for the first time — a fully automated instrument and

colorimeter as a turbidimeter at 600 nm to analyze low density lipopro-teins (1966) and compared the results thus obtained with more standard manual methods. When carefully performed, the three tech-niques — electroimmunodiffusion, the immunocrit, and the automated method — were in good agreement (Kahan and Sundblad, 1969). Further work by Thorp and Horsfall (1967) produced a new red-sensitive mi-cronephelometer that was used to study clinical variations of the low density lipoproteins (LDL) in normal and pathological states. In another study, light scattering low density lipoproteins and chylomicra were sep-arated by ultrafiltration and the fractions were analyzed by nephelom-etry to obtain an estimate of the LDL protein concentration and to perform phenotyping of hyperlipoproteinemic subjects (Werner *et al.,* 1970).

Measurement of the proteins in cerebrospinal fluid using turbidimetry (Ritchie, 1967) illustrated that the immunoprecipitates formed in a free liquid could be used to analyze low levels of individual proteins in dilute biological fluids. It was possible to analyze concentrations of im-munoglobulins as low as 0.5 μg per milliliter rapidly and with accuracy in an inexpensive instrument. Comparative results of this work and simi-lar studies of other investigators using different methods showed good correlation. A high quality fluorometer was modified to perform as a nephelometer by Alper and Propp (1968) to analyze for the first time, the third component of the complement system. The development of improved instrumentation for light scattering studies was aided by Wyatt (1968; Wyatt and Phillips, 1972) who used the method for microbio-logical studies and presented mathematical expressions describing various geometric shapes of materials such as microorganisms whose refractive index approximates that of the suspending medium. Unfortu-nately, none of this work was applied to study the geometry of immune precipitates. The description of a fully automated nephelometric im-munoassay system, using microgram quantities of antigen and microliter volumes of antibody, was presented in 1969 by Ritchie *et al.* Within a short span of time several workers described almost identical systems for the analysis of haptoglobin, C3, α_1-antitrypsin, transferrin, the im-munoglobulins, fibrinogen, and CSF proteins (Alper *et al.,* 1970; Eckman *et al.,* 1970; Ritchie and Graves, 1970; Killingsworth *et al.,* 1971; Killingsworth and Savory, 1971; Aitken, 1972; Halberstam and Derrico, 1972; Markowitz and Tschida, 1972; Fletcher *et al.,* 1972).

Efforts to improve the Automated Immunoprecipitation System or AIP,[1] as it has become known, produced an instrument capable of

[1] Technicon Instruments Corporation, Tarrytown, New York.

processing a variety of biological fluids in a multichannel mode at the rate of over 100 samples per hour, consuming extremely small volumes of antigen and antibody and yielding accurate results in the order of 3% (Ritchie *et al.,* 1973).

An extremely important step toward improved sensitivity was made through the work of Hellsing (1972). He showed that the addition of a polyanion such as polyethylene glycol markedly accelerated the reaction while improving sensitivity and achieved by chemical means results similar to those of MacDonald (1960) who had altered the angle of received light in his effort to move the point of equivalence to the right in the traditional precipitin curve.

Most work to the present has been devoted to analyzing antigens. However, the availability of a sensitive test system with clear, practical applications has stimulated several workers to reverse the format and analyze antibody rather than antigen (Vincent *et al.,* 1970; Davies, 1971; Larson, 1972; Ritchie, 1972b; Ebeling, 1974). This work becomes of significance in light of the critical need for standardization of immune reagents.

III. Methodology

A. Terminology

The term *nephelometry* and analysis by light scattering are essentially synonymous. They refer to the measurement of the intensity of light reflected from particles suspended in a medium. For the purpose of this chapter, the medium is an aqueous liquid and the suspended particles are composed of protein molecules usually complexed with their respective antibodies. From the analysis of the reflected light, conclusions can be drawn about the concentration of suspended material and if desired, the configuration and size of the particles.

Turbidimetry by contrast is the analysis of light which has successfully traversed the medium containing suspended protein particles.

B. Optical Considerations

Light entering a solution containing suspended particles is broken up into several general populations. In dilute solution, portions of the beam traverse the medium in parallel without interference and will be measured by the photosensitive surface in a turbidimeter and, therefore, will not be received at all in a nephelometer. Other portions of the beam's energy are totally lost within the medium, that is, absorbed to reappear as heat, in certain instances as new photoproduced chemical substances or to be reemitted at other wavelengths not received by the photomultiplier because of optical filters. A large portion of the beam's energy encounters reflecting particles. The secondary or reflected beam then encounters additional surfaces and so on. The concentration of the suspended particles directly affects the amount of light that traverses the medium. Very high particle concentrations will interrupt all incoming light, releasing little or none in any direction. Lower concentrations may allow some light to escape in the plane of the incoming beam but reflect or absorb the great bulk. Low concentrations interfere with very little light but also do not absorb secondary beams reflected from the small number of suspended particles. Turbidimetry, therefore, is applicable to analyzing a high concentration of suspended particles, while nephelometry is most valuable when the concentration is extremely low.

Both instruments become nonlinear when the concentration of particles is high (Yoe, 1928). There is an appropriately linear relationship among the concentration of suspended particles, the wavelength, and the intensity of the analytical beam. It can be expressed by Rayleigh's law:

$$\frac{I}{I_\lambda} = K \frac{dV^2}{\lambda^4} \sin^2 \theta$$

I, is the intensity of the scattered light received at angle θ, $I\lambda$ is the intensity of the analytical beam impinging on the medium, λ is the wavelength of the light, d can be either the depth of the illuminated medium or the number of particles, and V, is the volume of the medium.

Precipitates that are pigmented may produce serious errors due to selective absorption at certain wavelengths. However, precipitates involving proteins, even with intense colors such as transferrin or ceruloplasmin are gray/white to yellow/white. When suspended in clear, colorless solutions a quite linear relationship exists between the concentration of particles and the scattered light.

Many factors affect the analytical beam and therefore the results obtained. It will scatter or absorb more efficiently at shorter wavelengths. Particles of small dimensions, i.e., less than 1 μm, scatter light 16 times more efficiently for instance at 400 nm than at 800 nm, confirming that the relationship can be expressed as the inverse of the wavelength to the fourth power. As particle size increases, the relationship no longer holds. Ideally, nephelometric analysis should be performed on particles of uniform size, however, suspensions of antigen–antibody precipitates are not composed of such a population. Well-dispersed suspensions of immunoprecipitates, however, because of their wide and fairly even dis-

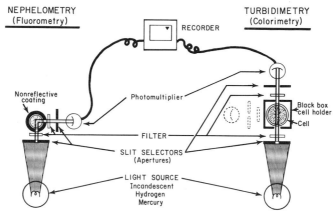

Fig. 1. Schematic diagram of a nephelometer (fluorometer) versus a turbidimeter (colorimeter).

tribution of particle size, exhibit what is known as internal compensation.

Figure 1 illustrates in its simplest form, the design of a nephelometer and a turbidimeter. *Turbidimetry* could be substituted for colorimetry or spectrophotometry in this diagram. The purpose constitutes the only difference. Turbidimetry is used for the analysis of turbid solutions as described above and the same instrument could be used as a colorimeter if light of different wavelengths were used in the analytical beam. Similarly, the nephelometer using reflected light to measure the concentration of suspended particles could be used as a fluorometer if the entering or exciting beam were of a narrow bandwidth produced by the use of filters or a monochromator and the emergent or excited light beam were limited by filters to another wavelength to exclude the exciting wavelength. In nephelometry, both incident and emergent beams are of the same wavelength. This ability for dual use of a single instrument has led to the term "fluoronephelometer."

In summary, the basic difference between nephelometry and turbidimetry is that the former measures the amount of light reflected, the latter the amount transmitted. The former is of greatest use at low particle concentrations while the latter is superior for high concentrations. Each embraces features of the other (Hach, 1970).

C. Instrumentation

Instruments in use today for nephelometric analysis are, in general, sophisticated fluorometers modified more or less for this relatively simple task. One instrument designed for lipoprotein and fibrinogen analysis[2] is an example of how small and simple the design of this system could be. Continuous flow analysis, when applied to nephelometry, requires that a flow-through cell be small, tubular, and devoid of shoulders or pocket areas where solutions can pool. It must also have an extremely light-tight cell holder. Small flow-through cells designed to meet the needs of miniaturization and minimization of sample and reagent consumption require that the analytical beam be of high intensity such as can be produced by a mercury arc lamp. Furthermore, the reduction in the internal dimensions of the flow cell reduces significantly the problems of attenuation or absorption of the incident beam by pigments in the samples such as hemoglobin or bile pigments. Despite the knowledge that greater sensitivity could be obtained with light at shorter wavelengths, most work has been restricted to above 460 nm, and in case of the instrument used for the measurement of lipoproteins, 600 nm was used.

The mercury burner used in the Technicon Automated Immunoprecipitin System (AIP) provides high intensity radiation in the 300- to 400-nm range. As illustrated in Fig. 2 the absorption of light by protein solutions remains considerable down to 300 nm, but at 357 nm absorption is negligible and thus was chosen as the analyzing frequency.

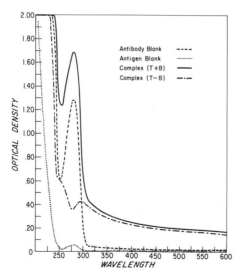

Fig. 2. Spectral absorption curves for solutions of antigen (human IgG)···, antibody (goat anti-human IgG)---, and a stable suspension of precipitates and complexes formed at a ratio near equivalence —,—·—. T (test) = combined optical density of antigen, antibody, and complex. B (blank) = combined optical density of antigen and antibody.

[2] Hach Nephelometer, Hach Diagnostics, P. O. Box 907, Ames, Iowa 50010.

Also shown in Fig. 2 is the fact that the absorption of light by antigen–antibody complexes is considerable at this frequency (Gitlin, 1949; Eisen, 1948).

In the AIP system, near ultraviolet light from the mercury burner is filtered prior to entry into the flow cell, is focused by a lens, enters a very small window in the cell apparatus, exits at 90 degrees through another window, is defocused by another lens, passes through a subsequent filter again at 357 nm, and impinges on the photomultiplier tube with high sensitivity at 357 nm.

The major difficulty with nephelometric cells is the entry of stray light from outside the analytical path. Such stray light can appear from minute cracks in the cell chamber, or in the case of the AIP system, could arrive at the photoelectric surface having been transmitted down the fluid column as though it were "a light pipe."

There are controls on the fluoronephelometer to alter sensitivity allowing the operator to vary recorder peak heights. Settings vary from one antigen–antibody pair to another. A baseline adjustment allows compensation for the intrinsic light scattering of the antibody solution itself. Different reagents may vary considerably in this property, particularly if they are not clarified or of sufficient potency to allow dilution of 30-fold or more.

There are a variety of fluoronephelometers that can be employed in the AIP format. Basically, however, the flow diagram remains the same with systems varying only in sensitivity and efficiency.

The *AIP flow diagram* can be presented in three basic forms. *The original,* shown in Fig. 3, is the most complex. A sample of whole serum is aspirated into the system through pump tubes of selected sizes that allow maximization of the amount of antigen present in the sample bolus. Successful tests have been run with sizes that aspirate 30 μl per minute to others that aspirate over 1 ml/min. The sample enters an already air bubble-segmented stream of prediluted antibody. During an average sample entry, a single bolus becomes subdivided into 15 individual subsegments that remain discrete throughout incubation and until optical analysis. Because the sample arm moves from a sequence of sample–air–saline wash–air–next sample, the serum is also segmented and prevented from mixing with the subsequent materials through laminar flow distortion. Once the sample has been introduced into the train of bubble-isolated antiserum segments, reaction with antibody begins. The time required in this manifold for light scattering to reach approximately 85% of maximum is about 15 min. A delay coil, fixing incubation to the proper time, is inserted into the stream. In the flow cell the bubbles that have insured individuality of subsamples are removed

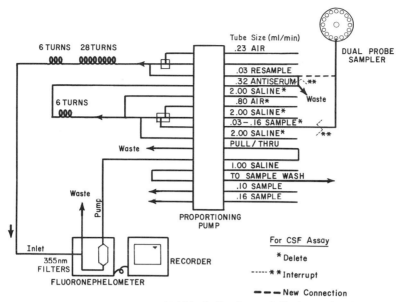

Fig. 3. Flow diagram of AIP manifold including internal dilution and option for testing solutions of low concentration such as cerebrospinal fluid and column effluents.

immediately prior to optical analysis of the uninterrupted stream. The steplike change in light scattering can be seen if chart speed and recorder sensitivity are high.

A *simplified version* of the original manifold (Fig. 4) has eliminated a considerable portion of the circuit designed to dilute the antigen concentration to the ideal range. In its place is a semiautomated dilution step outside the apparatus. While this might appear to be additional work, in practice it results in saving of time and materials. Whole serum frequently contains small pieces of coagulum that can plug the aspiration line partially or completely. By predilution of the sample to 1 : 100 the chance of plugging is reduced markedly. The chance of plugging is even further reduced since in the course of the semiautomated dilution step, the top of the sample can be aspirated rather than the portion near the bottom of the cone-shaped cup as does the automated sampler. Bits of fibrin tend to settle into the base of the sample cups, where they are easily encountered by the pick up probe. Plugging is infrequent with tube sizes above 0.1 ml/min, but is a major problem for the small sizes of 0.05 and 0.03 ml/min.

Predilution has three additional advantages. One is the reduction in sample consumption. In the original manifold, with automated cascade dilution, at least 95% of the diluted sample is discarded. In the semiau-

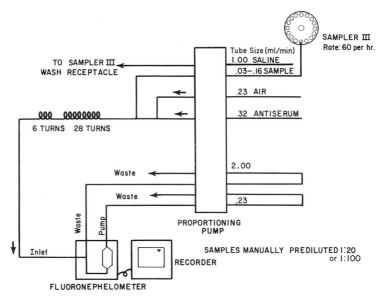

Fig. 4.   Flow diagram of a simplified manifold to accept prediluted samples ready for immunoanalysis.

tomated format, the entire portion can be reused for other analyses or further dilution if the concentration of antigen exceeds the accurate ranges. This feature is of particular importance in pediatric analysis where samples are frequently less than 1 ml. By predilution, samples as small as 10 μl can yield sufficient material for a dozen or more analyses. A second advantage is the ability of the operator to adjust easily the degree of dilution to better analyze a serum containing very high or very low levels of antigen. In practice, cord blood analysis for IgA and IgM are run at dilutions of 1 : 20 rather than at dilutions of 1 : 100, yielding far more accurate results. Furthermore, samples can be extensively diluted to accommodate very high concentrations.

A third and related advantage is that other body fluids such as cerebrospinal fluid, urine, pleural, and peritoneal fluids can be analyzed intermingled with serum samples. Cerebrospinal fluid requires no dilution for most protein analyses and only a 10-fold dilution for albumin and IgG.

A third design, shown in Fig. 5, is further simplified by the reduction of total processing time from 18 to 20 min to less than 3 min. High flow rates, rapid sampling, and increased wash to sample ratio from 1 : 1 to 3 : 1 have improved all features of operation. This advance has been made possible by the addition of a polyanion, polyethylene glycol 6000

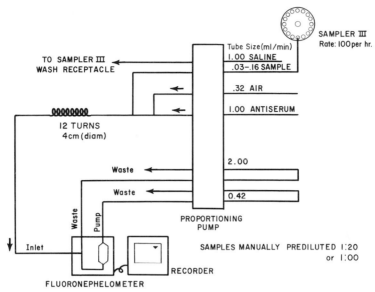

Fig. 5.   Flow diagram of simplified manifold (Fig. 4) further modified to use polyethylene glycol enhanced antibody for high-speed immunoanalysis.

(Hellsing and Laurent, 1964), as an accelerator to be discussed in another section. Antiserum flow rates have been increased 3-fold with the incubation time decreased by 75%. Total transit distance as well as time is greatly reduced. Moreover, the glass incubation coils have been replaced by a short length of transmission tubing wrapped about a plastic core, thus eliminating all glass with the exception of the flow-through optical cell.

D. Fluid Mechanics

Sample interaction through continuous flow systems is a major problem which was only solved by the introduction of a segmenting bubble by Skeggs (1957). As described by Chaney (1967) and Thiers *et al.* (1967), the success and efficiency of continuous flow systems depends entirely on the prevention of mixing of a sample with those immediately following and its contamination from samples that precede it. The further requirement, that samples be well mixed within themselves is extremely important lest they sediment and become completely unsuitable for optical analysis.

Fluid moving through tubing is subjected to shear forces that retard

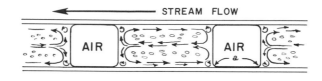

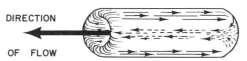

Fig. 6. Top: Saggital schematic representation of air-segmented fluid movement within tubing. Angle (*a*) is angle of contact. Bottom: Three-dimensional representation of segment between bubbles illustrating toroidal configuration of fluid movement with rapid streaming of core in the direction of actual flow.

the layers of fluid in contact with the wall. The core of the fluid stream is the least affected and, therefore, moves with the greatest ease and speed as pressure is applied to the end of the column. In only a few inches of wettable glass tubing this laminar flow will produce complete mixing of adjacent zones. If the fluid stream is segmented by air bubbles, the laminar flow pattern will be interrupted and converted to a toroidal flow with the fluid core moving in the direction of the total flow with a temporarily stationary shell of fluid exteriorly (Fig. 6). Relatively turbulent flow results in thorough mixing at both ends of the segment where the high velocity fluid core is either produced or dissipated. In practice, in an automated radioimmunoassay system (Johnston *et al.,* 1972), the design deliberately sought to produce large precipitates that were first seen at the forward end of the torus where fluid velocity falls abruptly. When wettable tubing such as glass is used, a thin fluid film remains as each bubble passes. On nonwettable surfaces such as Tygon or Teflon there is virtually no retained film and therefore no carryover to following samples. Changing the composition of the tubing may adversely alter the flow characteristics of the system to the extent that the bubble pattern breaks thereby compromising the reproducibility made possible by automation.

In addition to flow changes induced by the tubing materials, various wetting agents alter the surface tension and affect the overall system operation (Swartz *et al.,* 1964). Wettable tubing has a small contact angle (*a*) (Fig. 6), while unwettable materials have a large contact angle. The pressure developed during flow is inversely proportional to the angle of contact. Therefore, wettable surfaces or agents which lower surface tension tend to lower pressures and promote a more stable flow. In addition, a short fluid path is more stable than a long one. A balance must be struck between these variables to produce satisfactory performance. Operation of the AIP system is aided by several practical measures. A wetting agent, Tween-20, is used in all solutions. Perhaps of more importance is the use of whole animal serum at dilutions of approximately 1:40. Even with difficult-to-wet Tygon tubing, small wall contact angles are seen with minimal carryover and low flow pressures. It is quite likely that the superior performance of the simplest manifold (Fig. 5) is due to these above features combined with the extremely short transmission distance from sample probe to optical cell.

Proteins contained in both the antigen solution and the antibody have the ability to stick firmly to glass and to certain plastics. Glass is by far the worst offender. To minimize the problem of antigen and antibody loss onto the surface of the transmission channel, virtually no glass has been used in the newest manifold (Fig. 5). Moreover, the addition of polyethylene glycol and a high flow rate (Ritchie, 1972a) further decreases the contact angle about the segmenting bubble to promote a stable and predictable fluid flow.

For most human serum and spinal fluid samples, carryover between samples is minimal despite the low contact angles described above. Two circumstances, however, can produce difficulties. Samples with excessive levels of the protein being analyzed may disrupt laminar flow within the segment because of the number of macroscopic precipitates that adhere to the walls carrying fluid backward into following samples. At times, a single sample may completely disrupt the bubble pattern so that all following samples are unusable. The stream must be interrupted at this point and completely flushed.

Synovial fluids of high viscosity are characteristic of another difficulty that may disrupt flow dynamics. Because of the high molecular weight mucopolysaccharides wetting the channel surfaces, carryover problems for the subsequent one or two samples may occur. This problem, however, is minimized by the predilution of samples outside the continuous flow corridor.

Some carryover must occur even in the current automated system. However, because each segment constitutes only one of perhaps a dozen or more allied samples, much of the contamination of one segment with another is of a homologous nature. In addition, in the most recent manifold with a 3:1 wash:sample ratio, each group of subsegments is separated from the preceding and trailing samples by three times as many subsegments of saline and antibody. This alone virtually eliminates backward flow of any consequence.

E. Particles

The reaction of antigen and antibody in the continuously moving fluid medium produces fairly uniform particles, spheroidal in shape that remain unaggregated for a limited length of time. For this reason optical analysis must be carried out at a time compromising between the small amount of well-dispersed particles developed in the first few minutes of reaction and the increasing amount of inhomogeneous precipitate produced on longer incubation.

The ideal time varies with the antibody, the antigen, and whether or not an accelerating agent is present. The high speed polyethylene glycol-enhanced format produced some difficulty because of the great speed with which the reactions of high avidity antibody such as anti-albumin and anti-transferrin reach completion and go on to produce unacceptable flocculation. In these two instances, and perhaps with others in the future as antibody preparations improve in quality, the solution has simply been to remove the enhancing agent and retain all other features of the high speed system.

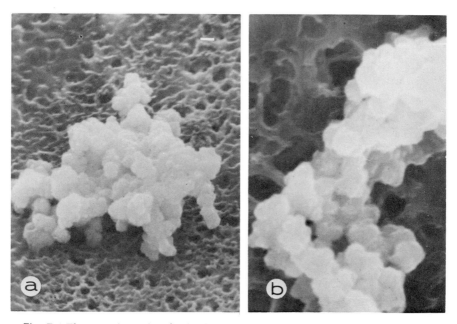

Fig. 7. Electron photomicrograph of antigen–antibody precipitates of the type developed in the AIP system. The average diameter of the spheroidal masses is about 0.5 μm. (a) C3 anti-C3, original magnification × 10,000, (b) × 20,000.

Automated management of the formation of antigen–antibody precipitates allows for precise examination of each facet of the reaction with little concern for technical variables. Therefore, by adjusting each of a host of variables, optima for sensitivity, stability, speed, and economy can be identified and combined for best overall performance (Goldberg and Campbell, 1951).

Electron microscopic examination of precipitates found in AIP effluents and those produced in a static or gently mixed fluid media discloses particles with dimensions of approximately 0.25 to 0.6 μm in diameter (Fig. 7) (Ritchie et al., 1973).

IV. Interference

As with any test system there are circumstances which may occasionally produce erroneous results. These errors are to be distinguished from those that occur through mechanical, electronic, or human failure in the system.

A. Pigments

Concern over the absorbing qualities of serum pigments in the 400- to 530-nm range has prevented the utilization of lower frequencies despite the knowledge that the intensity of scattered light is inversely proportional to the fourth power of the wavelength. In other words, approximately 16 times as much light will be scattered by a solution at 350 nm as at 600 nm. Three developments allowed the use of 357 nm light in the sensitive fluoronephelometer of the AIP system. The first was the combination of an intense mercury burner light source and a photomultiplier tube sensitive in the 350-nm range that produced an instrument sensitive to particle concentrations well below those possible in previous instruments. The second is the necessary low concentration of antigen allowing dilution of the sample to the point that intrinsic color is of little concern. Serum dilutions of 1:20 to 1:4000, depending on the antigen concentration, are usual. A third development was the availability of antisera with sufficiently high antibody content to allow extensive reagent dilution. In practice, the antibody solution is the limiting feature in that it represents the majority — sometimes as much as 99% — of the total protein present. For example, in the assay for IgG, the antibody is diluted 40-fold while the whole serum is diluted 2500 times.

Errors due to improper optical analysis may be seen with intensely jaundiced, hemolyzed or chylous samples. Management is simply to dilute the serum to a level that will reduce the level of pigment or light scattering material below the point of significant interference with the analytical beam. Attention must be paid to the extent of dilution used and to avoid extreme dilution where accuracy is compromised. Dilution is a much more serious problem in the analysis of proteins of low concentration, where the amount of serum required is relatively large, than for the analysis of IgG or albumin where dilution is extreme. As a rule, grossly hemolyzed, intensively jaundiced, or lactescent samples can be managed with only minor change in protocol. For the great majority of samples with a high concentration of pigment, dilution of two to four times will suffice. Despite the high levels of bile pigment seen in occasional samples, the immunological analysis yields accurate results in contradistinction to the dye-binding techniques where jaundice yields considerable error.

B. Turbidity

Samples with a large amount of chylomicra have a portion of their LDL protein closely associated with these large light scattering bodies. It would be anticipated that the removal of these bodies by centrifugation or filtration might adversely affect the accuracy of LDL protein analysis. A series of samples with high concentrations of chylomicra were examined to ascertain what fraction of the LDL protein was associated with the chylomicra and therefore removable with them by centrifugation. If the concentration of the LDL protein associated with chylomicra approximated the 2% previously reported (Fredrickson *et al.,* 1967), there would be little effect on the accuracy of LDL protein analysis. If, however, samples contained extremely high levels of chylomicra it might be anticipated that a very significant fraction of the total LDL protein would be lost through clarification by centrifugation. It was further important to know whether or not removal of these chylomicra might affect the concentration of other proteins and require correction such as is for instance common practice for the analysis of sodium in chylous samples. After removal of the chylomicra by centrifugation at 150,000 *g* for 1 hr, analysis of the floating fraction, infranatant, and the original material indicated that no significant change in the LDL protein level had occurred after the removal of chylomicra. The washed, floating fraction contained less than 1% of the total LDL protein present as analyzed in the AIP system. This value was not of sufficient magnitude to invalidate results obtained from clarified samples.

Chylous samples present two problems in nephelometry. One is the high level of blank produced by the light scattering chylomicra and large low density lipoprotein molecules. The second is the infrequent incorporation of certain plasma proteins into the lipoprotein–antibody complexes in such a fashion as to render them unassayable by specific immune reagents. The first problem can be solved simply by dilution or by centrifugation of the sample or passage through a filter membrane that will retard only chylomicra (Werner *et al.,* 1970).

The second problem affects the analysis of at least three plasma proteins. A test for the fourth component of the complement system, IgA and rarely IgM, may yield results indicating total absence of these proteins. The actual presence of the proteins can be documented by radial immunodiffusion or by immunoelectrophoresis. Nonspecific absorption of these proteins by the chylomicra surface is presumably the most common mechanism and may be similar to what is seen on addition of finely divided solids such as aerosilized silica or diatomaceous earth (Stephan, 1971). Ultracentrifugation or filtration of the sample to remove the light scattering particles results in the removal of the associated protein. The possibility also exists that the protein may be actively involved in an immune complex such as has been described by Lewis and Page (1965) in a syndrome characterized by the presence of an IgA–lipoprotein complex.

For practical purposes, samples obtained after an overnight fast as though they were to be processed for cholesterol and triglycerides, yield the best results with the smallest number of difficulties relating to lipoprotein–protein complexing.

C. Anti-ruminant Antibody

It is conceivable that because of the format of the automated analysis a reverse reaction could be observed. That is, precipitating antibody to goat or rabbit serum proteins could exist in the human serum being tested. Human antibodies to ruminant milk and serum proteins have been demonstrated (Huntley *et al.,* 1971; Leikola and Vyas, 1971) by gel diffusion and interfere with the method to detect an absence of IgA. Patients with IgA deficiency have a relatively high incidence of precipitating antibodies to ruminant IgM and lactalbumin. In RID the reaction of human anti-ruminant IgM would be indistinguishable from ruminant anti-human IgA. Fortunately, while these antibodies react well in gel diffusion techniques, the requirement of the AIP system to react strongly and rapidly appears to preclude interference with the automated system. Several individuals with high titers of anti-ruminant IgM, with either low or absent IgA, have been tested accurately in the AIP system.

D. Antibody Specificity

Many serum proteins display antigenic heterogeneity that may interfere with appropriate analysis. Antisera to the immunoglobulins may not be produced with adequate amounts or proportions of antibody to the four subclasses of IgG or to the two subclasses of IgA. Antibody to haptoglobin presents a similar problem. The determinants present on the type 1-1 species of molecules are also present on the type 2-1 and 2-2 forms. The latter two, however, have small portions of the molecules that are unique to them. Ideally, the antiserum for haptoglobin analysis should be prepared against type 1-1 molecules only.

E. Alteration of Antigen Molecular Weight

The physiological binding of hemoglobin to haptoglobin produces a complex of considerably larger molecular weight that reduces the diffusibility of the protein complex in gel films, thus giving an erroneously low value. It does not appear that the presence of hemoglobin complexed with haptoglobin alters the immunogenicity sufficiently to significantly alter the analysis. Although some masking of haptoglobin antigenic determinants by hemoglobin does occur, no data are yet available to indicate its effect on nephelometric analysis.

The alteration of molecular weight by the loss of large polypeptide fragments as occurs normally with the conversion of the native form of the third component of complement to C3c with the release of the C3d fragment which has been reported to affect nephelometric results by Davis (1972) but not by Alper (1970). Careful studies are underway to ascertain if antibodies of high affinity against many antigenic determinants can act to reassemble degraded molecules to approximate the correct total as though the protein were native.

A slightly different problem exists when the standard values used for curves have been produced with purified intact molecules whose concentration has been analyzed either by direct sample weighing or nitrogen analysis. IgG has been standardized in this fashion (Rowe *et al.,* 1970a). To properly analyze IgG, the antiserum must be γ chain-specific and be devoid of activity against the Fab portion of the intact molecule. If, however, a sample is tested containing free γ chain or the Fc fragment of IgG unassociated with light chain, an error in calculation occurs yielding a value approximately 40% higher than expected.

The analysis of IgA myeloma protein presents a particularly confusing situation in gel diffusion techniques. Because the IgA myeloma proteins often exist as a population of monomers and low and high polymers, values obtained by RID are often greatly disparate from those obtained by automated immunoanalysis in liquid media. Under these circumstances, an IgA myeloma protein may yield an incorrect and a much lower value by RID than by automated nephelometric analysis.

Comparison of IgM values determined by nephelometry and by RID incubated for the conventional 14 to 16 hr, may show the reverse situation when significant amounts of 7 S IgM are present (Markowitz and Tschida, 1972). Monomeric 7 S IgM, not restrained in its diffusion through gels like its 19 S counterpart, can produce a much larger diameter ring in RID than expected. The standard, however, will be 19 S IgM which when used to measure the amount of rapidly diffusing 7 S IgM results in an inordinately high value. The automated system, however, not being affected by diffusion properties, produces a precipitate proportional to the total mass of 7 S plus 19 S IgM and represents a more correct value. Comparison of the two methods of analysis can be used to calculate the amount of 7 S material present.

Other proteins that also exist as heterodisperse population such as an occasional polymeric monoclonal IgG and both type 2 haptoglobins diffuse at rates inversely proportional to their degree of polymerization. A more correct result is obtained in liquid analysis.

F. Rheumatoid Factor

There has been some concern that IgM with strong rheumatoid factor activity may produce aberrant nephelometric results. There are no data as yet to indicate that these 22 S complexes of IgM and IgG interfere with the analysis of either of the two immunoglobulins. If a serum contains sufficient amounts of these complexes to alter its light scattering qualities, baseline turbidity would be proportionately increased.

V. Antibody Characteristics

Development of laboratory equipment and new tests often does not take into consideration the quality and availability of the needed reagents. Furthermore, generally accepted standards for an individual test might be lacking for years — often indefinitely — and in the case of the analysis of plasma proteins are still lacking after "quantitative" procedures were introduced as a clinical tool.

The Medical Research Council of Great Britain presented recommendations for the manufacture and testing of antiserum for immunofluorescence and for gel diffusion techniques (Humphrey *et al.*, 1971). No

similar recommendations or guidelines for antisera to be used in nephelometric techniques have been proposed. However, in light of the fact
that an increasing portion of the antiserum now being produced is to be
used in the automated analysis of plasma proteins, guidelines for nephelometric grade antiserum and antigen standards usable in nephelometry are urgently needed.

The lack of quality control in immunologic reagents is due largely to
the inexactness of manual assay techniques. The worker who has become inured to errors of 15 to 20% under usual laboratory conditions
for RID considers the efforts needed to reduce this error to 7%, which
is believed to be the ideal, as impractical. Furthermore, he has had little
concern for the enormous errors that occur when a sample contains
either a very high or a very low concentration of a single protein (Hall,
1973). Phillips *et al.* (1971) and Reimer (1972) have underscored the
deficiencies that exist in commercial antisera to the immunoglobulins,
documenting that several major manufacturers actually distributed at full
cost, reagents devoid, or nearly so, of antibody activity. Until the AIP
system became available workers were faced with employing semiquantitative or qualitative methods to assess the specificity and potency of a
reagent. The automated system affords an accurate and quantitative
means of examining an antibody's reaction with a series of individual antigens, in virtually identical settings, thus, eliminating the variations due
to technical problems. With the wide range seen in the quality of commercially available antisera (Reimer, 1970; Phillips *et al.,* 1971; Ritchie
and Stevens, 1972; Hostey *et al.,* 1973) one is faced with a problem un-
paralleled in the field of health care or laboratory science. At the moment, the consumer has no idea of the specificity of his purchased antibody, from what source the antigen was obtained and how it was
prepared, what the antibody content is and what contaminant antibodies,
if any, remain and the manner in which the contaminants were removed.
Undoubtedly some of the manufacturing details are proprietary. However, most of this information could and should be made available as
product information.

The antibody content of antisera has been of little concern to most
users of manual immunoassay techniques. The concern over whether an
antibody "works" or how the results look has for the most part been sufficient. Introduction of the AIP system, however, has forced the beginning of the end to this unsophisticated characterization of immune
reagents by offering an accurate, numerical assessment of reagents to be
used for nephelometric testing.

For an antiserum to be acceptable for use in the AIP system it must
meet certain qualifications. It must be monospecific; for antisera to the
immunoglobulins this means that activity is limited to the heavy chain

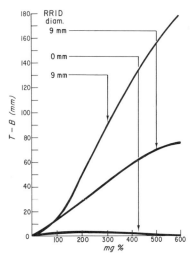

Fig. 8. Graphic illustration of three individual commercial antisera to human α_1-antitrypsin.

portion of the individual classes. Again, for the anti-immunoglobulins, they should have adequate activity against the four subclasses of IgG and to the two subclasses of IgA. They should have the ability to react avidly with their respective antigens to produce a precipitate with a reaction nearing completion within minutes (Boyd, 1947; Marrack and Richards, 1971). This latter quality supersedes the precipitin curve (Heidelberger and Kendall, 1935) which can be seriously misleading (Baier, 1947; Bolton, 1947). The amount of antibody may correlate well with the results of in-gel techniques. However, the same reagent may fail to perform satisfactorily in the AIP system. Figure 8 illustrates the analysis of three commercial preparations of anti-α_1-antitrypsin using the reverse radial immunodiffusion technique (RRID) (Reimer, 1970) and the AIP system. One clearly failed by all criteria; however, two produced equivalent results in RRID. Nevertheless, one of the latter failed to perform in the AIP system. A standardized means describing these three reagents could quite easily be generated for nephelometric qualifications. Of interest is that a "nephelometric grade" antibody preparation has never failed to be a superior reagent for RID, immunoelectrophoresis, or double diffusion.

A. Potency

Unlike manual reagents, a test:blank ratio is a needed parameter for nephelometry. For reagents to be acceptable the antibody should be capable of producing a test peak at least equal to the blank peak at approximately normal values. For instance, if a blank value of 25 mm is obtained with a fasting serum sample containing 100 mg% of IgM, the addition of antibody to the stream should produce an equivalent increase to a total of 50 mm of peak height. In practice, most nephelometric grade reagents produce test:blank ratios of 3 : 1 or greater and instances, such as with antibody to C3, of 15 : 1 are found and with anti-albumin or anti-transferrin ratios of 50 : 1 are usual when the high speed manifold is employed. For proteins of "low antigenicity," inverted test:blank ratios of 1 : 5 would be quite acceptable for investigative purposes.

High test:blank ratios are of particular importance when testing for antigens present in very low concentrations. The most common example is the testing for IgA and IgM in cord blood where mean concentrations are one-fifth to one-tenth the mean normal adult values.

B. Antigen Excess

Samples containing concentrations of specific antigen above the maximum working level established for the particular protein, produce peaks with abnormal configurations (Fig. 9). Analysis in far antigen excess produces a grossly distorted peak which not infrequently, as in the case of IgM, extends to disrupt the one or two immediately following. Samples with lower levels, but still in excess, produce less obvious distortions but are still recognizable by the operator as unsuitable. In prac-

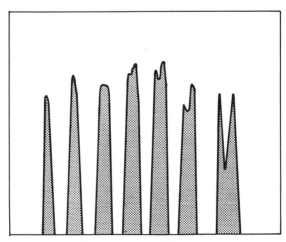

Fig. 9. Autoanalyzer peaks illustrating from left to right: two normals, one at equivalence, and four with increasing antigen excess.

tice, analysis of the three major immunoglobulins, haptoglobin, and α_2-macroglobulin display this difficulty. Samples at equivalence may be difficult to identify but if the proper operating protocol is followed, any peak exceeding the maximum peak height for the standard curve should be repeated at a modest dilution, i.e., $1:2$. Samples containing monoclonal proteins are the most frequently encountered clinical situations, with IgM presenting the most extreme elevation. Occasionally, samples from patients with Waldenström's macroglobulinemia may contain 100 times the mean normal value for IgM completely disrupting the sample stream flow. For other proteins, dilution of two to five times generally accommodates excessive antigen concentration. The extent of dilution required is rapidly learned by operating personnel.

Analysis of cerebrospinal fluid (CSF) protein may produce an analogous situation in view of the fact the extreme elevation of total CSF protein occurs frequently and may be unrecognized by laboratory personnel until the analysis has taken place.

C. Monospecificity

Unlike manual techniques where the presence of significant levels of contaminating antibodies appear to the user as a double ring in RID or an unconnected arc in immunoelectrophoresis, nephelometry produces a single value representing the amplitude of an electronic signal received as the result of light being scattered from an immune precipitate. No distinction can be made between a truly monospecific precipitate and one made up of many antibodies with their respective antigens.

Testing protocol using a standard serum for the generation of a curve does not obviate the problem unless the contaminant antibody cannot contribute to the total by virtue of the low concentration of the antigen under all conditions, or that the contaminating antibody is of such low potency as to preclude its contributing to the total nephelometric value under the test conditions. For example, a high titered antibody to C2 would have no effect if it were to contaminate an antibody to C3 since normal C2 concentrations are approximately two orders of magnitude lower than those for C3.

Certain situations can cause serious difficulties. Figure 10 illustrates such a situation where a relatively low level of an avid antibody B (to α_1-antichymotrypsin) is present as a contaminant in an antibody A (to α_1-antitrypsin). At low concentrations of protein B the error would go unnoticed. At high concentrations of protein B there would be no contribution of anti-B due to the situation of antigen excess. If, however, protein B is present at near ideal concentration, a very considerable frac-

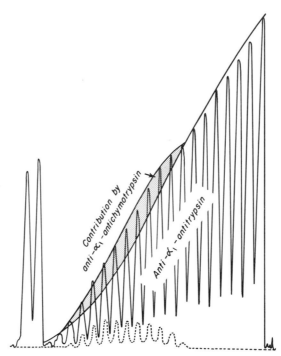

Fig. 10.   Autoanalyzer graph of an antibody to human α_1-antitrypsin containing antibody to human α_1-antichymotrypsin. Shaded area represents portion of recorder peaks contributed by contaminant. Dashed line represents α_1-antichymotrypsin peaks as they might be seen if separated from α_1-antitrypsin.

tion of the peak could be the result of the contaminant reaction. Such conditions can occur in the analysis of IgA and IgM in cord blood with a reagent containing significant amounts of anti-light chain antibodies. Because of the cross-reactivity with the light chain portion of IgG, a low or zero value would never be obtained except in true agammaglobulinemia. The analysis of haptoglobin frequently absent from cord blood or from the serum of patients who are hemolyzing would be erroneously high if antibody to α_2-macroglobulin were present. These two situations have actually been observed with commercial antisera that had not been standardized with procedures specifically designed to uncover the presence of contaminating antibodies.

The user of all immunological reagents should determine potency and specificity himself. It must be emphasized that the performance of antisera must be assessed in the system for which it is intended.

D. Species

Only antibodies produced in rabbits and goats have been extensively tested for nephelometry. The rabbit has been the most popular animal for antibody production and until recently, the volumes consumed the world over from multiple manufacturers seemed not to warrant the scale of production possible with the goat. There has been concern by many in the past that the goat was not the best producer of monospecific antisera because it was too sensitive to minute amounts of contaminants present in the immunogen. Nuttall (1904) suggested that quite the contrary was true as had Bordet before him (1899). Recent experience in several commercial operations indicates that the goat is an excellent animal for the economic production of high potency reagents. In 1975 the bulk of antibody reaching the marketplace will be produced in goats.

Testing in the AIP system of reagents made in various species uncovers no difference in performance. The limited experience with bovine and ovine antibody indicates that these two species also could be used but because of practical and economic reasons may never be employed to any great degree. Because of the presence of human antibodies to ruminant serum proteins, there might be danger of having a reverse antigen–antibody reaction occurring as described by Huntley *et al.* (1971) and Leikola and Vyas (1971) in testing of patients deficient for serum IgA by RID. While many samples with low or absent IgA have been found, a large percentage contain significant amounts of antibody to ruminant plasma proteins. Because of the AIP system's need for high potency antibody, it would seem unlikely that the relatively weak human anti-goat serum proteins could contribute to the nephelometric results. Horse antiserum has been used in the past for gel techniques, however, no experience in the AIP system has been collected to test whether or not the different precipitating qualities of equine serum interfere with automated use. It seems likely that most species, under proper management, could produce satisfactory reagents.

E. Clarity

For manual testing in gel, the clarity of the antisera has little more than aesthetic value. Turbid, hemolyzed, or lipemic antisera will work equally well. The strength of most antisera for nephelometric analysis allows for only modest dilutions of 1:20 to 1:50 which might be insufficient to prevent attenuation of the analytical light beam, therefore high levels of pigment are to be avoided. Turbid preparations are frequently due to the manufacturers combining isolated immunoglobulins from several units into a single small batch. The procedure of extracting the immunoglobulins, primarily IgG, whether by ammonium sulfate, Rivanol[3], alcohol fractionation, or exchange resins yields unstable proteins of reduced solubility.

Regardless of the apparent clarity of an antiserum, filtration immediately before use through membranes with a pore size no greater than 1 μm in diameter is important. Vigorous agitation and resultant aeration of the fluid, particularly if cold, can result in the release of small bubbles when the gas solubility falls as the fluid stream is warmed on passage through the manifold. Small bubbles often do not fuse during transit with the large segmenting bubbles and present a problem in the nephelometer by escaping the debubbling process and rising into the optical portion of the flow cell. Sharp recorder peaks result that can severely hamper the proper analysis of the graphic data. To prevent these problems, diluent saline should be used at room temperature, dilution of the antiserum should be by gentle repeated inversion rather than shaking to avoid foaming, filtration should not be pressurized, and finally, the solution can be briefly degassed by a low vacuum pump (20 to 35 lb vacuum) for 5 to 10 sec.

VI. Accelerating Agents

Chemicals that increase the amount of antigen–antibody precipitate or accelerate the immunological reaction are of increasing practical importance to nephelometric testing. The use of agents that promote the precipitation of antigen–antibody complexes began with the work of Ogston and Phelps (1961) who found that gels of high uronic acid content affected the solubility of proteins in proportion to the protein's molecular weight and concentration but apparently independently of ionic strength and pH. Laurent (1963a,b) found that dextran also exerted the same effect upon the solubility of proteins. Hellsing and Laurent (1964; Hellsing, 1966) showed that the solubility of immune complexes was much more affected than that of the individual components as predicted from their increasing molecular weight. The effect is believed to be the result of steric exclusion from an area called a domain surrounding the polysaccharide. The addition of polymers, therefore, appears to decrease the effective volume that is available to a given molecular species or

---

[3] 6,9-Diamino-2-ethoxyacridine lactate.

configuration. Antigens, antibodies, and especially their complexes, therefore, find themselves in smaller and smaller volumes as the immune reaction progresses, increasing and accelerating the possibility of reaching the point of insolubility (Hellsing, 1969). The ability of certain polymers to increase the amount of light scattered by a given suspension of antigen–antibody complexes was first described by Hellsing (1972) and Lizana and Hellsing (1974a) in an albumin–anti-albumin system. The use of this enhancing agent, polyethylene glycol (PEG), with a molecular weight of approximately 6000 has been confirmed in several laboratories and is in routine use for the analysis of 12 proteins in our department (Ritchie, 1972a). An additional assay of β_2-microglobulin in urine has been recently reported (Lizana and Hellsing, 1974b).

PEG has been used previously as a protein-precipitating agent (Polson *et al.*, 1964). Fibrinogen precipitates readily at 6% concentration; other species begin to precipitate at 3% and are not fully insolubilized until 20%. Exposure of whole goat antiserum to 4% PEG buffered to near neutrality for over 30 min is the recommended procedure. The solution becomes slightly turbid or even occasionally flocculent and must be filtered before use. The solution then appears to be stable and only after 48 hr or more does additional precipitate become noticeable. The precipitate produced by this maneuver contains small amounts of unclottable fibrinogen or its split products and unstable immunoglobulins. Removal of this material, therefore, has a salutary effect on the stability of the reagents. Exposure of the human serum sample to the PEG containing antiserum does not produce precipitation during the short time from incubation to optical analysis. In fact, the addition of PEG lowers the light scattering ability of serum samples as measured during the blank run. A series of samples had an average reduction in blank peak height of 40% with very turbid or chylous samples being most noticeably affected. Addition of PEG appears to significantly increase sensitivity of the assay of at least 14 of the major proteins in the AIP device. Although Hellsing's work was with an anti-albumin–albumin system, experiments with other protein species and their respective antibodies confirms that an increase in sensitivity of 3- to 8-fold can be expected. In the AIP system, modified to use PEG with a high speed format (Fig. 5), the increased sensitivity and accelerated reaction rate made it impossible to use PEG in the analytical system for the determination of albumin and transferrin in human serum. The extreme increase in light scattering, even at the lowest of clinically expected serum albumin concentrations could not be compensated for by the practical dilution of whole serum. The enhancing agent was, therefore, deleted from this assay. However, the use

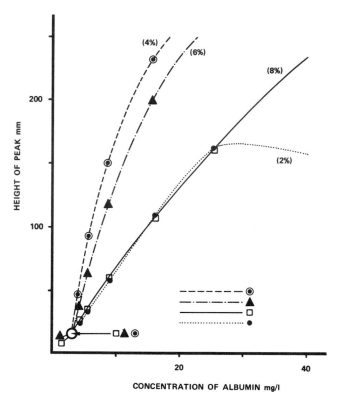

Fig. 11. The effect of increasing amounts of polyethylene glycol 6000 on the curve of antigen concentration versus peak height. From Hellsing (1972).

of PEG made it possible to analyze albumin in human urine at concentrations as low as 5 mg/liter (Hellsing, 1972; Lizana and Hellsing, 1974a).

The practical effect of polyethylene glycol is believed to be due to the rapid precipitation of complexes that might eventually have been analyzed nephelometrically after prolonged incubation. It is also possible that relatively weak antibody with low avidity becomes functional in the AIP format when exposed to PEG. The point of equivalence is essentially moved up and to the right, increasing the range of an individual assay (Fig. 11).

The addition of this polyanion has, in addition, made it possible to reduce the concentration of both antibody and antigen with a net increase in sensitivity. The reduction in processing time from 20 min to 2 to 3 min in the AIP system eases the problem of assay on a large scale. Recently Killingsworth and co-workers (1974) described the effect of another commonly used agent 0.01% Tris-Cl buffer with nearly as much enhancement effect as PEG. The mechanism for this action was attributed in part to the low ionic strength in the face of effective buffering at pH 7.4.

VII. Limits of Sensitivity

All laboratory tests are limited by what can loosely be called background, noise, or blank readings. Theoretically, low concentrations of a substance can be compensated for by the addition of increasingly large volumes of sample. In this manner, ranges of slightly more than one order of magnitude can easily be spanned. However, when a range of two to three orders of magnitude is desirable or necessary the blank or background reading may become a serious problem. In other words, the test:blank ratio becomes the deciding factor. In nephelometry, background is generally called the blank and represents the light scattering by the sample itself. For most proteins, an effort is made to keep the test:blank ratio above three when the values are in the normal ranges. However, for many proteins important values are frequently seen in abnormal samples that are in the 10 to 25% of a mean, normal value where the test:blank ratio falls to less than unity and actually may be as low as 0.2. This problem is frequently encountered in, for instance, the testing of human cord blood for the levels of IgA and IgM where expected values are one or more orders of magnitude lower than that of the normal adult population.

In addition to the normally low levels of several serum proteins in the first year of life, very low levels of many other proteins may be the result of genetic variations or accompany adult disease. Compounding the problem of low levels is the fact that the test:blank ratio may be further compromised by the increase in the level of serum lipoproteins as a reflection of serious illness.

Normally fasting samples allow for an adequate test:blank ratio ($\geqslant 3$) when the protein under scrutiny is present in concentrations of 50 mg% or more. For IgG and albumin, the very high concentrations allow great dilution where test:blank ratios of over 50 are usual. Recent work with enhancing agents described elsewhere in this chapter has allowed a significant increase in the amount of light scattering immunoprecipitates in the antibody excess range, i.e., the low end of the analytical curve, while also reducing the intrinsic light scattering of a sample by 40 to 60%. It has been possible to markedly increase the test:blank ratio, for instance, for the analysis of IgM at the 20 mg% range from 0.2 to 1.4.

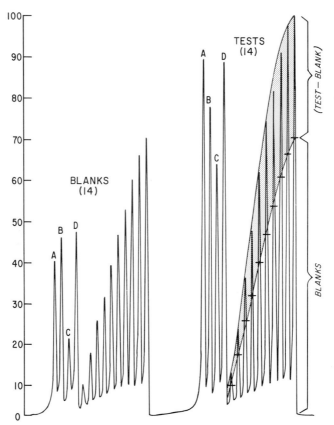

Fig. 12. Low concentration analysis of human ceruloplasmin. Nephelometric blanks shown on the left; combined test and blank on the right. Shaded area represents portion of peaks contributed by antigen–antibody complexes. Largest peak contains 1 mg/dl of ceruloplasmin. The smallest 0.1 mg/dl. Actual specific protein content is 600 ng and 60 ng, respectively, per aspirated sample.

In general, the simple and successful format for analysis of plasma proteins requiring only a single dilution has discouraged the manipulation of the sample to alter the optical properties by clarification or concentration by salt fractionation. The reluctance to employ sample manipulation has been strengthened by the successful analysis of several serum proteins at concentrations much below the 5 mg% range. Analysis of the C1 inhibitor with a mean value of 18 mg% yields test:blank ratios comparable to those seen for haptoglobin with mean concentrations 5 to 8 times higher. Analysis of the Gc globulin yields test:blank ratios an order of magnitude higher than expected. While the reasons for this success at low concentrations in unprocessed serum is not clear, it lends impetus to efforts to reach below the 1 mg% range or lower with many additional protein species (Fig. 12) and to reexamine the properties of antisera and their antigens that permit high test:blank ratios.

As yet not practical on a commercial scale is the production of immune reagents that contain only high avidity antibody, all other immunoglobulins having been removed (Cambiaso *et al.,* 1974a). Such materials have been produced in small volumes and may be of great importance in the future analysis of proteins that are present only at very low concentrations.

A. Sample Clarification

The lower limit of nephelometric sensitivity is largely set by the light scattering ability of the serum itself. About 60% of a normal serum's light scattering ability is due to lipoprotein–triglyceride complexes. Removal of these, therefore, would be a desirable procedure if practical. Several maneuvers can be carried out to eliminate these materials. As will be seen, each presents some serious problems.

The most convenient is the reduction of the number of chylomicra and the amount of triglyceride–lipoprotein complexes that exist in a sample. This can be at least partially accomplished by requesting the patient to fast for at least 14 hr prior to venipuncture and in addition, requesting that he completely abstain from alcoholic beverages for 24 hr prior to the test.

The addition of Aerosil (Degussa) to human plasma for the preparation of a stable lipid-free protein infusate, free of hepatitis virus was described by Stephan (1971). Aerosil is composed of finely divided or aerosilized silica with particle sizes ranging from a few tenths of a micrometer up to several micrometers in diameter. This material when added to whole serum or plasma and incubated for 4 hr at 37°C removes the great majority of high density and low density lipoproteins, producing a crystal clear solution. The original authors considered that only these proteins were removed. Analysis of the material before and after processing did actually appear to have no effect on the level of the 10 major proteins with the exception of a modest increase in total protein concentration, presumably due to the hydration of the silica and removal of water from the original material. When trace proteins were analyzed, however, it was noted that the fourth and fifth components of the complement system were removed as was most of the esterase inhibitor and β_2-glycoprotein I. Other unidentified trace proteins of undisclosed nature were found in the eluent from the Aerosil when the material was tested by immunoelectrophoresis against a good quality anti-whole human serum. Therefore, while the material may perform quite well as an osmotically active infusion and be potentially of superior optical quality, it lacked at least some of the proteins of current interest to protein analysts.

Dextran sulfate has also been used as a precipitant for lipoproteins but like Aerosil-treated samples, some trace proteins are also removed.

Removal of low density lipoprotein and chylomicra can be accomplished by ultracentrifugation of the whole serum. The amount of LDL protein lost by the removal of chylomicra and particles with flotation constants of 1.06 and below appeared to have no significant effect on the total level of LDL protein analyzed in the whole sample versus that of the clear infranatant. This, however, requires the availability of expensive, specialized equipment and is not designed to handle even modest numbers of samples.

Lipase has been used by workers at the University of Louvain to clarify serum (Riccomi et al., 1972b). However, its greatest use appears to be on chylous samples and therefore it does not aid in achieving the highly clarified samples required for analysis at concentrations below 10 mg%.

Filtration through membranes with pore sizes of 50 to 100 nm can also markedly reduce the light scattering ability of pathological samples (Werner et al., 1970) by removing the larger light scattering particles.

The additional manipulation needed for clarification is a serious problem in the handling of large numbers of samples. However, for the present, the ability to process a modest number of samples for the automated analysis of certain trace proteins will be incentive enough for many workers. Outside the research laboratory the indication for immunoanalysis of trace proteins is as yet small. However, should the direct nephelometric analysis of thyroxine-binding globulin or cortisol-binding globulin for instance become possible, methods for handling large numbers of samples would undoubtedly be devised. Certain body fluids are already well suited to nephelometric analysis but their components exist at very low levels. Cord blood, cerebrospinal fluid, and urine all contain extremely low levels of light scattering materials. Spinal fluid and urine, in particular, can be processed at extremely high concentrations because of the lack of large molecular species (Lizana and Hellsing, 1974b). Cord blood can be processed easily at five times the concentration normally used for whole adult serum. This is of particular importance to the worker interested in measuring immunoglobulins A and M in cord blood.

B. Inhibition Technique

Because of the simplicity of nephelometric analysis and the absence of radioactive, enzymatic, or fluorescent labels, investigation into the possibility of increasing its sensitivity by additional immunological maneuvers is justified. Riccomi and co-workers (1972a) introduced the Automated Inhibition Immunoassay (NINIA) as a procedure with sensitivity nearly on a par with radioimmunoassay.

This work was amplified upon by Cambiaso *et al.* (1974b) who added to the work of Riccomi the use of PEG as an enhancing and accelerating agent as described previously.

The NINIA technique makes use of the fact that antisera contain a fraction of the total immunoglobulins that represent molecules with high affinity or avidity (Pauling *et al.*, 1944; Pressman and Siegel, 1953, Cambiaso *et al.*, 1974a). Even relatively weak antisera contain a population of very active molecules. A small amount of antigen, therefore, can involve this highly active population and effectively remove it from the reaction, significantly reducing the precipitating properties of the antiserum. Riccomi *et al.* (1972a) used anti-dinitrophenol (DNP) and DNP-lysine as the test system, whereas Cambiaso and co-workers (1974b) used progesterone–anti-progesterone as the test system. The former group added 1.2 to 11 ng of DNP-lysine to batches of anti-DNP, diluted 1:67 in saline. These extremely small doses of hapten are incapable of causing precipitation of antibody of their own; however, as previously noted above, the high affinity antibody molecules are preferentially rendered less reactive or completely inactive by their presence. To test the residual reactivity of the antiserum batches to which DNP-lysine had been added, the exposed or absorbed antisera were used to test the reaction with an antigen that would produce a precipitin reaction in nephelometric analysis. The antigen used was BSA linked to nine molecules of DNP and has been referred to as the developer antigen. In testing various concentrations of the developer antigen it was found that the maximal effect and therefore sensitivity was in the 0 to 2 ng/ml range of DNP-lysine. With a developer antigen composed of IgG, coupled to 23 residues of DNP, 200 pg of DNP-lysine hapten produced significant decrease in peak height. Again, as in the direct nephelometric assay intrinsic turbidity of serum is a limiting factor at low sensitivities. In Cambiaso's estimation, the lower limit for a progesterone assay is in the neighborhood of 10 ng of progesterone per milliliter of whole serum.

VIII. Standards

The development of a new, more accurate means of measurement often generates a flurry of activity with the proponents of the new technique fending off and parrying outcries from the "old school." When the established techniques were politely labeled as "approximate" or "semiquantitative," and the reagents often frankly unsuitable for any form of use, the introduction of an accurate automated instrument for the analysis of human plasma proteins not unexpectedly loosed a flood of anxiety by user and manufacturer alike as to the viability of the new approach. The destruction of the crude status quo, so much more comfortable than after automation opened the Pandora's box, released a seemingly endless sequence of problems of increasing complexity. Nevertheless, the box is opened and the first pair of serious problems has emerged in the form of standards for serum proteins and its much more elusive counterpart, standards for antiserum. The development of the AIP system, with accuracy and repeatability in the order of $\pm$ 2 to 3%, makes it possible for the first time to analyze and compare antigen and antibody in a mode almost completely free from human and unpredictable variations.

A. Antigen

A great deal of effort has been expended in developing standard sera for distribution to interested parties. The International Union of Immunologic Societies with support from the World Health Organization have made available large amounts of a lyophilized pool of serum with known amounts of IgG, IgA, IgM (Rowe *et al.,* 1970a), IgD (Rowe *et al.,* 1970b), and IgE (Rowe *et al.,* 1970c). The values for these proteins were determined chiefly by RID, in 13 laboratories throughout the world. These ampules of International Reference Preparation have been widely distributed and have contributed greatly to stabilization in this difficult area.

Two schools of thought have developed concerning standards for serum proteins: (a) The amount of a protein present in a given sample is analyzable and can be reported in absolute values of weight/volume and (b) the absolute amount in a sample is of little meaning, and for most proteins unattainable, and all analyses should be expressed as a percentage of an internationally accepted standard. Whatever the reader's proclivity, a few points must be accepted. Plasma proteins are unstable moieties that suffer serious alteration at the hands of their neighbors, let alone those who desire to "purify" them for use as standards. Some proteins begin degradation almost immediately on being withdrawn from the donor, others lose their biological activity rapidly with change in temperature or pH. High concentration serum proteins, such as the 3 major immunoglobulins and albumin, have survived quite well in the hands of careful workers but those workers capable of isolating in an unaltered state for accurate absolute measurements, proteins such as the complement components, clotting factors, etc., must indeed be rare. Once isolated, the problem of transport of such fragile "purified" components in their pristine state into the hands of other workers for parallel and cooperative analysis seems overwhelming.

Perhaps some indication of the magnitude of the task can be drawn from the fact that as yet, even serum albumin has not achieved the status of possessing an international standard although the International Union of Immunologic Societies (IUIS) and the American Association of Clinical Chemists in concert with the National Committee for Clinical Laboratory Standards are nearing completion of that project.

Compounding the problem is the heterogeneity of the proteins themselves, especially those whose genetic variations have as yet to be studied in sufficient numbers to draw conclusions as to their reactivity in various test systems.

Distributed standards by the World Health Organization have gone a long way toward establishing the logistics for distribution of an internationally accepted reference material. Stabilization of the plasma or serum preparation has proved to be a serious problem when the lyophilized IUIS Standard for immunoglobulins was used in the nephelometric system. The extreme turbidity of the reconstituted lyophilate impeded analysis, although for IgA and IgG values agreed quite well because of the high dilution possible. Analysis of IgM, however, proved to be a more serious problem mitigated recently only by the introduction of the PEG enhancement. An effort is underway by the IUIS to prepare another International Reference Preparation suitable for nephelometry.

B. Antiserum

As mentioned above, careful control of the immune reagents is required for nephelometric immunoanalysis. The inexactness of manual techniques is chiefly to blame for the poor quality of most commercial reagents. However, the striking contrast in antiserum potency that can be obtained by testing in the AIP system (Fig. 8) has induced several manufacturers of immune reagents to use this instrument for quality control. This can only work to the consumer's benefit and indeed, since the introduction of the automated device the quality of some commercial antisera, has shown a slow trend toward improvement (Ritchie, 1972a).

C. Intralaboratory

Sensitive electronic instruments are subject to a variety of sudden, intermittent, and chronic changes that silently alter overall operations. When these changes occur during the processing of a series of unknowns, gross inaccuracies for at least a part of the run can occur. Traditionally, samples of known concentration are inserted at intervals during testing to identify the occurrence of such changes. In the nephelometric system that employs high intensity lamps and photoreceptors with operational characteristics that may change considerably, yet remain usable, this monitoring is of particular importance. Loss of peak height can be due to several problems. The two most commonly observed are a loss in sensitivity of an electronic nature or changes that reflect on the ratio of antigen to antibody within the fluid stream. As we have discussed before, serum itself has an intrinsic light scattering ability due largely to triglyceride–lipoprotein complexes. This property can be utilized to test the sensitivity of the system during the blank run or prerun without antiserum. Later, however, when antiserum is added such monitoring is not possible. During this phase of testing the appropriateness of the antigen–antibody reaction can be analyzed and monitored. The use of a pool of whole normal serum to measure the nephelometric efficiency of the system must take into consideration that regardless of the temperature at which the pool is stored, changes do occur with time even at $-100°C$.

To properly answer both questions we employ two materials. The first, as before, are samples of a large, sterile, filtered pool of normal serum stored at less than $-20°C$ to follow the immune reaction and second, a stable light scattering chemical that can be made up and stored at room temperature. An aqueous solution of 6% Ficoll is inserted either before or after each normal pool control and acts to monitor the electronic sensitivity of the system. In practice these controls are inserted as pairs every 10 to 18 samples. Comparison of the measured peak height of both during blank and test runs gives an indication of operational efficiency and drift. Undoubtedly, as nephelometry becomes more sophisticated, internal standards will be developed to allow monitoring of equipment efficiency similar to what is available for spectrophotometric instruments.

IX. Assay of Other Biological Fluids

Analysis of specific proteins is usually performed on serum. Nevertheless, other body fluids, as well as solutions of partially purified proteins, can be analyzed with only minor adjustments in the testing protocol.

Analysis of blood components involved in the clotting mechanism requires the use of plasma. Certain components can be analyzed in the automated instrument before and after clotting, for example anti-thrombin III and prothrombin. Nonclottable fibrinogen or fibrin split-products can be analyzed readily by nephelometry (Fletcher *et al.*, 1972). Plasma is not as ideal a fluid as serum for nephelometry owing to the presence of the large light scattering molecules of fibrinogen. For the analysis of fibrinogen the slight increase poses no-problem because of the high dilution of reagents used for this avid antigen–antibody reaction. The buffer system need only be altered to contain 0.1% EDTA to prevent the formation of fibrin during the procedure.

Cerebrospinal fluid is almost ideal for nephelometric analysis since it lacks large molecular species such as LDL protein, IgM and α_2-macroglobulin, and chylomicra. Serum samples are routinely prediluted (Fig. 4 or 5). Spinal fluid samples can be analyzed neat interspersed with diluted serum samples without special handling. The high dilution required for serum is usually unnecessary with cerebrospinal fluid, except for the analysis of IgG and albumin which may require dilution of the fluid. Minor problems may result if analysis is attempted of spinal fluids containing large numbers of white cells or talcum powder particles from the physician's rubber gloves. A simple step of employing a Millipore filter of 0.8 to 1.2 μm suffices to remove these interfering particles. Certain laboratories still sterilize instruments in colored solutions of aqueous Zephiran. Samples contaminated with these solutions cannot be quantitated with any degree of accuracy because of the apparent loss of antigenicity of all proteins by exposure to the sterilizing chemicals. Despite the availability of excellent stoppered containers for CSF, some hospitals still use corks. These render spinal fluid virtually useless for any analysis, in particular for proteins. Cork has a high affinity for CSF protein and will, after a few hours of contact, remove most of the proteins from the solution while adding a yellowish color suggesting xanthochromia. Samples submitted in this fashion should not be analyzed.

Tears, like CSF, can easily be analyzed. The small volumes required for analysis make nephelometry an ideal tool for the investigation of this fluid. Pleural, pericardial, abdominal, or blister fluids can be analyzed as though they were serum and only require filtration or centrifugation to remove white or red blood cells before analysis. Amniotic, joint, and enteric fluids present problems of a hyperviscous solution. They can be managed as though they were serum if attention is paid to careful dilution of the viscid material followed by filtration or centrifugation. Thoracic duct lymph is analogous to chylous serum samples in that it contains extremely high levels of chylomicra. These particles must be removed if accurate values are to be obtained. Prostatic or seminal fluid proteins can be analyzed in the same fashion as described above for joint fluids. Clarification by centrifugation or filtration is very important with these fluids and is best carried out following dilution with suitable buffers. Urine presents a unique and extremely interesting fluid for nephelometric analysis. Like tests for total CSF protein, measurement of total urinary protein is an estimate at best. Several interfering materials exist in urine which are not found in CSF. The high concentration of urea may significantly inhibit the antigen–antibody reaction unless dilution of the sample is carried out. In addition, many samples contain large amounts of particulate matter such as white blood cells, various crystals, and mucous shreds that must be removed prior to analysis. Despite these problems, a fresh, early morning specimen is an even better medium for nephelometric analysis than is cerebrospinal fluid where light scattering materials are at extremely low levels. Hellsing has found that 10% PEG allows the analysis of albumin in urine samples down to concentration of 1 mg/liter. β_2-Microglobulin has also been analyzed in a like fashion (Hellsing and Lizana, 1974) using 10% PEG.

Any fluid of sufficient clarity can be analyzed for specific proteins. The protein to be analyzed should be brought into an optimum range that for most proteins is something greater than one order of magnitude wide. This range allows a reasonable latitude and frequently makes it possible to analyze many proteins in extremely small samples.

X. Correlations

Correlations of results obtained by automated nephelometric analysis and other more familiar immunological techniques present a dilemma to the critical evaluator. Because of the much improved repeatability and reproducibility of AIP analysis and its relative freedom from interference by variation in a protein's molecular weight and degree of polymerization, correlation between values obtained by manual immunochemical analysis and the automated nephelometric method may be poor. Coefficients of variation with automated nephelometric analysis are in the 2 to 3% range, while with radial immunodiffusion values they can rarely be brought to below 7% even under the most ideal conditions.

Albumin is an excellent species of protein on which to obtain optimum testing results because of its stability in whole serum and its high concentration. The immunoglobulins or the complement components with higher molecular weights, molecular asymmetry, tendency toward aggregation, and not infrequently, multiple populations of various molecular weights present many more difficulties in analysis by diffusion techniques. With nephelometry, these variables appear to have little effect on the end result. This escape from inherent inaccuracy of manual methods by nephelometric analysis, has actually been used by Markowitz and Tschida (1972) to estimate the levels of 7 S IgM in human serum. When accurate manual techniques are compared to the AIP system, correlation coefficients of better than 0.9 are usually obtained (Watson *et al.*, 1974; Marcroft and Newland, 1973; Ebeling, 1973). Comparison with a dye-binding method for albumin (Ritchie *et al.*, 1973), also yields *r* values exceeding 0.9. A recent comparative study by Killingsworth *et al.* (1974) documents the stability of this form of analysis and showed good correlation between values obtained by analysis under various buffer systems.

Correlation with serum protein electrophoresis is exceedingly difficult except at the grossest level. The six major electrophoretic fractions are so heterogeneous that major changes may occur within them without any detectable alterations in the protein pattern. Attempts to correlate quantitative data with densitometric scans of electrophoresis patterns provide no more information than what can be observed with the naked eye. The dye-binding capacities of various serum proteins varies considerably and occasionally to great extremes. Automated nephelometric immunoassay may serve not only to open new areas of study but to sharply focus attention, if only briefly, on how inaccurate the manual immunochemical methods have been.

XI. Normal Values

Perhaps the most common question concerning new laboratory tests is "what are the normal ranges?" Despite the fact that protein analysis is not a new laboratory test, the imminence of mass population screening with the recovery of valuable diagnostic, genetic, and therapeutic data has emphasized the need for setting limits for human plasma protein data.

As noted elsewhere, plasma proteins exhibit a bewildering array of genetic variations, changes with age, with sex and ethnic background, and of course, with pathological change, preclinical or overt. The "normal range" may, for plasma proteins, be of little value when a population's data are applied to an individual. While a "range of normal" can be applied to a population, it may be much more valid to refer to an individual's range of normal, allowing excursions during a state of health. Nevertheless, some information of quite significant medical use can be obtained from comparison of an individual's data to a population even ignoring the variations of age, sex, etc. (Laurell *et al.*, 1970; Weeke *et al.*, 1971; Dotchev *et al.*, 1973).

Table I describes the limits that were established after modifying basic statistical data to fit clinical experience. The table is in no way intended to exemplify a population other than that for a northern New England, White population. Alterations would have to be made for different ethnic and racial groups.

TABLE I

Normal Values for 14 Human Serum Proteins[a]

	Mean (mg/dl)	Range (mg/dl)
Albumin	4000	3200–5500
α_1-Antitrypsin	240	160–360
α_1-Acid glycoprotein (orosomucoid)	100	40–150
C1 inhibitor	18	11–26
Ceruloplasmin	32	18–45
α_2-Macroglobulin	550 pediatric	200–700[b]
	300 female, adult	120–540[b]
	240 male, adult	90–400[b]
Haptoglobin	108	25–180[c]
Transferrin	280	200–350
Low density lipoprotein	105	40–140[d]
C3	165	90–220[e]
C4	30	10–40
IgA	240	60–360[f]
IgM	105	25–170[f]
IgG	1100	700–1500[g]

[a] Values derived from a large northern New England White population.

[b] Varies markedly during and about the time of puberty.

[c] Varies from 0 to normal adult during first 2 weeks of life.

[d] Varies from 10% of normal to normal adult during first year of life.

[e] Varies from 50% of normal to normal adult during the first month of life.

[f] Varies from 0 to normal adult during first year of life.

[g] Varies from adult normal at birth to 25% of normal at about 3 months, returning to adult normal during next several years.

XII. Data Reduction

Conversion of data recovered from immunochemical testing for all practical purposes cannot be done with simple conversion factors, although limited portions of the ranges of data under scrutiny closely approximate the linear. Generally, curves are drawn on graph paper or transparent masks from actual data recovered during testing a series of standards. This method is tedious for large studies and affords great opportunity for error. With the availability of small and powerful electronic calculators, much of the tedium of converting actual data such as

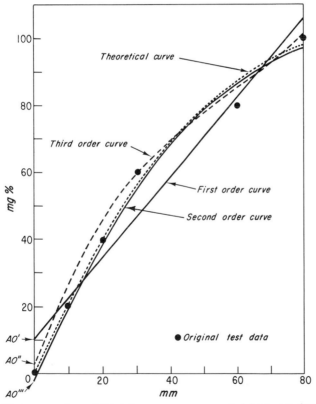

Fig. 13. First-, second-, and third-degree curves computed from raw data in Table II. Note that the second-order curve more closely approximates the theoretical curve while the third-order more closely approximates the test data. A fourth-order curve would fit the test data exactly.

that retrieved from nephelometric testing can be relegated to easily performed curve fitting programs.

First-order curves can not be used to express immunological data. However, at times first-order calculations can be used with good approximation over a considerable range. Figure 13 illustrates five points from a standard curve for the measurement of the protein orosomucoid (α_1-acid glycoprotein) by nephelometry. The first point is zero on both dimensions and should be included in all curves. A third-order curve may be a closer fit for perfect data. However, if points are aberrant, a high order curve fit could cause a serious localized problem. A lower order curve spreads the error over the entire span and minimizes the error as shown in Fig. 13.

The following paragraphs summarize a simple stepwise form for producing the first-and second-order equations needed to generate curve fitting programs for small programmable calculators.

To generate a *first-order* line that best fits N points, certain preliminary calculations must be made from the original data. In this example, a first-order line that best fits the X (mm) and Y (mg) for the five test values and zero is calculated from the hypothetical data in Table II. Before proceeding to Eqs. (1) and (2), the five values (1–5) listed in Table III must be calculated. The numbers in parentheses are correct calculations for assistance.

To calculate the Y intercept for the first-order line (A0') use Eq. (1) and to arrive at the value for the slope of A1', use Eq. (2). The line is illustrated in Fig. 13. With these two values and the peak height in mm ($X?$) the mg% ($Y?$) for that peak can be calculated.

$$A0 = \frac{(\Sigma Y \Sigma X^2) - (\Sigma X \Sigma XY)}{(N \Sigma X^2) - X^2} \tag{1}$$

TABLE II

List of Hypothetical Test Values for Practice Calculations

Sample number	mm peak height (= X)	mg% of specific protein (= Y)
1	0	0
2	10	20
3	20	40
4	30	60
5	60	80
6	80	100

TABLE III

List of Values from Practice Calculations

(1) N	(	6)
(2) $\Sigma\, X$	(	200)
(3) $\Sigma\, Y$	(	300)
(4) $\Sigma\, XY$	(	15,600)
(5) $\Sigma\, X^2$	(	11,400)
(6) $\Sigma\, X^2Y$	(	1,000,000)
(7) $\Sigma\, X^3$	(	764,000)
(8) $\Sigma\, X^4$		(54,900,000)

$$A1 = \frac{(N\Sigma XY) - (\Sigma X \Sigma Y)}{(N\Sigma X) - \Sigma X^2} \tag{2}$$

$$Y? = A0 + (A1\ X?) \tag{3}$$

For a *second-order* curve that best approximates the data, two simultaneous equations with three unknowns are needed. Eight preliminary calculations are used (Table III, 1–8). To simplify the final equation proteins have been reduced to single characters [Eqs. (4)–(9)]. Values in parenthesis indicate correct calculations for each.

After the preliminary and condensing equations are completed, Eqs. (10) through (12) generate the four curve functions that are needed to convert millimeters to milligrams with Eq. (13).

If the standard curve for a protein produces a sigmoid curve, a third-order equation with four simultaneous equations is needed; however, a sigmoid curve generally indicates that the tests are being run in antibody excess. A small increase in antibody dilution will generally flatten the lower portion of the standard curve to look more like Fig. 13.

$$\text{Set A} = (N\Sigma XY)\quad - (\Sigma X \Sigma Y)\quad =\quad 33,600 \tag{4}$$

$$\text{Set B} = (\Sigma X \Sigma X^2 Y) - (\Sigma X^2 \Sigma XY) =\quad 22,160,000 \tag{5}$$

$$\text{Set C} = (N\Sigma X^2)\quad - (\Sigma X)^2\quad =\quad 28,400 \tag{6}$$

$$\text{Set D} = (\Sigma X \Sigma X^3)\quad - (\Sigma X^2)\quad =\quad 22,840,000 \tag{7}$$

$$\text{Set E} = (N\Sigma X^3)\quad - (\Sigma X \Sigma X^2)\quad =\quad 2,304,000 \tag{8}$$

$$\text{Set G} = (\Sigma X \Sigma X^4)\quad - (\Sigma X^3 \Sigma X^2)\quad = 2,270,400,000 \tag{9}$$

$$A0 = \frac{\Sigma Y}{N} - \frac{\dfrac{BE - AG}{DE - GC}\Sigma X}{N} - \frac{\dfrac{BC - AD}{CG - DE}\Sigma X^2}{N} = 1.197 \tag{10}$$

$$A1 = \frac{BE - AG}{DE - GC} \qquad\qquad = 2.128 \tag{11}$$

$$A2 = \frac{BC - AD}{CG - DE} \qquad\qquad = 0.01165 \tag{12}$$

$$Y? = A0 + (A1\ X?) + [A2(X?^2)] \tag{13}$$

While higher order or polynomial equations can be used to improve the fit to collected data, this is generally unnecessary and may actually lead to diminished accuracy as illustrated in Fig. 13 in the third-order curve.

A program to accommodate the 18 steps in the second-order curve calculation can easily be accommodated with a desk top programmable calculator with 1K of memory. The task for technical personnel is markedly simplified and made more accurate.

ACKNOWLEDGMENTS

We gratefully acknowledge the advice and criticism of Chester Alper on this review and the conscientious support of Sandra Christiansen in preparation of the manuscript.

REFERENCES

Aitken, J. (1972). *Colloq. A.I.P., Brussels, 1972* p. 33.
Aladjem, F., and Liebermann, H. (1952). *J. Immunol.* **69,** 117.
Alper, C. A. (1970). *Advan. Automat. Anal.* **1,** 105.
Alper, C. A., and Propp, R. P. (1968). *J. Clin. Invest.* **47,** 2181.
Alper, C. A., Abramson, N., Johnston, R. B., Jandl, J. H., and Rosen, F. B. (1970). *J. Clin. Invest.* **49,** 1975.
Baier, J. G. (1947). *Physiol. Zool.* **20,** 172.
Bloor, W. R. (1914). *J. Biol. Chem.* **7,** 377.
Bloor, W. R. (1915). *J. Biol. Chem.* **22,** 145.
Bolton, E. T. (1947). *J. Immunol.* **57,** 391.
Bolton, E. T., Leone, A., and Boyden, A. A. (1948). *J. Immunol.* **58,** 169.
Bordet, J. (1900). *Ann. Inst. Pasteur, Paris* **14,** 257.
Boyd, W. C. (1947). *J. Exp. Med.* **74,** 369.
Boyden, A. (1942). *Physiol. Zool.* **15,** 109.
Boyden, A., and DeFalco, R. J. (1943). *Physiol. Zool.* **16,** 229.
Boyden, A., Bolton, E., and Gemeroy, D. (1947). *J. Immunol.* **57,** 211.
Cambiaso, C. L., Masson, P. L., Vaerman, J. P., and Heremans, J. F. (1974a). *J. Immunol. Methods* **5,** 153.
Cambiaso, C. L., Riccomi, H. A., Masson, P. L., and Heremans, J. F. (1974b). *J. Immunol. Methods* **5,** 293.
Chaney, A. L. (1967). *Automat. Anal. Chem. Technicon Symp. 1967* p. 115.

Chow, B. F. (1947). *J. Biol. Chem.* **167,** 757.

Davies, G. E. (1971). *Immunology* **20,** 779.

Davis, N. C. (1972). *Colloq. A.I.P., Brussels, 1972* p. 39.

Denis, W. (1921). *J. Biol. Chem.* **47,** 27.

Dotchev, D., Liappis, N., and Hungerland, H. (1973). *Clin. Chim. Acta* **44,** 431.

Ebeling, Von H. (1973). *Z. Klin. Chem. Klin. Biochem.* **11,** 209.

Ebeling, Von H. (1974). *Z. Klin. Chem. Klin. Biochem.* **12,** 54.

Eckman, I., Robbins, J. B., Van den Hammer, C. J., Lentz, J., and Scheinberg, I. H. (1970). *Clin. Chem.* **16,** 558.

Eisen, H. N. (1948). *J. Immunol.* **60,** 77.

Fletcher, A. P., Alkjaersig, N., Roy, L., and Owens, O. (1972). *Colloq. A.I.P., Brussels, 1972* p. 1.

Fredrickson, D. S., Levy, R. I., and Lees, R. S. (1967). *N. Engl. J. Med.* **276,** 34, 94, 148, 215, and 273.

Gitlin, D. (1949). *J. Immunol.* **62,** 437.

Gitlin, D., and Edelhoch, H. (1951). *J. Immunol.* **66,** 67.

Goldberg, R. J., and Campbell, D. H. (1951). *J. Immunol.* **66,** 79.

Hach, C. C. (1970). *Med. Electron. & Data* **1,** 104.

Halberstam, D., and Derrico, G. (1972). *Colloq. A.I.P., Brussels., 1972* p. 43.

Hall, C. T. (1973). "Non-Syphilis Serology Quantitative Immunoglobulins." NCDC, DHEW, Atlanta, Georgia.

Heidelberger, M., and Kendall, F. E. (1932). *J. Exp. Med.* **55,** 555.

Heidelberger, M., and Kendall, F. E. (1935). *J. Exp. Med.* **62,** 697.

Heiskell, C. L., Fisk, R. T., Florsheim, W. H., *et al.* (1961). *Amer. J. Clin. Pathol.* **35,** 222.

Hellsing, K. (1966). *Acta Chem. Scand.* **20,** 1251.

Hellsing, K. (1969). *Biochem. J.* **114,** 145.

Hellsing, K. (1972). *Colloq. A. I. P., Brussels, 1972* p. 17.

Hellsing, K., and Laurent, T. (1964). *Acta Chem. Scand.* **18,** 1303.

Hellsing, K., and Lizana, J. (1974). *Z. Klin. Chem. Klin. Biochem.* **12,** 245.

Hostey, J. A., Hollenbeck, M., and Shane, S. (1973). *Clin. Chem.* **19,** 524.

Humphrey, J. H., Anderson, S. G., Bangham, D. R., *et al.* (1971). *Immunology* **20,** 3.

Huntley, C. C., Robbins, J. B., Lyerly, A. D., *et al.* (1971). *N. Engl. J. Med.* **284,** 7.

Johnson, P., and Ottewill, R. H. (1954). *Discuss. Faraday Soc.* **18,** 327.

Johnston, H. H., Brann, B. H., Ritchie, R. F., and Graves, J. (1972). *Advan. Automat. Anal.* **1,** 69.

Kahan, J., and Sundblad, L. (1966). *Eur. Technicon Symp., Paris, 1966* p. 361.

Kahan, J., and Sundblad, L. (1969). *Scand. J. Clin. Lab. Invest.* **24,** 61.

Killingsworth, L. M., and Savory, J. (1971). *Clin. Chem.* **17,** 936.

Killingsworth, L. M., Savory, J., and Teague, P. O. (1971). *Clin. Chem.* **17,** 374.

Killingsworth, L. M., Buffone, G. J., Sonawane, M. B., and Lunsford, G. C. (1974). *Clin. Chem.* **20,** 1548.

Kober, P. A. (1912–1913). *J. Biol. Chem.* **8,** 485.

Kober, P. A. (1917). *J. Biol. Chem.* **29,** 155.

Kober, P. A., and Klett, R. E. (1921). *J. Biol. Chem.* **47,** 19.

Kraus, R. (1897). *Wien. Klin. Wochenschr.* **10,** 736.

Larson, C. (1972). *Advan. Automat. Anal.* **4,** 67.

Laurell, C.-B., Kullander, S., and Thorell, J. (1970). *Scand. J. Clin. Lab. Invest.* **26,** 345.

Laurent, T. C. (1963a). *Biochem. J.* **89,** 253.

Laurent, T. C. (1963b). *Acta Chem. Scand.* **17,** 2664.

Leikola, J., and Vyas, G. N. (1971). *J. Lab. Clin. Med.* **77,** 629.

Leone, C. A. (1960). *Trans. Kans. Acad. Sci.* **63**, 147.

Lewis, L. A., and Page, I. H. (1965). *Amer. J. Med.* **38**, 286.

Libby, R. L. (1938a). *J. Immunol.* **34**, 71.

Libby, R. L. (1938b). *J. Immunol.* **34**, 269.

Lizana, J., and Hellsing, K. (1974a). *Clin. Chem.* **20**, 415.

Lizana, J., and Hellsing, K. (1974b). *Clin. Chem.* **20**, 1181.

MacDonald, J. Y. (1960). *Bull. Serol. Mus.* **23**, 1.

McDuffie, F. C., and Kabat, E. A. (1956). *J. Immunol.* **77**, 193.

Marcroft, J., and Newland, I. M. (1973). *Clin. Chim. Acta* **46**, 399.

Markowitz, H., and Tschida, A. R. (1972). *Clin. Chem.* **18**, 1364.

Marrack, J. R., and Grant, R. A. (1953). *Brit. J. Exp. Pathol.* **34**, 263.

Marrack, J. R., and Richards, C. B. (1971). *Immunology* **20**, 1019.

Nishi, H. H., and Kestner, J. S. (1974). *Clin. Chem.* **20**, 895.

Nuttall, G. H. F. (1904). *In* "Blood Immunity and Blood Relationship," pp. 5–19 and 96–102. Cambridge Univ. Press, London and New York.

Ogston, A. G., and Phelps, C. F. (1961). *Biochem. J.* **78**, 827.

Pauling, L., Pressman, D., and Campbell, D. H. (1944). *J. Amer. Chem. Soc.* **66**, 330.

Phillips, D. J., Shore, S. L., Maddison, S. E., Gordon, D. S., and Reimer, C. B. (1971). *J. Lab. Clin. Med.* **77**, 639.

Polson, A., Potgieter, G. M., Largier, J. F., *et al.* (1964). *Biochim. Biophys. Acta* **82**, 463.

Pope, C. G., and Healey, M. (1938). *Brit. J. Exp. Pathol.* **19**, 397.

Pressman, D., and Siegel, M. (1953). *Arch. Biochem. Biophys.* **45**, 41.

Reimer, C. B., Phillips, D. J., Maddison, S. E., and Schur, S. L. (1970). *J. Lab. Clin. Med.* **76**, 749.

Reimer, C. B., (1972). *Health Lab. Sci.* **9**, 178.

Riccomi, H., Masson, P. L., Vaerman, J. P., and Heremans, J. F. (1972a). *Colloq. A.I.P., Brussels, 1972* p. 9.

Riccomi, H., Masson, P. L., and Heremans, J. F. (1972b). *Colloq. A.I.P., Brussels, 1972* p. 53.

Richards, T. W. (1895). *Z. Anorg. Chem.* **8**, 253.

Ritchie, R. F. (1967). *J. Lab. Clin. Med.* **70**, 512.

Ritchie, R. F. (1972a). *Protides Biol. Fluids., Proc. Colloq.* **21**, 593.

Ritchie, R. F. (1972b). *Colloq. A.I.P., Brussels, 1972* p. 59.

Ritchie, R. F., and Graves, J. A. (1970). *Technicon Int. Congr., New York, 1972* p. 117.

Ritchie, R. F., and Stevens, J. (1972). *Advan. Autom. Anal.* **4**, 9.

Ritchie, R. F., Alper, C. A., and Graves, J. A. (1969). *Arthritis Rheum.* **12**, 693.

Ritchie, R. F., Alper, C. A., Graves, J., Pearson, N., and Larson, C. (1973). *Amer. J. Clin. Pathol.* **59**, 151.

Rowe, D. S., Anderson, S. G., and Grab, B. (1970a). *Bull. W.H.O.* **42**, 535.

Rowe, D. S., Anderson, S. G., and Tackett, L. (1970b). *Bull. W.H.O.* **43**, 607.

Rowe, D. S., Tackett, L., Bennich, H., Ishizaka, K., Johansson, S.G.O., and Anderson, S. G. (1970c). *Bull. W.H.O.* **43**, 609.

Savory, J., Buffone, G., and Reich, R. (1974). *Clin. Chim.* **20**, 1071.

Schultze, H. E., and Schwick, G. (1959). *Clin. Chim. Acta* **4**, 15.

Skeggs, L. T., Jr. (1957). *Amer. J. Clin. Pathol.* **28**, 311.

Stephan, W. (1971). *Vox Sang.* **20**, 442.

Stone, M. C., and Thorp, J. M. (1966). *Clin. Chim. Acta* **14**, 812.

Swartz, A. M., Rader, C. A., and Hueg, E. (1964). *Advan. Clin. Chem.* **43**, 250.

Tchistovitch, T. (1899). *Ann. Inst. Pasteur, Paris* **8**, 406.

Thiers, R. E., Cole, R. R., and Kirsch, W. J. (1967). *Clin. Chem.* **13**, 451.

Thorp, J. M., and Horsfall, G. B. (1967). *Med. Biol. Eng.* **5,** 51.

Tiffany, T. O., Parella, J. M., Johnson, W. F., and Burtis, C. A. (1974). *Clin. Chem.* **20,** 1055.

Vincent, W. F., Harris, E. W., and Yaverbaum, S. (1970). *Immunology* **18,** 143.

Watson, A., Young, P., Davidson, J. F., and Fleck, A. (1974). *Med. Lab. Technol.* **31,** 63.

Weeke, B., Weeke, E., and Bendixen, G. (1971). *Acta Med Scand.* **189,** 113.

Werner, M., Montgomery, C. K., Jones, A. L., and Nussenbaum, S. (1970). *Clin. Chem.* **16,** 573.

Wyatt, P. J. (1968). *Appl. Opt.* **7,** 1879.

Wyatt, P. J., and Phillips, D. T. (1972). *J. Colloid Sci.* **39,** 125.

Yoe, J. H. (1928). *In* "Photometric Chemical Analysis," Vol. I. Wiley, New York.

Subject Index

A

N-Acetylgalactosamine
  linkage with serine or threonine in glyco-
    proteins, 182
  in plasma glycoproteins, 172
N-Acetylglucosamine
  aspartic acid linkage with, in glycopro-
    teins, 180
  in plasma glycoproteins, 172
Acetylhexosamines
  in ceruloplasmin, 73, 74
  in glycoproteins, 172
N-Acetylneuraminic acid, in glycoproteins,
  173
α_1-Acid glycoprotein
  carbohydrate-aspartic acid linkage in,
    180–182
  maternofetal transfer of, 276
  number and sites of oligosaccharide
    units in, 195
  synthesis in liver, 297
Afibrinogenemia, total absence of fibrinogen, 143–145
Agammaglobulinemia
  adult, 352
  clinical implication of, 353
  clinical variants, 351
  congenital, 352
  immunoglobulin deficiency in, 347
  metabolic defect and its genetic implica-
    tions, 354–358
Alanine
  in ceruloplasmin, 73
  in fibrinogen α chain, 121
Albumin
  copper complex, 98
  dimeric variants, 329
  distribution in body fluids, 267
  half-life of, in analbuminemia, 331–333
  maternofetal transfer of, 276–279, 282
  nephelometric analysis of, and correla-
    tion with other analyses, 417
  structural and quantitative variants, 324

synthesis in the conceptus, 296
  by yolk sac, 290
turbidimetric determination of plasma,
  379
Albumin A, 325–329
Albumin B, 325–329
Albuminemia, double, 324, 325
Alloalbuminemia, 324
Amidohydrolase, in linkage determination
  between aspartic acid and carbohydrate, 182
Amino acids
  of ceruloplasmin, 71–73
  of fibrinogen, 119–121
    sequence of, 128
  of fibrinopeptides, 122, 123
  of haptoglobins, 3, 18, 19, 23
Amniotic fluid
  ceruloplasmin levels in, 80
  plasma proteins in, sources and fate of,
    272–274
  plasma protein turnover in, 270–272
Analbuminemia
  clinical and physiological implication of,
    333, 334
  nature of defect, 331–333
  occurrence of, 330
Anhaptoglobinemia, 35, 39
Antibodies
  animal species, for automated im-
    munoprecipitation analysis, 403
  antigen reaction with, effect of particles
    on immunoprecipitation analysis,
    392
  anti-ruminant, effect on automated im-
    munoprecipitation on, 395
  characteristics and automated im-
    munoprecipitation analysis,
    397–399
  potency, effect on automated im-
    munoprecipitation analysis, 399
  specificities, effect on automated im-
    munoprecipitation analysis, 396,
    401

427

A 5
B 6
C 7
D 8
E 9
F 0
G 1
H 2
I 3
J 4